Landmark-Based Image Analysis

Computational Imaging and Vision

Landmark-Based Image Analysis

Using Geometric and Intensity Models

by

Karl Rohr

Department of Computer Science,
University of Hamburg,
Hamburg, Germany

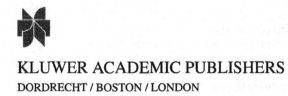

KLUWER ACADEMIC PUBLISHERS
DORDRECHT / BOSTON / LONDON

A C.I.P. Catalogue record for this book is available from the Library of Congress.

ISBN 978-90-481-5630-6

Published by Kluwer Academic Publishers,
P.O. Box 17, 3300 AA Dordrecht, The Netherlands.

Sold and distributed in North, Central and South America
by Kluwer Academic Publishers,
101 Philip Drive, Norwell, MA 02061, U.S.A.

In all other countries, sold and distributed
by Kluwer Academic Publishers,
P.O. Box 322, 3300 AH Dordrecht, The Netherlands.

Printed on acid-free paper

To
Andrea, Katharina, and Viktoria

Contents

Preface   xi

1 Introduction and Overview   **1**
  1.1   Image Analysis as a Knowledge-Based Process   4
  1.2   Model-based and Knowledge-Based Approaches   7
  1.3   Image Analysis and Image Synthesis   13
  1.4   Geometric Models and Intensity Models   16
  1.5   Differential Models and Deformable Models   19
  1.6   Parametric and Nonparametric Models   21
  1.7   Feature- and Landmark-Based Image Analysis   26
  1.8   Overview of Our Work   28
      1.8.1   General Characterization   29
      1.8.2   Feature Extraction   31
      1.8.3   Performance Characterization   32
      1.8.4   Elastic Image Registration   33

2 Detection and Localization of Point Landmarks   **35**
  2.1   Motivation and General Approach   36
      2.1.1   3D Anatomical Point Landmarks   36
      2.1.2   A Framework for Developing Landmark Operators   39
      2.1.3   Semi-Automatic Landmark Extraction   40
  2.2   Definition and Characterization of Anatomical Point Landmarks   41
      2.2.1   Problems   42
      2.2.2   2D Landmarks   43
      2.2.3   3D Landmarks   45
  2.3   Mathematical Description of Anatomical Point Landmarks   47
      2.3.1   General Mathematical Descriptions   47
      2.3.2   Applicable Approaches to Landmark Extraction   50
  2.4   3D Differential Operators Based on Curvature Properties of
      Isocontours   52
  2.5   3D Generalization of Differential Corner Operators   58
      2.5.1   2D Operators   60
      2.5.2   3D Operators   63
      2.5.3 nD Operators   68
      2.5.4   Experimental Results   70
      2.5.5   Statistical Interpretation   78
      2.5.6   Interpretation as Principal Invariants   81

	2.5.7	Multi-step Approaches for Subvoxel Localization	84
2.6	Parametric Approaches		87
	2.6.1	Radiometric Model and Imaging Process	90
	2.6.2	Parametric Intensity Models of Landmarks	93
	2.6.3	Model Fitting	100
	2.6.4	Experimental Results	102
2.7	Summary and Conclusion		106

3 Performance Characterization of Landmark Operators — **109**

3.1	General Approach		110
3.2	Analytic Studies		112
	3.2.1	Localization Accuracy	112
	3.2.2	Localization Precision in 2D Images	117
	3.2.3	Localization Precision in 3D Images	143
3.3	Experimental Studies		151
	3.3.1	Operator Responses	151
	3.3.2	Statistical Measures for the Detection Performance	152
	3.3.3	Detection Performance Visualization and Measure ψ	156
	3.3.4	Number of Corresponding Points	168
	3.3.5	Localization Accuracy	169
	3.3.6	Affine Registration Accuracy	171
	3.3.7	Projective Invariants	172
3.4	Summary and Conclusion		176

4 Elastic Registration of Multimodality Images — **179**

4.1	Background and Motivation		183
	4.1.1	General Registration Scheme	183
	4.1.2	Point-Based Elastic Registration	186
4.2	Clinical Applications		188
4.3	Interpolating Thin-Plate Splines		191
4.4	Relation to Elasticity Theory		198
	4.4.1	Bending of a Thin Plate	198
	4.4.2	Relation to the Navier Equation	201
4.5	Approximating Thin-Plate Splines with Isotropic Errors		205
	4.5.1	Theory	206
	4.5.2	Experimental Results	211
4.6	Approximating Thin-Plate Splines with Anisotropic Errors		216
	4.6.1	Incorporation of Weight Matrices	217
	4.6.2	Special Cases of 2D and 3D Images	221
	4.6.3	Combination of Weight Matrices	224
	4.6.4	Estimation of Landmark Localization Uncertainties	226
	4.6.5	Experimental Results	232
4.7	Orientation Attributes at Landmarks		241
4.8	Biomechanical Modelling of Brain Deformations		247
4.9	Related Work		250
4.10	Conclusion and Future Work		255

Bibliography **259**

Index **301**

Preface

Landmarks are preferred image features for a variety of computer vision tasks such as image mensuration, registration, camera calibration, motion analysis, 3D scene reconstruction, and object recognition. Main advantages of using landmarks are robustness w.r.t. lightning conditions and other radiometric variations as well as the ability to cope with large displacements in registration or motion analysis tasks. Also, landmark-based approaches are in general computationally efficient, particularly when using *point landmarks*. Note, that the term landmark comprises both artificial and natural landmarks. Examples are corners or other characteristic points in video images, ground control points in aerial images, anatomical landmarks in medical images, prominent facial points used for biometric verification, markers at human joints used for motion capture in virtual reality applications, or in- and outdoor landmarks used for autonomous navigation of robots.

This book covers the *extraction of landmarks* from images as well as the use of these features for *elastic image registration.* Our emphasis is on *model-based* approaches, i.e. on the use of explicitly represented knowledge in image analysis. We principally distinguish between *geometric models* describing the shape of objects (typically their contours) and *intensity models,* which directly represent the image intensities, i.e., the appearance of objects. Based on these classes of models we develop algorithms and methods for analyzing *multimodality images* such as traditional 2D video images or 3D medical tomographic images. The book describes theoretical foundations, computational and algorithmic issues, as well as practical applications, particularly in medicine (neurosurgery, radiology), remote sensing, and industrial automation.

In the first chapter we give some background on model-based computer vision and point out relations to computer graphics as well as artificial intelligence. Then, in the second chapter we present different classes of approaches for the detection and localization of landmarks comprising differential and parametric schemes. A separate chapter of the book is subsequently devoted to detailed analytic and experimental studies on the performance of landmark extraction schemes. Both geometric and intensity models of landmarks are utilized, and the focus is on 3D anatomical point landmarks of the human brain. In the final chapter, we consider the use of point landmarks for elastic image registration, i.e. the computation of locally adaptive geometric transformations between corresponding image data. Here, we present a nonparametric spline-based approach. Image registration is a fundamental task in computer vision and allows for image fusion, i.e. to integrate multimodality images. In medicine, fused image data can improve diagnosis, surgery planning and simulation, as well as intraoperative navigation. Other application areas are, for example, remote sensing, cartography, geographic information systems (GIS), geology, morphometrics, computer graphics (warping, morphing), and virtual reality (VR).

The intended audience are all readers interested in an introduction and overview of *landmark-based image analysis,* in particular, graduate students and researchers in computer science, engineering, computer vision, and medical image analysis.

Acknowledgement

This book is based on the author's Habilitation thesis submitted in April 1999 at the Computer Science Department of the University of Hamburg.

I'm particularly grateful to Prof. Dr.-Ing. H. Siegfried Stiehl for many discussions, for his experience in medical image analysis issues and beyond, and, most of all, for encouraging support and enthusiasm within the last six years. Working with him was a pleasure. I also thank him for valuable comments on a draft version of this monograph.

I'm also very grateful to Prof. Dr. Bernd Neumann for support and advise since I joined his Cognitive Systems Group (KOGS) in 1992, for providing a stimulating research environment with a rather broad spectrum of topics, and for always finding time for discussions. I also thank him for valuable comments on the manuscript.

I sincerely thank Prof. Dr. Karl Heinz Höhne, Prof. Dr. Heinrich Müller, and Prof. Dr. Max A. Viergever for kindly acting as Habilitation referee. I'm grateful to Max A. Viergever for inviting me to publish this monograph in the Computational Imaging and Vision Series of Kluwer Academic Publishers as well as for constructive and helpful comments.

For discussions and collaboration I particularly thank Dr. Christian Drewniok, Mike Fornefett, Sönke Frantz, Alexander Hagemann, Thomas Hartkens, Dr. Anders Heyden, Dr. Wladimir Peckar, Prof. Dr. Joachim Rieger, Prof. Dr. Christoph Schnörr, Dr. Carsten Schröder, Dr. Rainer Sprengel, and Dr. Rafael Wiemker.

For providing a constructive and pleasant working atmosphere I thank the current and former members as well as the students of KOGS (Arbeitsbereich Kognitive Systeme) and the LKI (Labor für Künstliche Intelligenz). I thank Dieter Jessen, Jörn Tellkamp, and Sven Utcke for technical support, and the librarians of the FBI (Fachbereich Informatik), E. Criegee and M. Obernesser, for making available a rather large number of the cited literature.

A major part of this work has been supported since 1994 by Philips Research Laboratories, Hamburg, within the project IMAGINE (IMage- and Atlas-Guided Interventions in NEurosurgery). For cooperation and discussions I thank Dr. T.M. Buzug, Dr. M.H. Kuhn, Dr. K. Ottenberg, Dr. J. Weese, and Dr. T. Zängel. Parts of this work have been supported by the DFG (Deutsche Forschungsgemeinschaft) and the EU (European Union), ESPRIT project VIVA (Viewpoint Invariant Visual Acquisition). I also acknowledge the administrative support of the MAZ (Mikroelektronik Anwendungszentrum) Hamburg GmbH, particularly Dr. H. Marburger.

The tomographic image data used in this work have kindly been provided by Philips Research Hamburg, the AIM project COVIRA (COmputer VIsion in RAdiology) of the EU, the IMDM of the University Hospital Eppendorf (UKE) as well as W.P.Th.M. Mali, L. Ramos, and C.W.M. van Veelen (Utrecht University Hospital) via ICS-AD of Philips Medical Systems Best. I also thank Dr. F.J. Schuier and T. Wittkopp, Dept. of Neurology at the Rheinische Landes- und Hochschulklinik Düsseldorf, for making available the SAMMIE atlas developed within the EU project SAMMIE as well as for the CT images shown in Figures 2.29,2.33. The pre- and postoperative MR images in Figure 4.53 have kindly been provided by Dr. U. Spetzger and Prof. Dr. J.-M. Gilsbach, Neurosurgical Clinic, University Hospital Aachen of the RWTH.

Chapter 1

Introduction and Overview

Computer vision is the scientific field that is concerned with the processing, analysis, and interpretation of *visual information* represented by *images*. The term *image* here refers to digital images, i.e. arrays of intensity values or also other values (e.g., range data). Such discrete representations are the basis for processing by a computer.

Generally, images are two-dimensional (2D) and represent a projection of a three-dimensional (3D) scene. Elements of such *2D images* are called *pixels* (from picture elements). Alternatively, 2D images may directly represent 2D aspects of an object. Examples are images which are slices of a 3D object as is the case with tomographic images. If we acquire spatially contiguous slices, we obtain a spatial image sequence which actually is a *3D image* or a *volume image* (Figure 1.1). Such 3D spatial images are particularly relevant in the medical area, but are also important in other areas such as geology or industrial inspection. The elements of such images are called *voxels* (from volume elements). On the other hand, if we acquire 2D images over time for the purpose of depicting dynamic processes, then we obtain a temporal image sequence, which can be also considered as a 3D image. An example are video images of street traffic scenes. Even further, if we acquire 3D spatial images over time, then we obtain a 4D image, which is relevant, for example, for analyzing the behavior of the beating human heart. Moreover, all these images may be color images or, more generally, multispectral images. Such images are vector images representing the different spectral bands. Images may not only be classified w.r.t. their dimension as above, but also w.r.t. the underlying imaging technique. Actually, there exists a large variety of different imaging techniques that generally depict different aspects of a scene, e.g., one can distinguish between video images, microscopy images, infrared images, ultrasound images, X-ray images, X-ray Computed Tomography images (CT),

1

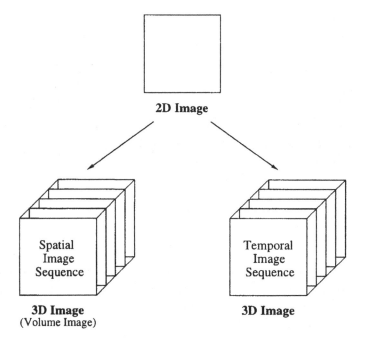

Figure 1.1.   2D and 3D images.

Magnetic Resonance images (MR), functional MR images (fMRI), Positron Emission Tomography images (PET), and temporal tomographic images.

Given these different kinds of images the general aim of computer vision is to develop algorithms and methods to *construct symbolic descriptions* (e.g., Marr [328], Ballard and Brown [22]). An important aspect is that computer vision systems have to be seen as active systems in the sense that they interact with the environment and should have the possibility to control the image acquisition process. This paradigm is known as *active vision* (e.g., Bajcsy [17], Aloimonos [5]). With an active system certain tasks can greatly be facilitated and it enables to design more efficient algorithms. However, in certain branches of computer vision, e.g., in medical image analysis, active systems currently have no importance. Note, that in the following we use the terms *computer vision* and *image analysis* synonymously. Both terms subsume the field of *image processing* (in a more narrow sense) dealing with pure image-to-image transformations such as image enhancement. More or less alternative terms for computer vision are *machine vision, image understanding*, and *scene analysis*, where the latter two emphasize higher interpretation levels.

One emphasis of scientific research in computer vision is the development of *generic methods* that are applicable to a large variety of different kinds of images, different scenes as well as different application tasks. The central question is: What are the *general principles* of analyzing and interpreting (digital) images? The aim of early work in computer vision has been the development of fully automatic computer vision systems. Currently, however, there is also a trend to design computer vision systems as support systems within a human-computer interaction environment. On the one hand, such systems have the advantage that the user has the possibility to control the system and thus its output. This is important, for example, in medical applications related to brain surgery since the possibility to control the system generally increases the user acceptance and thus the applicability of computer vision technology. On the other hand, about 40 years of experience in computer vision research and application has shown that for not too restricted applications fully automatic and reliable systems are currently beyond the state-of-the-art. The reasons for this fact seem to be the large spectrum of objects and phenomena encoded in visual information, the large variety of tasks, as well as the computational complexity of vision problems. It seems that we currently do not have the principles and the knowledge required for building more general and reliable computer vision systems.

This book is concerned with *model-based analysis* of images, particularly 2D and 3D images, and describes contributions towards the introduction of explicitly represented knowledge in computer vision. We mainly focus on two fundamental tasks in computer vision, namely feature extraction and image registration. As image features, we here consider *landmarks*, which are prominent geometric image features. On the one hand, we are concerned with the accurate and reliable extraction of landmarks from image data, and, on the other hand, we describe an image registration method based on such landmarks. Other tasks for *landmark-based image analysis* are, e.g., image mensuration, camera calibration, motion analysis, 3D scene reconstruction, and object recognition. Central to our work are model-based approaches using a certain class of models, namely *geometric and intensity models*. These models are very effective in representing generic knowledge as well as allow rather direct exploitation for analyzing images. The key problem here is to find such models, that are realistic enough, but at the same time can efficiently and reliably be used for image analysis. Within the field of computer science the closest relationships to our work exist to knowledge representation in artificial intelligence and to computer graphics. In this introductory chapter, we discuss these relationships and describe the context in which our work is embedded. We also classify different models used in model-based image analysis and characterize our work on the basis of this classification.

The remainder of this introductory chapter is organized as follows. In the next section, we consider image analysis from the point of view of a knowledge-based process and we also discuss its relation to other scientific fields. Then, in Section 1.2 we describe in more detail what we mean by model-based and knowledge-based approaches and discuss related views in computer vision. In Section 1.3 we summarize relationships between computer vision and computer graphics, which are particularly relevant in the context of model-based approaches to computer vision. After that, we characterize in more detail different classes of models used in model-based approaches. The main distinctions we make are between geometric models and intensity models (Section 1.4), between differential models and deformable models (Section 1.5), as well as between parametric and nonparametric models (Section 1.6). Then, in Section 1.7, we consider in more detail the image information utilized in computer vision approaches and focus on the use of landmarks as image features. Finally, on the basis of the classifications in the previous sections, in Section 1.8 we characterize our work on landmark extraction and image registration, point out our contributions in comparison to previous work, and give an overview of the subsequent chapters.

1.1   Image Analysis as a Knowledge-Based Process

When analyzing images we generally have to make idealized assumptions about the real world while disregarding irrelevant, accidental, and disturbing information. Moreover, we have to utilize prior knowledge about objects and processes. Thus, image analysis and interpretation is a *knowledge-based process*. One main question in developing computer vision systems concerns the knowledge which is necessary to accomplish a given task. Second, we have to find means to adequately represent this knowledge, and third, we need methods to utilize this knowledge for analyzing visual data. In summary we have to pose three main questions:

- Which knowledge ?

- Which knowledge representation ?

- How to utilize the knowledge ?

   Due to the fact that knowledge representation and utilization plays a central role, computer vision can be considered a subfield of *artificial intelligence (AI)*. Actually, computer vision is one of the largest and most difficult subfields of AI. On the other hand, image processing (in a more narrow sense) as a subfield of image analysis, has close relations to *signal processing* which is a subfield within *electrical engineering*. Additionally, techniques from the field of *pattern recognition*, dealing primarily with object classification, are important in computer vision. The general goal in computer vision is to design and implement complex information processing systems, which is central in *computer science*. Generally, the functionality of these systems can be related to aspects of intelligent behavior of humans, which motivates the use of the term *intelligent systems* and also constitutes the connection to *cognitive science* dealing with the perception and reasoning of human beings. To develop intelligent systems, where it is central to cope with the complexity of a given task, we have to develop formal models. This requires a theoretical analysis of the problem, i.e. we have to structure the problem and find a *mathematical description*. This description may be either more signal-oriented or more symbolic-oriented. For signal-oriented descriptions often models from *physics* are used. Since the aim of computer vision is the development of systems that work and interact with the environment, techniques from the areas of *software engineering, computer architectures,* and *robotics* are also important. A very close relationship exists to the field of *computer graphics* (or *image synthesis*), particularly in the case of model-based approaches to computer vision. This concerns, for example, geometric models of 3D objects or models of image formation. The relationship between image analysis and image synthesis will be discussed in more detail below. To summarize, computer vision has a truly interdisciplinary character with a large number of related disciplines while model building and knowledge representation are central issues (see also, e.g., Shapiro [482], Winston [564], Brauer and Münch [63], Wilhelm [562]).

One problem in the field of computer vision is the lack of awareness that image analysis and interpretation actually is a knowledge-based process as discussed above. A consequence is that currently too little knowledge is employed (e.g., Jain and Binford [262], Neumann [370],[369]; see also Christensen [94]). Another lack is that often knowledge is only *implicitly* encoded in certain image operators. Thus, although knowledge is used, it is not represented *explicitly*. The consequences are that the assumptions behind these algorithms are not clear, adaption to other circumstances is hardly possible, and the performance of the algorithms is hardly predictable. Recently, however, *performance characterization* of computer vision algorithms has gained increased attention. On the one hand, such characterizations are a major step towards the scientific foundation of the field of computer vision which hopefully will reduce the number of *ad hoc* approaches. On the other hand, performance characterizations serve a clear practical need. Since often existing algorithms are integrated into a computer vision system, central questions are which algorithms should be selected and how good these algorithms perform (see also, e.g., Jain and Binford [262], Haralick [224], Christensen and Förstner [95], Bowyer and Phillips [58], Klette et al. [281]).

We now discuss in more detail the knowledge which can be utilized for image analysis. Certainly, the knowledge required in a computer vision system depends on the considered domain as well as the given task. Generally, there is a hierarchy of knowledge ranging from very general to rather specific knowledge. Such a hierarchy comprises knowledge about, e.g., the geometry and other properties of objects, the imaging process, the spatial relations between objects, or the motions of objects. Examples for *general knowledge* are assumptions about object symmetries, about the smoothness of the intensity variations of images, or about the smoothness of motions. Algorithms based on such assumptions can be applied to a wide spectrum of images. However, on the basis of such knowledge only a very restricted class of tasks can be solved. To solve more complex tasks more *specific knowledge* is necessary. Such knowledge includes specific geometric models about the form of objects, specific physical knowledge about object motion, or specific models about the intensity variations based on photometric or radiometric models. Note, that the degree of specificity of each of these models can be rather different depending on the admissible degrees-of-freedom. For example, a geometric model of an industrial working piece may be defined by fixed dimensions or may also have some flexibility by introducing size and shape parameters. In the latter case we speak of a *generic model*. Note also, that there is no clear distinction between general and specific knowledge, but the transition between these types of knowledge is continuous. Also, it is generally not easy to judge which knowledge is more specific than other knowledge. An advantage of specific knowledge is that the *predictive value* is rather high. This property allows to generate expectations about the scene content with rather hard constraints and thus enables to focus image analysis on restricted parts of the image. By this, the solution space can significantly be reduced, which generally leads to a significant reduction of the computation time. The use of very specific knowledge allows to reduce the solution space to a minimal extent. However, such an approach is only feasible in a limited number of applications with rather controlled environments. For an approach, which can be applied to a wider range of applications it is required to use not too specific knowledge. Thus, the general task is to find a good compromise between the specificity of the knowledge, the range of potential applications, and the size of the solution space.

Both general and specific knowledge can be utilized at different levels of processing ranging from *low-level vision* to *high-level vision* (Figure 1.2). Starting out from the raw image data to end up with conceptual descriptions one can distinguish the following main *abstraction levels* in image analysis: Extraction and description of image features (image structures), recognition and description of objects in the scene, and recognition of object configurations, situations, as well as events. While in low-level vision knowledge is often represented in image-like, i.e. *analogical* form, in higher levels *propositional* (or *conceptual*) descriptions dominate. Each form is useful for different purposes, e.g., propositional descriptions are often better suited to represent motion events. With propositional descriptions the connection to the given visual data is not direct, thus it is generally more difficult to utilize the represented knowledge for analyzing images than with analogical representations. In general, it seems

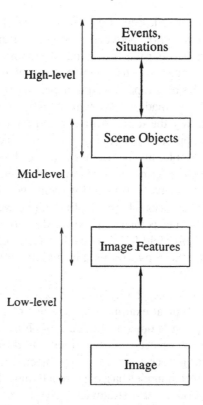

Figure 1.2. Different abstraction levels in image analysis.

that both analogical and propositional representations are necessary (see also, e.g., Kanade [269], Marr [327], Ballard and Brown [22], Rosenfeld [453], Jain and Binford [262], Neumann [369]).

1.2 Model-based and Knowledge-Based Approaches

Computer vision approaches utilizing explicitly represented knowledge are generally denoted as model-based or knowledge-based approaches. In this section, we discuss the meaning of these two terms and also describe some principal views related to these approaches. For surveys as well as books dealing with model-based or knowledge-based approaches see also, e.g., Kanade [269], Marr [327],[328], Ballard and Brown [22], Binford [44], Besl and Jain [39], Niemann [376],[377], Chin and Dyer [89], Shirai [484], Rao and Jain [412], Rosenfeld [453], Neumann [368],[369], Shapiro [482], Stiehl [502], Haralick and Shapiro [226], Suetens et al. [506], Arman and Aggarwal [10], McInerney and Terzopoulos [337], Crevier and Lepage [108], Graham and Barrett [201],

Schröder [476], as well as Niessen and Viergever [381]. Note, that in most of these references a distinction between model-based and knowledge-based is not made. Thus, concerning the formation of technical terms in computer vision, one possibility would be to use the two terms synonymously. However, when going through titles of computer vision papers, for example, it seems that an 'intuitive' distinction is made. For example, when conceptual knowledge is involved, then generally the term knowledge-based approach is used. On the other hand, for an approach where a geometric cylinder model is fitted to the image data, for example, always the term model-based approach is used and one would not use the term knowledge-based. Thus, there seems to be a distinction between these two terms and it seems worthwhile to work on a characterization. For references where a distinction between model-based and knowledge-based approaches is made and where definitions of these two terms are given, we refer to Rosenfeld [453] as well as Haralick and Shapiro [226]. Below, we characterize these two terms and mainly follow the definition of Haralick and Shapiro [226].

In *model-based approaches* the utilized knowledge for image analysis is formulated explicitly. Typical examples are the use of geometric models for 2D or 3D shape description of objects or the use of physical models to describe possible deformations of objects. Often, these models are employed in a *top-down* (model-driven) process by matching object representations to image representations. However, a model-based approach may also comprise *bottom-up* (data-driven) or *hybrid* control strategies. The use of both bottom-up and top-down strategies is generally performed within a *hypothesize-and-test* cycle. Note, that the knowledge typically is represented in a *generic model*, which defines a model class, while the comparison with the image data is performed with *instantiated models*, i.e. representatives of the model class.

Knowledge-based approaches are also based on a model of the real world, formulate this knowledge explicitly, and use it for image analysis. However, main features of a knowledge-based approach are a separate and well-structured knowledge base together with an inference (or reasoning) component. Typically, the inference component is rule-based. Recently, also logic-based approaches have been proposed, e.g. description logic systems with the general goal of providing decidable inference services (e.g., Möller et al. [349]). Knowledge-based approaches typically represent knowledge by conceptual descriptions in comparison to model-based approaches. An emphasis of knowledge-based approaches is to represent knowledge in a rather task-independent manner and to access the knowledge with generic mechanisms. Knowledge-based approaches generally comprise bottom-up as well as top-down control strategies. In Figure 1.3 the general architecture of a knowledge-based system has been depicted (Neumann [368]). In comparison to a conventional system architecture the program part is much smaller. The

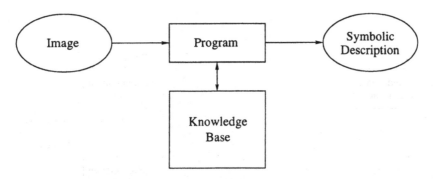

Figure 1.3.   General architecture of a knowledge-based computer vision system (from [368]).

reason for this is that the domain-specific knowledge has been transferred into the knowledge base and now the program is essentially an interpreter, which is (as far as possible) application-independent and requires less programming effort.

A common characteristic of model-based and knowledge-based systems is that (at least) three principal components are necessary: image features, a generic model (generic knowledge), and a similarity measure. *Image features* may be, for example, image edges or corners, Fourier descriptors, or also the image intensities directly. The *generic model* (*generic knowledge*) explicitly represents the available knowledge. Finally, a *similarity measure* is needed to perform a comparison of the model (knowledge) with the extracted image description.

Central to model-based and knowledge-based approaches is the utilization of *explicitly represented knowledge*. This view has particularly been emphasized by Marr [327],[328]. He suggested an overall framework for visual information processing that distinguishes three *levels of representation:* 2D (elementary image structures such as curves and regions; also denoted as primal sketch), $2\frac{1}{2}$D (discontinuities, depth and orientation of surface elements), and 3D descriptions (shape representation of 3D objects as well as their spatial organization). At each of these levels information is made explicit. The intention of this framework has been the derivation of 3D shape descriptions from images. Higher abstraction levels in computer vision, where, e.g., events and situations are represented, have not been taken into account (but see, e.g., Neumann [369], Niemann [376]). Also, the conception that computer vision systems have to be seen as active systems in the sense that they interact with the environment and should have the possibility to control the image acquisition process, did not play an important role at that time (e.g., Bajcsy [17], Aloimonos [5]; see also [372]). Note, that the framework of Marr [327],[328] has been established for 2D projection images. Particularly in the case of 3D spatial

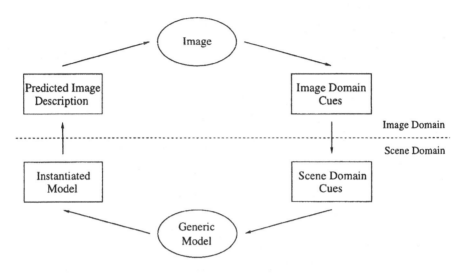

Figure 1.4.   Image interpretation cycle according to Kanade [269].

images the introduction of a $2\frac{1}{2}$D description has no relevance. However, the main point is to distinguish different levels of abstraction in image analysis.

Kanade [269] suggested a cyclic scheme as a general model for an image analysis process (Figure 1.4). Given an image, image domain cues (e.g., edge segments and texture properties) and scene domain cues (e.g., depth and reflectance) are computed and used to access the generic model to generate hypotheses. The generic model describes the generic shape of objects and relations among them. Selecting a specific situation we obtain an instantiated model from which a predicted image description (denoted as view sketch in [269]) can be derived, which is then matched with the input data. This framework makes a clear distinction between the image domain and the scene domain. Also, the scheme is well-structured in the sense that corresponding descriptions from the image and the model also visually correspond in the scheme. For a summary and discussion of different control structures in image analysis, see also Tsotsos [534].

Another main contribution of Marr [327],[328] is to emphasize the importance of a *computational theory*. The computational theory is considered as the first level of understanding an information processing task, and is concerned with the goal of computation, its appropriateness, as well as the logic of the strategy by which it can be carried out. The second level is the level of *representation and algorithms*, which is concerned with the design of algorithms for implementing the computational theory. Finally, the third level is the *hardware* level, where the problem is addressed of how representation and algorithms can be realized physically. Particular emphasis is on the distinction between the first and the second level. An example for the first level is the theory of Fourier transform, while algorithms like the Fast Fourier Transform (FFT) belong to the second level. Marr writes: *"The theory of a computation must precede the design of algorithms for carrying it out, because one cannot seriously contemplate designing an algorithm or a program until one knows precisely what it is meant to be doing"*. Furthermore he states: *"... to write plausible constraints directly into an algorithm ... (has) ... nothing to do with the theory of vision"*.

This view can be seen as a motivation to put strong efforts in the development of computational theories. These theories have to be formulated mathematically. Actually, when consulting recent work in computer vision, see, e.g., the recent proceedings of international conferences such as ICCV (International Conference on Computer Vision), ECCV (European Conference on Computer Vision), and CVPR (Computer Vision and Pattern Recognition), one observes an emphasis on mathematically well-founded approaches and mathematical rigor. On the one hand, the currently often high mathematical level in computer vision can be seen as an indication that computer vision problems are rather difficult. On the other hand, one might get the impression that computer vision is only a branch of *applied mathematics*. A comment w.r.t. this issue has been given by Faugeras in the introduction of his book [149]: *"We have stressed the mathematical soundness of our ideas in all our approaches at the risk of scaring some readers away. We strongly believe that detailing the mathematics is worth the effort, for it is only through their use that computer vision can be established as a science. But there is a great danger that computer vision will become yet another area of applied mathematics. We are convinced that this danger can be avoided if we keep in mind the original goal of designing and building robotics systems that perceive and act."* While Faugeras' focus is on building robotics systems, this comment applies also to other computer vision systems not connected to physical actuators, e.g., computer vision based support systems in the medical area or computer vision systems for image retrieval. Generally, the systems interact with the human or the environment, and a prerequisite for building systems that work reliably is the development of algorithms based on a sound mathematical theory (see also Florack [155]).

Others, in particular Horn [254], emphasize the importance of better *physical models* particularly in the case of image formation: *"Machine vision should be based on a thorough understanding of image formation"*. He advocates *physics-based vision* and the use of *continuous mathematics* for describing physical and geometric models. While physical models for image formation describe a forward process (from scene elements to image elements), the task of computer vision is the inverse process (see also Kanade and Ikeuchi [270]). Physical models are also very relevant in modelling deformable shapes, which can be applied for image segmentation and tracking. The utilized *deformable models* rely on the use of elasticity theory dealing with elastic deformations of bodies under applied forces. These models are able to represent the variability of object form (either man-made objects or biological structures). Note, that in this case the primary focus is often not on modelling the real physical behavior of observed objects, but to use the physical knowledge to constraint the solution. Starting from the well-known snake models of Kass et al. [274], i.e. *deformable contour models,* this research area has evolved very much in the last years (see McInerney and Terzopoulos [337] for a survey). Recently, elastic models play an important role in image registration, i.e. matching whole images with each other, while theses images generally have been acquired from different sensors (multimodality images). Main applications are within the medical area. Very recently, in the medical area there is also a growing interest in modelling soft tissue deformations (e.g., see a recent workshop on this topic organized by Székely and Duncan [509]). In this case one is interested in modelling the real physical behavior of objects. Modelling soft tissues such as the human brain and heart is important for surgery simulation and intraoperative navigation (see also Section 1.3 below). For further literature on physics-based vision, see also Shafer et al. [479] as well as Metaxas and Terzopoulos [341].

Having described characteristics and principal views concerning knowledge-based and model-based approaches, we now summarize the advantages and problems of these approaches. One advantage is certainly that the assumptions of such approaches are made explicit. Thus, the domain of application can be stated precisely. Also, in a concrete application task it is possible to recognize whether there are significant deviations from the model as well as to determine how large these deviations are. In addition, model-based and knowledge-based approaches can more easily be adapted to different circumstances than approaches, where the utilized knowledge is incorporated implicitly. Moreover, formal investigations of the performance of the algorithms are generally easier. This allows to predict the performance in a certain application task, e.g., as a function of perturbations such as image noise. On the other hand, there are certainly also problems with model-based and knowledge-based approaches. A principal problem is often to find models that are realistic enough but at the same time are not too complex so that the problem remains tractable and that reliability is guaranteed. For example, when describing the generic shape of an object with a nonlinear parametric model, there is generally a limit on the number of parameters which can reliably be estimated from images. Thus, the real task in designing model-based and knowledge-based approaches is to find realistic models which allow reliable as well as efficient use in image analysis.

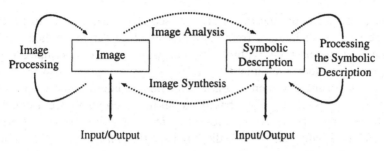

Figure 1.5. Relation between image analysis and image synthesis.

1.3 Image Analysis and Image Synthesis

This book is concerned with model-based approaches to computer vision. As already mentioned above, particularly in this context there exist close relationships to computer graphics. Often, models developed in this field are rather relevant for model-based image analysis. Thus, it is important to study related methods from computer graphics. In this section, we discuss relationships between *computer vision (image analysis)* and *computer graphics (image synthesis)* and emphasize areas common to both fields, which are particularly relevant in the context of model-based approaches to computer vision (see also, e.g., Eklundh and Kjelldahl [140], Besl [38], Witkin et al. [567], Pun and Blake [408], Lengyel [306]).

The general relation between image analysis and image synthesis has been depicted in Figure 1.5 (see also, e.g., Voss [544], Leister and Rohr [305], Calvert and Chapman [78]). Whereas the aim of image analysis is the derivation of a symbolic description from real images, it is the aim of image synthesis to produce realistic images from a symbolic description. Besides that, image processing denotes pure image-to-image transformations and, analogously, symbolic descriptions may be transformed into new symbolic descriptions. Figure 1.5 clearly makes explicit that computer vision is the inverse process of computer graphics. Thus, these two fields have completely different goals. However, to achieve these goals often techniques from the other field are needed. As already mentioned above, for image analysis we generally have to employ knowledge of the depicted scene. For example, we may model objects by geometric models and this task is actually a central topic within computer graphics. Another example concerns the validation and evaluation of computer vision algorithms. Here, it is generally important to generate synthetic images for testing the algorithms. Doing this, we are very flexible to incrementally increase the complexity of the images (e.g., simple vs. complex objects, small vs. large number of objects, consideration of occlusions, incorporation of highlights or image noise). In contrast to real images, *ground truth* is available in this case, i.e., we know the correct result (see also Chapter 3). To generate synthetic images, techniques from computer graphics can be applied. On the other hand, a current topic within computer graphics is, for example, to generate geometric models automatically from camera images or also from other data, e.g., depth measurements from a laser range finder. To accomplish this task, which is known as image-based modelling, techniques from computer vision have to be applied. Another recent topic in computer graphics is image-based rendering, where images are directly used to synthesize new views of the scene without employing geometric models of objects. A central task here is to compute image correspondences, which actually is a central task in computer vision. A central characteristic of image analysis is that we have to deal with measurement errors, particularly due to image noise, and also with incomplete information. This is a main difference to computer graphics. Below, we now describe areas common to both fields.

One common topic of computer vision are models of *image formation*. These models include geometric and physical models, e.g., projective geometry models or illumination models such as the one of Phong [402]. In the case of image synthesis it is clear that the better the models for image formation are, the more realistic are synthetically generated images. Note, however, that often a compromise has to be made between the complexity of the models and the computation time, to allow their use in practical applications. In the case of image analysis the same holds true, while here the emphasis is on exploiting image formation models to develop approaches for deriving descriptions of the depicted scene, e.g., approaches that allow a comparison between the image and the model. In Section 1.2 we already mentioned that particularly Horn [254] emphasized the need for better physical models of image formation. Traditionally, computer graphics deals with the synthesis of projection images (camera and video images), i.e. images as usually perceived by humans. However, there are a lot of other imaging modalities, particularly in the medical domain. Recently, there is a growing interest in image formation models for medical images such as MR (Magnetic Resonance) images or PET (Positron Emission Tomography) images (e.g., Kwan et al. [294]). Whereas in camera or video images the intensities represent the brightness due to light emission, in the case of MR images, for example, the intensities represent the magnetic effect of the spin of atomic nuclei (see also Sections 1.4 and 2.6.1 below). Image formation models for such radiological images can be used to produce simulated images, which is important for evaluating image analysis algorithms. Particularly in the medical domain there is a lack of ground truth data, and also the number and range of imaging parameters is rather large (e.g., T_1- vs. T_2-weighted MR images, intensity inhomogeneity, resolution, slice thickness, noise). Instead, by using simulated data the correct result is known and also the imaging parameters can be controlled independently to study the performance of algorithms. Interestingly, image formation models for such imaging modalities are (currently) studied within the field of medical image analysis and not within computer graphics.

The most important common area of computer vision and computer graphics are *geometric models* of 3D objects. Here, a main distinction can be made between stick figures (skeletons), surface and volume representations. Examples of primitive shapes are cylinders, ellipsoids, or superquadrics. Shapes may mathematically be described in explicit, parametric, or implicit form (e.g., Hoffmann [249], Hoschek and Lasser [256], Bolle and Vemuri [48]). Particularly, surface representations of scattered data play an important role in both fields. Scattered data may be directly acquired using a range finder but may also be computed from images, e.g., by computing sparse depth values from stereo images. In computer graphics main criteria for geometric models are that they are flexible, efficient, and easy to use. In computer vision, geometric models are often used for matching them with features from image data (e.g., with image edges) for the purpose of locating and recognizing objects. Thus, flexibility, efficiency, and ease-of-use are relevant criteria, but additionally their suitability for matching is important (see, e.g., Stiehl [502] for a synopsis of criteria). A principally different approach to object recognition is to use a view (or aspect) graph of a 3D object (e.g., Koenderink and van Doorn [285], Rieger [417]). In this case, the shape of 3D objects is represented by a finite number of characteristic views, and on the basis of these views and their invariant features, objection recognition is performed. Here, a main class for 3D shape description are piecewise algebraic surfaces, i.e., surfaces subdivided into surface patches that are described by polynomials and where certain continuity conditions are imposed. In the ideal case one would like to directly employ 3D model representations from computer aided (geometric) design (abbreviated by CA(G)D) as a subfield of computer graphics, while using view graph algorithms developed within computer vision. However, there are a number of fundamental problems that still have to be solved (see also, e.g., Rieger and Rohr [420],[419]).

Another important common topic of image analysis and image synthesis, which recently gained increased attention particularly in computer vision, is the *modelling of movements*. Here, one distinguishes between kinematic and dynamic models of movements. This includes articulated movements of bodies, e.g., locomotion of the human body, where the body parts are treated as moving rigid objects which are connected by joints (e.g., Zeltzer [576], Tost and Pueyo [532], Calvert and Chapman [78], Rohr [429],[435], Cédras and Shah [82], Shah and Jain [480], Aggarwal et al. [3], Gavrila [186]). But also elastic deformations are included, e.g., modelling of skin deformations in facial expressions or modelling of brain deformations. In the latter case the aim is to simulate deformations of real objects under applied forces and the approaches are generally based on elasticity theory from physics. Applications are, for example, training and planning systems in the medical area or the simulation of car crash tests. Within computer vision, elastic models are particularly used for image segmentation and registration (see also Section 1.5 below). In the case of registration, one wants to find a geometric transformation that maps one image as good as possible onto another image. A major distinction can be made between rigid, affine, piecewise algebraic, and elastic transformations. These types of transformations represent different types of movements, e.g, rigid, piecewise rigid (articulated), and elastic movements. For further classifications of motion see the literature in computer graphics (e.g., Wilhelms [563]) and computer vision (e.g., Kambhamettu et al. [268], Aggarwal et al. [3]).

Finally, we mention *human-computer interaction* as a common topic of computer vision and computer graphics. Currently, there is a focus on the development of virtual (or augmented) reality systems for improved human-computer interaction. Central to this topic is the combination of information from different sensors (e.g., images, speech, tactile information) and generally real-time manipulation is necessary. From the field of computer graphics, interactive techniques and methods for 3D visualization are very relevant. Computer vision techniques are necessary, for example, to allow automatic recognition of human gestures.

Since computer vision and computer graphics have a larger number of common areas, there are also a larger number of mathematical subfields which are relevant for both of these fields, particularly geometry, differential geometry, approximation theory, estimation theory, functional analysis, and numerics.

1.4   Geometric Models and Intensity Models

We now describe in more detail which types of models are used in computer vision to represent object shapes together with their variability. We distinguish between geometric models and intensity models.

Geometric models are generally used to describe the shape of objects in a depicted scene, i.e. they represent their *geometry*. Examples for objects are man-made objects (e.g., houses, chairs, and industrial working pieces) but also natural objects (e.g., the human body and its organs).[1] Usually we have to deal with the shape of 3D objects, where mostly surface representations are

---

[1]Note, that also natural objects such as trees or meadows can be adequately described by geometric models. For example, each leaf and branch of a tree has a geometric form which can well be modelled by existing geometric models. The problem is that usually trees are viewed at a scale where the whole tree (or a large part of it) is visible and for an adequate model of the appearance of a tree it would be necessary to model each leaf and branch of the whole tree. This, however, would result in such a complex geometric model, which would be very unsuited for computer vision applications. Therefore, in this case other models are better suited, e.g., texture models or fractal models for describing natural objects.

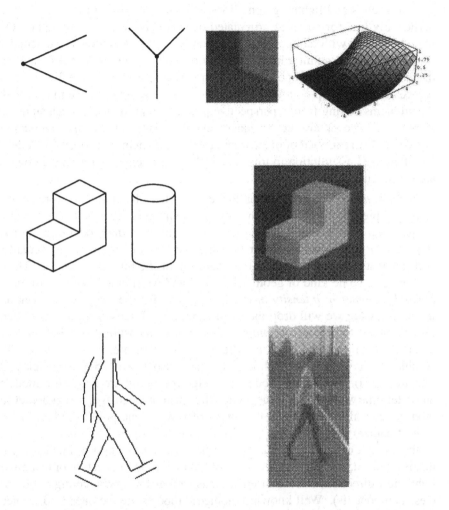

Figure 1.6. Geometric models (left) and corresponding intensities or intensity models (right) for corners (top row), single objects (middle row), and articulated objects (bottom row).

applied (e.g., generalized cylinders, superquadrics, algebraic surfaces, generalized splines). In the case of projection images (e.g., video images) these models are often projected onto the image (typically using perspective projection) and are compared with image features. A principal approach is to compute the contours of the object model and to compare them with image edges or other geometric image features (Figure 1.6 on the left). The fundamental advantage of such an approach is that we only have to deal with object boundaries, but we do not have to care directly about the corresponding intensity variations. Finding models that directly represent the intensity variations for rather general viewpoints and lightning conditions is in many cases not possible. This is particularly true for complex articulated objects (Figure 1.6 on the right). On the other hand, with an approach based only on object contours, we actually do not take into account a lot of information that is encoded in the image. In the case of 3D spatial images the situation is analogous. Here, the 3D shape of objects is directly represented by the image, thus, we do not have to deal with the problems arising from a perspective projection, particularly, occlusions do not occur. However, also here a general approach is to consider the contours of objects (e.g., the surface of organs) and to describe them by geometric models. An often used assumption in this case is that the intensities for single objects are homogeneous.

Intensity models, in comparison to the geometric object models from above, directly represent the image intensities. These models describe the systematic intensity variations of imaged objects. An example is the model of a blurred step edge or of a blurred corner (see the top row in Figure 1.6). Actually, such intensity models represent the geometry of the intensity surface. Thus, they are also some kind of geometric model and we should denote them more precisely *geometric intensity models*. However, for the sake of abbreviation in the following we will drop the word geometric. Intensity models are often closely related to *radiometric models*. Radiometry measures the radiant energy incident on or radiated from a surface patch or an area. If we deal with (visible) light we speak of photometry (see also Horn [254], Haralick and Shapiro [226]). Projection models of image formation are geometric models and determine where some scene point will appear in the image, and radiometric models determine how bright the image of some scene point will be. In the case of camera and video images, for example, image brightness depends on (i) the amount of light that falls on a surface, (ii) the fraction of incident light that is reflected, and (iii) the geometry of light reflection (direction of incoming light, view direction, surface orientation as well as the spatial configuration of these components). Well-known radiometric models are the ones by Torrance and Sparrow [530] and Phong [402] (see also Newman and Sproull [374], Claussen [97]). Based on such models and under certain assumptions it is possible to determine the geometry of surfaces in the scene directly from the image intensities. This approach is known as shape-from-shading (e.g., Horn [254]). In the case of other imaging modalities (e.g., X-ray CT, MR, PET, range finders) the laws that determine the image intensities are different and thus the meaning of the intensities is different (see also Section 2.6.1 below). Nevertheless, by intensity models we here denote models that directly describe the systematic variations of the intensities, regardless of the sensor by which the images have been acquired.

Recently, in computer vision there is a major trend to use intensity information for direct matching, e.g., in object recognition tasks such as face recognition. Schemes of this type are denoted *appearance-based* approaches, since they directly model the appearance of objects. Partly, geometric shape models are combined with intensity models to improve robustness (e.g., Murase and Nayar [360], Nastar et al. [365], Black et al. [45], Cootes et al. [103], Hager and Belhumeur [222], Jones and Poggio [264], Negahdaripour [366], and Sclaroff and Isidoro [477]).

1.5 Differential Models and Deformable Models

Geometric models and intensity models as described above may generally be represented by the same mathematical formalisms. One principal approach is to use concepts from *differential geometry* (e.g., Lipschutz [311], do Carmo [121]). Here, the shape of 3D objects, the corresponding intensity variations or also the image contours are described locally. This approach relies on partial derivatives of the models or of the images, and often curvature properties are exploited. Note, that in 2D images the term *contour* refers to a curve whereas in 3D spatial images the term contour generally refers to a surface. Analogously, we use the term *edge* for 2D and 3D images to refer to curves and surfaces, respectively. Main focus in the case of 2D images is on the description of contour curves and the intensity surface. In the case of 3D spatial images main focus is on 3D ridge (or crest) curves and on contour surfaces, and these features are often defined on the basis of isointensity surfaces within an image (see also, e.g., Koenderink [284], Haralick et al. [227], Monga et al. [352], Eberly et al. [137],[136], Florack et al. [154],[155]).

Another principal approach in computer vision, which we have already mentioned above, is based on *deformable models*. In comparison to differential approaches, deformable models integrate larger regions of an image, often complete objects. Also here, differential measures are often involved. Currently, deformable models are one of the main topics in computer vision (see also the survey by McInerney and Terzopoulos [337] as well as the book by Singh et al. [487]). These models in general combine geometry, physics, and approximation theory and are effective in exploiting image features in the bottom-up direction and a priori knowledge in the top-down direction. The aim in designing deformable models is to describe local and global deformations of depicted objects, e.g., the deformations of a beating human heart, but also the shape variability of objects from the same class. The main applications are image segmentation and tracking, but also image registration and simulation of object deformations. A broad range of object models and deformation models has been proposed. Most object models are either 2D or 3D contour models, i.e., geometric models. The exploited a priori knowledge ranges from very general assumptions to rather domain-specific models. The intention is to represent a large variety of shapes by using only a small number of parameters. One tries to find a compromise between generality and efficiency of the description. In the following, we classify the existing approaches into three categories: deformable generalized splines, deformable primitive shapes, and deformable template models. Approaches to elastic registration are discussed separately in Chapter 4.

Deformable generalized splines include curve and surface models. The possible deformations are modelled by physically-motivated energy functions. Curves of this kind are named *snakes* or *active contours* (e.g., Kass et al. [274]). Surfaces of this kind are used to describe 3D shapes (e.g., Terzopoulos et al. [518], Cohen and Cohen [99]). *Deformable primitive shapes* are more specific than deformable generalized splines, i.e., they describe a more restricted class of shapes and can generally be represented by a smaller number of parameters. Examples for primitive shapes are cylinders, spheres, or superquadrics. The deformations of the primitives may be global, for example, stretching, bending, and tapering (e.g., Barr [25],[26], Pentland [399], Solina and Bajcsy [493]), or may be both global and local (e.g., Terzopoulos and Metaxas [519], Pentland and Sclaroff [401], Vemuri and Radisavljevic [536]). *Deformable template models* are generally more domain-specific than the above mentioned two model classes. Models of this third class are often hand-crafted, partly they are based on theoretical considerations. Most of theses models can be regarded as rigid templates with added flexibility specified by a set of parameters. One can distinguish between contour models and models of image intensities. In the latter case, a main distinction can be made between discrete templates and analytic models. *Discrete templates* directly consist of the (noise perturbed) intensities within an image region and are used particularly in photogrammetry (e.g., Förstner [170]). *Analytic models* use analytic descriptions to represent the systematic intensity variations. These models have several advantages over discrete templates, e.g., increased descriptive power and larger independence of discretization and filtering effects when matching those models with the image data (see also Drewniok and Rohr [127],[129]). Examples for deformable templates are face templates, human chromosome templates and human eye templates (e.g., Fischler and Elschlager [153], Widrow [560], Yuille et al. [575], Jain et al. [261]). Deformable template models have also been designed for extracting low-level image features, namely edges (e.g., Hueckel [258], Nalwa and Binford [364]), corners (e.g., Rohr [427]), and circular landmarks (e.g., Drewniok and Rohr [128]).

Most deformable models use a finite difference (FD) scheme or the finite element method (FEM) for numeric computation (e.g., Terzopoulos et al. [518], Cohen and Cohen [99], Pentland and Sclaroff [401]). For 3D surface models using a Fourier parameterization see, e.g., Staib and Duncan [498] as well as Székely et al. [508]. Discrete deformable curve and surface models have been described by, e.g., Miller et al. [348], Lobregt and Viergever [313]. Statistical models, where deformations are only allowed in accordance with some training data, have been proposed by, e.g., Cootes and Taylor [102], Nastar et al. [365], and Martin et al. [332]. Besides explicitly defined deformable models, an emerging topic is the development of implicitly defined deformable models (level set methods, geometric or geodesic active contours). A main advantage of implicitly defined models is that topology changes can be handled naturally (e.g., Caselles et al. [80],[81], Malladi et al. [322], Yezzi et al. [573], Niessen et al. [380], Lorigo et al. [316]).

1.6   Parametric and Nonparametric Models

Above we have argued for *generic models* to represent knowledge in computer vision. Generic models are defined over a class and represent the spectrum of variations of prototypes. By instantiation we obtain a representative of the model class (e.g., [562]). A prominent example of generic models are deformable models as described in Section 1.5 above.

One principal approach to represent generic knowledge is to use *parametric models*. In this case, the spectrum of variations of a model is defined by a set of parameters $\mathbf{p} = (p_1, ..., p_n)$. For such a model we can write $f_M(\mathbf{p})$ and an instantiated model is obtained by assigning certain values to the parameters. Thus, the problem of image analysis is reduced to estimating the parameters $\mathbf{p}$ from images. For example, the length and width of an object may be specified by parameters and some shape prototype may be assumed, e.g., a cylinder or a superquadric. Also, one can use a parameter to specify the number of objects or object parts. While in the first example, real-valued parameters are appropriate, in the second example an integer-valued parameter is required. Note, that this distinction leads to principally different mathematical approaches for parameter estimation. In most cases a parametric model is given in *explicit form*. For example, in the case of an object surface in 3D we can write $f_M = f_M(\mathbf{x}, \mathbf{p})$, where $\mathbf{x} = (x, y)$ denote spatial coordinates. Alternatively, a parametric model of an object surface may be given in *implicit form*, i.e., $F_M(\mathbf{x}, \mathbf{p}) = 0$, $\mathbf{x} = (x, y, z)$, or also in *parametric form*, i.e., $\mathbf{x}(u, v, \mathbf{p}) = (x(u, v, \mathbf{p}), y(u, v, \mathbf{p}), z(u, v, \mathbf{p}))$. Note, that conversion from one form to another is not always possible (e.g., Hoffmann [249], Hoschek and Lasser [256], Bolle and Vemuri [48]).

A central problem in computer vision is the fact that we have discrete measurements (the image is sampled and quantized) and that these measurements are perturbed, particularly they are corrupted by noise. If we can assume additive noise $\mathbf{n}$, then the relation between the measurements f and the parametric model f_M can be stated as

$$f(\mathbf{x}_i) = f_M(\mathbf{x}_i, \mathbf{p}) + \mathbf{n}(\mathbf{x}_i), \qquad i = 1...m, \tag{1.1}$$

where x_i may represent spatial or temporal coordinates or both. Now, the aim is to estimate those parameters which optimize some criteria. Usually, the aim is to minimize the deviation between the (instantiated) model and the measurements. An often used similarity measure is the (squared) l_2-norm (Euclidean distance), which is well-suited for stochastic errors and where large errors are weighted strongly:

$$S(\mathbf{p}) = \sum_{i=1}^{m} (f(\mathbf{x}_i) - f_M(\mathbf{x}_i, \mathbf{p}))^2 \rightarrow min, \qquad (1.2)$$

which can also be written as $S(\mathbf{p}) = |\mathbf{f} - \mathbf{f}_M(\mathbf{p})|_2^2$ with $\mathbf{f} = (f(x_1), ..., f(x_m))^T$ and $\mathbf{f}_M(\mathbf{p}) = (f_M(x_1, \mathbf{p}), ..., f_M(x_m, \mathbf{p}))^T$. This approach is well-known as *least-squares method*. If we weight the errors in (1.2) then this approach is known as weighted least-squares. For the parameters we have $\mathbf{p} = (p_1, ..., p_n) \in \mathbb{R}^n$, i.e., the solution space is the space of dimension n of the real numbers. If f_M depends linearly on the parameters $\mathbf{p}$, i.e., $f_M(\mathbf{p}) = \mathbf{X}\mathbf{p}$, then the solution to (1.2) can be stated analytically as $\mathbf{p} = \mathbf{X}^{\#}\mathbf{f}$ using the generalized inverse $\mathbf{X}^{\#} = (\mathbf{X}^T\mathbf{X})^{-1}\mathbf{X}^T$. If there is a nonlinear relationship, then the solution can generally be computed only numerically. Besides the l_2-norm other important norms are the l_1-norm and the l_∞-norm. The l_1-norm measures the absolute deviation and is suited in the case of outliers. The l_∞-norm, which measures the maximal deviation, is more appropriate if we have no stochastic errors, i.e. in the case of approximating analytically given functions.

For the least-squares method there is also a statistical interpretation. If we have no statistical a priori knowledge about the parameters, and if we can assume additive zero-mean white Gaussian noise, which is independent of the parameters, then the least-squares approach in (1.2) is equivalent to *maximum-likelihood estimation* and it shares the same properties. In the linear case, the estimate is unbiased, efficient (minimal variance), and Gaussian distributed. In the nonlinear case, these properties hold in the limit of a large number m of measurements, i.e. the estimate is asymptotic unbiased (consistent), asymptotic efficient, and asymptotic Gaussian distributed (e.g., Sorenson [494]). In computer vision, parametric models have been applied, for example, for 3D object recognition (e.g., Pentland [399], Solina and Bajcsy [493]) and for extracting 2D image features (cf. Section 2.6).

In temporal image sequences the images and thus the measurements are acquired sequentially over time. Therefore, particularly in real-time applications, it is advantageous to incrementally estimate the model parameters. A standard method to do this is known as *Kalman filter* (e.g., Gelb [190], Sorenson [494]). Actually, this filter can be regarded as a sequential least-squares approach. Movement models can be incorporated by using time-dependent parameters. Based on the parameter values $\mathbf{p}_{k-1}$ of the previous image and the movement model, it is possible to make a prediction $\mathbf{p}_k^*$ for the current image to be analyzed. This generally reduces the search space significantly. In the linear case $f_M(\mathbf{p}_k) = \mathbf{X}_k \mathbf{p}_k$, an estimate of the parameters $\mathbf{p}_k$ of the current image can be obtained using the prediction $\mathbf{p}_k^*$ and the current measurements $\mathbf{f}_k$ by

$$\mathbf{p}_k = \mathbf{p}_k^* + \mathbf{K}_k(\mathbf{f}_k - \mathbf{X}_k \mathbf{p}_k^*), \qquad (1.3)$$

where the matrix $\mathbf{X}_k$ denotes the measurement model and the matrix $\mathbf{K}_k$ weights the deviation between the current measurement and the predicted model. In addition to estimating $\mathbf{p}_k$, we obtain an estimate of the current covariance matrix, which represents information about the reliability of the estimated parameters. If there is a nonlinear relationship between f_M and the parameters $\mathbf{p}$, then by linearization we arrive at the recursive formulas of the extended Kalman filter. In computer vision, Kalman filter approaches have been applied, for example, for tracking rigid objects from measured image points (e.g., Broida and Chellappa [67]), for tracking edge lines (e.g., Faugeras [149]), or for tracking articulated objects (e.g., Rohr [429],[435]).

In the case of a parametric model the form is known except for finitely many unknown parameters. Thus, these models are well-suited if detailed knowledge is available and they have a relatively high level of specificity. One main advantage is that the parameters generally have a direct physical meaning, e.g., they may be used to specify the length and width of an object. This means that the estimated parameter values can directly be used for further analysis. Additionally, estimation methods for parametric models have nice efficiency properties.

A principally different approach in comparison to using parametric models is based on *nonparametric models* (see also, e.g., Eubank [146], Wahba [545], Green and Silverman [202]). These models are not defined on the basis of a finite set of parameters and they are generally more suited in the case of little or no prior knowledge. Thus, the central question for choosing one of these two models is the question, which assumptions can be made about the model? Since nonparametric models do not require to specify a parametric form they have a greater flexibility. It is only assumed that the model belongs to some infinite dimensional space of functions. This space is usually motivated by smoothness properties the model can be assumed to possess. Often we have a Hilbert space $\mathcal{H}$, which is a complete space and the norm of which is defined on the basis of a scalar product. A Hilbert function space is an extension of the Euclidean space and the members of this space are functions instead of n-tuples (vectors). In the case of estimating the parameters of parametric models we have to minimize *functions*. Instead, in the case of nonparametric models we have to minimize *functionals*, i.e., mappings from functions to real numbers, which can be seen as a generalization of functions. A disadvantage of nonparametric models is that the physical interpretation of the solution is generally not as direct as is the case with the estimated parameters of parametric models. Also, nonparametric approaches are often less efficient. The basis is usually a minimizing functional, and often a finite difference (FD) scheme or the finite element method (FEM) is used for numeric solution. Only in certain cases, the solution can be stated analytically. In these cases, the models are denoted also as nonparametric regression models (e.g., [146]). Note, that here we use the term nonparametric model to refer to both kinds of approaches, i.e. approaches based on numeric as well as analytic solutions of minimizing functionals.

An example, where the solution to a minimizing functional can be stated analytically, is the thin-plate spline functional

$$J_\lambda(f_M) = \frac{1}{m} \sum_{i=1}^{m} (f(\mathbf{x}_i) - f_M(\mathbf{x}_i))^2 + \lambda \int_\Omega f_{M,xx}^2 + 2f_{M,xy}^2 + f_{M,yy}^2 \, d\mathbf{x}$$

$$\rightarrow \; min, \tag{1.4}$$

where discrete (generally scattered) measurements $f(\mathbf{x}_i)$ are given and certain boundary conditions are assumed. Note, that the additional subscripts to f_M denote second-order partial derivatives w.r.t. the space coordinates. Using this functional we are searching a surface that is close to the data according to the first term (data term), but which is also sufficiently smooth according to the second term (smoothness term). The relative weight between the two terms is determined by the parameter λ. Since the formulation in (1.4) is identical to the regularization method for solving ill-posed problems, λ is often denoted as regularization parameter (e.g., Tikhonov and Arsenin [527], Poggio et al. [404], Terzopoulos [517], Bertero et al. [34], Szeliski [511]). In computer vision, functionals of the type in (1.4) have been used, for example, for surface reconstruction of depth maps and for elastic image registration (cf. Chapter 4). Note, that the first term in (1.4) agrees (up to a constant factor) with (1.2) in the case of parametric approaches besides the fact that in (1.4) no parameters are involved. Since the solution to (1.4) can be stated analytically we yield an efficient computational scheme. Interestingly, we here obtain a parametric model as the solution:

$$f_M(\mathbf{x}) = \sum_{\nu=1}^{M} a_\nu \phi_\nu(\mathbf{x}) + \sum_{i=1}^{n} w_i U(\mathbf{x}, \mathbf{x}_i), \tag{1.5}$$

with linear monomials ϕ and certain radial basis functions U (for details see Chapter 4). The parameters can be summarized by $\mathbf{p} = (a_1, ..., a_M, w_1, ..., w_n)$ and for the model we can write $f_M(\mathbf{x}) = f_M(\mathbf{x}, \mathbf{p})$. Thus, the nonparametric problem is reduced to a parametric problem. However, a difference to usual parametric models is that here the number of the parameters increases with the

	Parametric models	*Nonparametric models*
Prior knowledge	detailed	little
Model form	known, except for finite number of parameters	only smoothness properties known
Specificity	high	low
Flexibility	low	high
To be minimized	functions	functionals
Type of solution	parameter vectors	functions
Solution space	finite parameter space $\mathbb{R}^n$	infinite function space $\mathcal{H}$
Existence of solution	generally exists	has to be clarified
Physical interpretation of the solution	often direct	generally not direct
Computation time	efficient	in general less efficient
Mathematical subfield	estimation theory, approximation theory	calculus of variations, approximation theory

Table 1.1.   Properties of parametric and nonparametric approaches.

number of measurements. Additionally note, that the solution to the nonparametric problem (1.4) is identical to the constrained minimization problem

$$S(f_M) = \frac{1}{m} \sum_{i=1}^{m} (f(\mathbf{x}_i) - f_M(\mathbf{x}_i))^2 \rightarrow min, \qquad J(f_M) \leq \rho \qquad (1.6)$$

where $J(f_M) = \int_\Omega f_{M,xx}^2 + 2f_{M,xy}^2 + f_{M,yy}^2 \, d\mathbf{x}$ denotes the smoothness term and $\rho \geq 0$ is a constant that places a bound on the smoothness (Eubank [146]). By introducing a Lagrange multiplier we find this equivalent to minimizing $S(f_M) + \lambda(J(f_M) - \rho)$, which is essentially (1.4). If we specify $\rho = 0$, i.e. $J(f_M) = 0$, then we obtain linear polynomials as the solution.

Nonparametric approaches are theoretically investigated in the mathematical subfields of calculus of variations, approximation theory, and functional analysis (e.g., Courant and Hilbert [106], Eubank [146], Wahba [545], Heuser [240]). The mathematical subfields devoted to the estimation of parametric models are (parameter) estimation theory and approximation theory (e.g., Sorenson [494], Gelb [190]). In Table 1.1 we have summarized the properties of parametric and nonparametric approaches. In computer vision, parametric and nonparametric approaches have a wide spectrum of applications, e.g., image segmentation, surface approximation of depth values, 3D object recognition, image registration, and optic flow estimation.

1.7   Feature- and Landmark-Based Image Analysis

Above, we have characterized different classes of models used for model-based image analysis. In this section, we consider in more detail the utilized image information. Principally, one can distinguish between feature-based and intensity-based schemes. In *feature-based approaches* features are first extracted from the images and then these features are exploited for subsequent processing. Examples for image features are moments, Fourier descriptors, edges or corners. In comparison, *intensity-based approaches* directly exploit the image intensities. Note, that the notion *image feature* is very general. Actually, one can even consider the intensities as some kind of feature. However, for a characterization of approaches, a distinction between features and intensities is generally helpful.

An important class of feature-based approaches relies on the use of landmarks. *Landmarks* are prominent geometric image features, which are sparsely scattered over the image and are distinguishable. These features have a defined position, thus a prerequisite is their explicit extraction from images based on some kind of non-maximum suppression scheme. This is in contrast to edgeness or cornerness features, for example, which represent continuous values over the whole image. Depending on the domain and application the complexity of landmarks may vary largely from relatively simple features to rather complex structures or objects. In the latter case, these landmarks are often represented by a combination of simple features. Originally, the meaning of landmark refers to visually prominent reference 'points' in a landscape, e.g. a characteristic hill, a steeple, a smokestack, or a heap of stones. Such landmarks have particularly been used for navigation of ships and airplanes. Examples for relevant landmarks in computer vision are: prominent facial points, points at human joints, anatomical landmarks of the human brain, corners or other characteristic points of man-made objects, ground control points in aerial images, or in- and outdoor landmarks used for autonomous navigation of robots or for computer-assisted orientation of blind people. A main distinction can be made between *already existing (natural)* landmarks and *artificial* landmarks. Examples for the latter case are ground or wall signs and skin or cloth markers.

Landmarks are preferred features for a variety of computer vision tasks, e.g., image mensuration, registration and camera calibration, motion analysis, 3D scene reconstruction, as well as object recognition (Figure 1.7). The main tasks in *landmark-based image analysis* are (i) the detection and localization of landmarks, and (ii) the use of these features for the above-mentioned tasks. Note, that the term landmark is primary used for *point landmarks*, e.g., prominent points of anatomy or of man-made objects. These landmarks have a unique position which can be deduced from a sufficiently large neighborhood around the prominent point. However, there are also other classes of landmarks. In

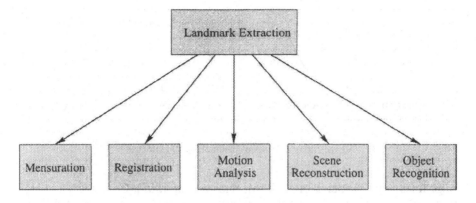

Figure 1.7. Landmark-based image analysis.

the case of 2D images one can principally distinguish between *point, curve,* and *region landmarks* (Figure 1.8). Examples for 2D curve landmarks are characteristic edge or ridge lines. Examples for 2D region landmarks are circular landmarks or characteristic blobs. Note, that for region landmarks often a distinguished point is determined, e.g., the center point or the center of gravity, which is then used for further processing. In this case, the landmark can also be regarded as point landmark. For applications of 2D landmarks we refer to the following references using point landmarks (e.g., Barnard and Thompson [24], Dreschler [122], Förstner [168],[170], Sethi and Jain [478], Bookstein [49], Ansari and Delp [9], Rohr [427], Shi and Tomasi [483], Wiskott et al. [565], Noelker and Ritter [384]), curve landmarks (e.g., Faugeras [149], Zhou et al. [579], Wyngaerd et al. [571]), and region landmarks (e.g., Goshtasby [198], Drewniok and Rohr [128], Dulimarta and Jain [133], Sim and Dudek [485], Zitova and Flusser [580]). In the case of 3D images we can classify *point, curve, surface,* and *volume landmarks* (Figure 1.9). Examples for these landmarks are prominent points in 3D tomographic images of the human brain (e.g., Evans et al. [147], Hill et al. [244], Dean et al. [114], Thirion [521], Rohr [434]), 3D

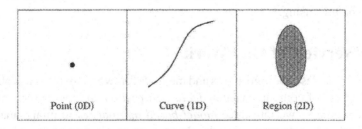

Figure 1.8. Classes of landmarks in 2D images.

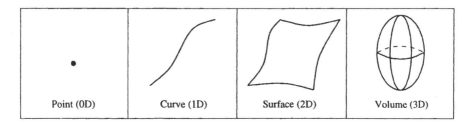

Figure 1.9.   Classes of landmarks in 3D images.

ridge lines (e.g., Declerck et al. [115], Subsol et al. [505], Collins et al. [101], Rangarajan et al. [410]), characteristic 3D organ surfaces (e.g., Szeliski and Lavallée [513], Davatzikos et al. [111], Thompson and Toga [524]) or characteristic volume structures. There are also approaches, where a combination of different landmark types are used, e.g., point and surface landmarks (e.g., Collignon et al. [100], Meyer et al. [342], Christensen et al. [93], Maurer et al. [335], Morris and Kanade [355], Tang and Medioni [515]). As mentioned above, main characteristics of landmarks are that they are scattered over the image and that they are distinguishable. Usually, landmarks in the depicted scene correspond to landmarks in the image, but this need not necessarily be the case. Consider, for example, a T-junction, which is a prominent image point in a video image where three edges intersect. This landmark results from an occlusion of objects in the scene but does not correspond to a prominent scene point. In this work, we primarily use the word landmark to denote prominent structures in images.

A main advantage of landmark-based approaches in comparison to intensity-based approaches is that they are less sensitive to lightning conditions or other radiometric variations. Also, when applied to compute image correspondences, larger displacements are allowed. In addition, the computational complexity is often significantly lower, particularly in the case of using point landmarks. On the other hand, with landmark-based approaches the full image information is not taken into account. Therefore, to profit from the strengths of both approaches, a combination of landmark-based and intensity-based schemes seems to be promising.

1.8   Overview of Our Work

In this book, we describe algorithms and methods for two fundamental problems within the field of computer vision: *feature extraction* and *image registration*. For these problems we introduce *model-based approaches* to image analysis. The key problem in developing such schemes consists in finding models which sufficiently well describe the entities of interest, but at the same time allow efficient and reliable use in image analysis. The work in this monograph describes contributions in this direction.

Concerning the problem of *feature extraction* we have developed approaches for the detection, localization, and characterization of geometric image features, particularly *point landmarks,* in 2D and 3D multimodality images. We introduce three principally different approaches: differential-geometric approaches, statistical approaches, and schemes based on parametric models. Our approaches are based on geometric models (contour models) and intensity models. Given the extracted image features there is a wide spectrum of direct applications, e.g., camera calibration and mensuration tasks in industrial automation. The extracted point landmarks are used in our case as features for *image registration*, i.e., for computing a geometric transformation between two corresponding multimodality images, which allows to map one image onto another. One main application is remote sensing (photogrammetry). In our case, we deal with 2D aerial images, where often affine transformations are used for registration. Another main application area is medicine, particularly radiology and surgery. Here, we deal with 2D and 3D spatial images and investigate elastic transformations based on a nonparametric model which allows to cope with local differences between images. Note, that the notion of image registration is very general and actually subsumes a number of classical tasks in computer vision, e.g., motion analysis, stereo-reconstruction, and structure-from-motion (e.g., Szeliski and Coughlan [512]). There, typically 2D images of the *same* modality (monomodal images) are analyzed and a central task is to determine image correspondences, i.e., also there a geometric transformation has to be computed. Besides the above-mentioned two main topics we also deal with the topic of *performance characterization* in computer vision. We consider the extraction of landmarks and perform theoretical as well as experimental investigations to characterize the performance of existing approaches.

In the subsections below, we describe more details of our work concerning these main topics and also point out our contributions in comparison to previous work. These subsections also reflect the structure of the subsequent chapters. The chapters have been written in a self-contained manner such that they can be read rather independently. Prior to detailing our work, we give a more general characterization of it.

1.8.1 General Characterization

Central to our work are model-based approaches to computer vision with emphasis on *geometric models*. Primarily, we consider geometric models of objects, geometric transformation models between corresponding images, as well as geometric models of the image intensities. In the latter case, we speak of *(geometric) intensity models*. Geometric models are very effective in representing generic knowledge as well as allow rather direct exploitation for image analysis. On the one hand, they are more specific in comparison to rather general assumptions. On the other hand, since with geometric models flexibility can be integrated in various form, these models are more general in comparison to rather specific knowledge. In comparison to knowledge in propositional (or conceptual) form, the connection to visual data is more direct. Actually, geometric models can be considered as a means to link different levels of knowledge, starting out from the raw image data to end up with conceptual descriptions. In comparison to approaches where knowledge is only implicitly encoded, in our approaches the assumptions are made explicit. Therefore, it is generally easier to predict the performance of the algorithms. Another advantage is that in practical applications it is easier to recognize deviations from the model and to quantify how large these deviations are. Additionally, the approaches can more easily be adapted and extended to different circumstances and tasks.

As already mentioned in Section 1.1 above, explicitly represented knowledge can be exploited at different levels of processing ranging from low-level to high-level vision (see Figure 1.2). Starting out from the raw image data to end up with conceptual descriptions one can distinguish the following main abstraction levels in image analysis: Extraction and description of image features, recognition and description of objects in the scene, and recognition of object configurations, situations, as well as events (e.g., Kanade [269], Marr [327], Neumann [369]). Within this hierarchy our approaches to image analysis can be embedded as follows. The work on *feature extraction* comprising differential and parametric approaches belongs to low-level vision. With differential schemes the images are analyzed locally and the incorporated knowledge is rather general. In comparison, the parametric schemes analyze larger image regions (semi-global regions) and utilize more specific knowledge about the image structure. Thus, within low-level vision these schemes are located above differential schemes. The work on *image registration* is devoted to finding a global geometric mapping between images and is based on extracted image features, their correspondences as well as a rather general nonparametric transformation model. Within the hierarchy of abstraction levels this approach is located somewhat above feature extraction and it can provide additional cues for subsequent object recognition tasks, for example.

A main aspect of our work is the *modelling step*. As mentioned above, the problem is to find realistic and flexible models, which allow efficient and reliable use for image analysis. The modelling part together with a sound mathematical description is in our opinion crucial. Emphasis in our work is therefore on the *computational theory*. Our aim is to assure certain theoretical properties of the approaches, which is the basis to arrive at algorithms with a predictable performance. Our focus is on *continuous models*. These models, in comparison to discrete models (e.g., Latecki [300]), are in our opinion a more natural way to describe the observed entities. Based on such continuous descriptions a second step is *discretization*, so that we end up with algorithms for the underlying discrete images. As already mentioned above, we deal with *2D* and *3D images*, either spatial or temporal images, and our focus is on video images, Magnetic Resonance images (MR), and X-ray Computed Tomography images (CT). However, the algorithms and methods we describe are *generic* in the sense that they can be used for other images as well as other domains.

1.8.2 Feature Extraction

The first main topic of our work is the detection and localization of point landmarks in 2D and 3D images (Chapter 2). Landmarks are geometric image features and our work is devoted to the extraction of prominent point features, particularly corners and anatomical point landmarks. Our focus is on point landmarks in 3D tomographic images (MR, CT) of the human brain.

Based on a detailed analysis of the brain anatomy and a differential-geometric characterization, we propose 3D differential operators for landmark extraction. The geometric characterization concerns the contours of 3D anatomical structures but not directly the image intensities. Since this characterization is based on the standard classification in differential geometry, which includes the generic point types of tips and saddle points, our approaches are also applicable to other 3D spatial images from different domains, e.g., geology and industrial inspection. Additionally, we propose 3D differential operators that have a statistical interpretation. These operators extract prominent points with minimal localization uncertainty. We also show that these operators form a complete set of principal invariants under similarity transformations. Since the operators depend only on first order derivatives of an image, they belong to the most efficient differential operators that exist. Our 3D differential operators for point landmark extraction are among the first that have been proposed in the literature.

Besides differential operators, we also describe a parametric approach to landmark extraction. This approach is based on a radiometric model and directly represents the image intensities. The approach is more specific than differential operators. Since it integrates more global information of the image it is more robust against image noise. The parametric model is nonlinear and it is defined by geometric and radiometric parameters that have a direct physical meaning, e.g., the landmark's position or the image contrasts in the neighborhood of the landmark. Using a least-squares method the parameters are estimated simultaneously by fitting the model directly to the image intensities. Under the assumption that the model well describes the observed intensities, the estimated parameters are very accurate. For example, for the location of a landmark (for which a subpixel position is obtained), there is no systematic localization error as is generally the case with differential operators. Concerning the precision of the estimated parameters the lower uncertainty bound in estimation theory can be achieved (Cramér-Rao bound). In this work, our focus is on corners in 2D images of 3D polyhedral objects, on planar circular landmarks in 2D aerial images, and on anatomical point landmarks in 3D tomographic images. Note, however, that our approach is also applicable to other domains. Central to our work is that we directly model the image intensities by semi-global models with physically interpretable parameters. In comparison to that, existing work on deformable models used to segment image structures, is often based only on the contours of objects and the estimated model does not comprise parameters with a direct physical interpretation. Discrete templates in comparison to our analytic models are not as flexible and also have other disadvantages that result from necessary discretization and filtering.

1.8.3   Performance Characterization

The topic of performance characterization has recently gained increased attention in computer vision. As already sketched above, on the one hand, validation and evaluation studies are a major step towards a sound characterization of algorithms as well as the foundation of computer vision as a scientific field. On the other hand, it serves a clear practical need when we have to choose a certain algorithm for some application given a list of requirements.

Our work on performance characterization is mainly concerned with approaches for extracting point landmarks (Chapter 3). The general approach we employ consists of three steps: (i) modelling the signal structure of landmarks, (ii) analysis of the degrees-of-freedom, and (iii) performing theoretical as well as experimental studies. Also in this part of work the modelling step plays a central role. We utilize both geometric and intensity models of landmarks.

Our theoretical studies are based on analytic models of the intensity variations at landmarks, and we have derived new closed-form expressions for the performance of existing algorithms. We consider both the localization accuracy for extracting corners in 2D images and the localization precision of general landmarks in 2D and 3D images. Thus, we theoretically analyze both the systematic localization errors and the stochastic errors due to image noise. In the latter case, the investigated landmark types include point landmarks (e.g., corners, blobs) and also other landmarks (e.g., edges, lines).

In our experimental studies we have investigated a large number of existing 3D differential operators for extracting point landmarks in tomographic images of the human brain. These studies are based on geometric models of landmarks as well as real image data. We have analyzed both the detection performance and the localization accuracy utilizing, e.g., statistical measures as well as other performance measures. Additionally, other performance criteria have been investigated such as the image registration error under affine transformations and the number of matched points under elastic transformations. Experimental studies on the performance of 3D operators are really rare. Our study is actually the broadest and most detailed one. Previously, only a relatively small number of different operators and a limited set of performance criteria have been utilized.

1.8.4 Elastic Image Registration

A fundamental problem in computer vision, which recently has well been recognized, is the problem of finding optimal geometric transformations between corresponding images. This task is known as image registration and the emphasis here is on images of different modalities. The aim is to integrate images from different sensors and from existing image databases (e.g., digital atlases) into one representation, i.e., one coordinate system, such that complementary information can more easily and accurately be exploited. The central problem here is that we generally have to deal with multidimensional and multimodality images and that the spectrum of the geometric variations between images is rather broad. For example, we have to cope with different objects, with distortions, or also with time-varying phenomena.

In the medical domain, image registration is important for diagnosis, for planning and simulation of surgical interventions, as well as for intraoperative navigation. A main application is the registration of 3D tomographic images (e.g., MR, CT). From these images an integrated 3D model can be established, which can be viewed under different (virtual) viewpoints using 3D visualization techniques. If additionally biomechanical models are incorporated, then also deformations due to, e.g., surgical interventions, can be simulated. Actually, such virtual reality (VR) applications are currently of high relevance (e.g., Rosen et al. [452], Völter [542], Astheimer et al. [15], Ellis and Begault [141], Satava and Jones [461]). Other applications of image registration are in geology, cartography, and photogrammetry (remote sensing). For example, to establish geographic information systems (GIS) it is necessary to integrate and visualize different image data of the world such that, e.g., the planning of streets, railway tracks, and landscapes as well as environmental protection can be performed more effectively (e.g., Burrough and McDonnell [77]).

In our work, we have developed an approach to elastic image registration which allows to cope with global as well as local geometric differences between multidimensional and multimodality images, particularly 2D and 3D images (Chapter 4). The approach is based on a nonparametric model and as image features we use anatomical point landmarks which can be localized by applying the operators described in Chapter 2. The basis of the model are certain splines, namely thin-plate splines. These splines have a physical motivation and are mathematically well-founded. A main feature of our approach is that the solution to the underlying minimizing functional can be stated analytically. Thus, we obtain an efficient computational scheme to compute the transformation. In comparison, approaches based on finite differences (FD) or the finite element method (FEM), that numerically solve a minimizing functional, are computationally much more expensive (e.g., Bajcsy and Kovačič [20]). Our main contribution concerns the extension from an interpolation to an approximation scheme and is a step towards fault-tolerance of image registration algorithms. In comparison to previous work, our approach allows to integrate isotropic as well as anisotropic landmark errors. This is important in practical applications, since landmark extraction is always prone to error. Another main contribution is that we estimate the landmark localization uncertainties directly from the image data based on a statistical scheme.

The application we mainly consider here is the registration of 2D and 3D tomographic images of the human brain. Also, we have applied this approach to 2D aerial images (Wiemker et al. [561]). Besides that, there are a lot of other application areas and related tasks, e.g., image warping and morphing in computer graphics (e.g., Wolberg [568],[569], Beier and Neely [29]) or morphometrics (e.g., Dean et al. [114]). Another application is human face recognition, where partly elastic graphs are used (e.g., Lades et al. [295], Wiskott et al. [565]). Prior to using thin-plate splines for elastic registration, these splines have been applied in computer graphics and computer vision for surface reconstruction from scattered data (e.g., Hoschek and Lasser [256], Boult and Kender [56], Terzopoulos [517]). While in the latter case mappings $u : \mathbb{R}^2 \to \mathbb{R}$ are considered, in image registration mappings $\mathbf{u} : \mathbb{R}^d \to \mathbb{R}^d$, where d is the image dimension, are relevant. Note, that thin-plate splines can be implemented as a neural network composed of radial basis functions with regularization properties. Thus, parallelization is directly possible (e.g., Szeliski [511]).

Chapter 2

Detection and Localization of Point Landmarks

Geometric image features denoted as *landmarks* are preferred features for a variety of computer vision tasks, e.g., camera calibration, mensuration, image registration, scene reconstruction, object recognition, and motion analysis (see also Section 1.7 above). Since higher-level descriptions directly depend on the quality of the low-level information, accurate and reliable extraction of these features from images is a central topic. Note, that the original meaning of landmark refers to visually prominent reference 'points' in the scene. This includes prominent objects in a particular landscape and also prominent anatomical structures. These landmarks often have been given a name. In addition, landmark also refers to prominent structures in images, particularly 2D and 3D images. Usually salient points in the scene correspond to salient points in the image, but this need not necessarily be the case. In this work, we primarily use the word landmark to denote prominent structures in images.

Among the different types of landmarks (points, curves, surfaces, and volumes) we here primarily consider *point landmarks*. These landmarks have a unique position which can be deduced from the intensity variations in a sufficiently large neighborhood around the prominent point. Examples for point landmarks are corners of 3D polyhedral objects depicted in 2D images (i.e., intersections of edge lines), centerpoints of circular features in 2D aerial images, or prominent anatomical points in 2D and 3D medical images. While *detection* means to establish whether there is a landmark, the task of *localization* is to determine its position. Actually, these two tasks are coupled since detecting a landmark usually implies that we also determine a (probably coarse) position of it. Moreover, landmarks may be *characterized* by additional attributes, e.g., by the image contrasts in their neighborhood.

In this chapter, we are primarily concerned with anatomical point landmarks in 3D tomographic images of the human brain, e.g., MR (Magnetic Resonance) and CT (X-ray Computed Tomography) images. The primary application we have in mind is 3D medical image registration (cf. Chapter 4). However, our approaches are also applicable to other volume image data and could also be used in other applications, e.g., motion analysis in 3D spatio-temporal images. Partly, we also deal with 2D point landmarks such as corners and circular symmetric landmarks. In the following, we give some further motivation and describe our general approach to the problem of extracting 3D anatomical point landmarks (Section 2.1). As a prerequisite to develop computational schemes, we then consider the modelling of anatomical landmarks (Section 2.2). After that, we discuss mathematical descriptions of point landmarks (Section 2.3) and then describe two principally different classes of approaches to the detection and localization of point landmarks. We introduce differential operators (Sections 2.4 and 2.5) and describe parametric approaches to landmark extraction (Section 2.6). Among the class of differential operators we consider both differential-geometric approaches and statistical approaches.

2.1   Motivation and General Approach

The usage of *point landmarks* in comparison to other types of geometric landmarks has several advantages. First, since the imaged objects are represented by a relatively small number of coordinates this representation is very efficient. Also, if the points are suitably selected they represent substantial image information. On the other hand, points are very general, i.e., curves, surfaces, and volumes can in principle be represented by (a sufficiently large number of) points. Moreover, with a semi-automatic approach to feature extraction, user-interaction is most easily when using point landmarks. In addition, establishing correspondences between different datasets is usually easier than with other geometric landmarks, and for the task of image registration simpler and more efficient algorithms can be used.

2.1.1   3D Anatomical Point Landmarks

In medical image analysis different types of *3D point landmarks* are used for image registration. One can distinguish between (i) point markers at a stereotactic frame and head screws, (ii) skin markers, and (iii) anatomical landmarks (e.g., Viergever et al. [539]). A stereotactic frame or head screws are directly fixed at the patient's head. The accuracy obtained with these markers is very high, however, they are fixed to the patient for several hours under examination which is very unpleasant. Also, these markers can only be placed outside the brain and thus no information about internal structures can be included. In comparison, skin markers are more patient-friendly but have a lower accuracy since the skin can deform and displace, and thus the markers can move. Skin markers can also be placed only outside the brain. *Anatomical landmarks,* in compar-

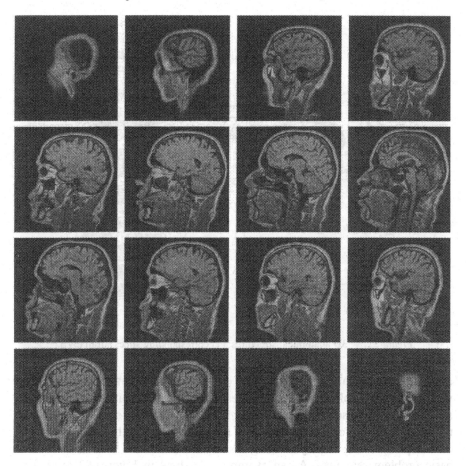

Figure 2.1. Sagittal slices of a 3D MR image of the human head.

ison to the above mentioned fiducial markers, are most patient-friendly and can be located also inside the brain which generally increases the registration accuracy in these regions. Additionally, a retrospective match is possible while with the other markers only such images can be processed which have been acquired together with the markers. However, the problem with anatomical point landmarks is their reliable and accurate extraction from 3D images.

Usually, *3D anatomical point landmarks* have been selected manually (e.g., Chen et al. [87], Schiers et al. [466], Evans et al. [147], Hill et al. [244],[245], Ende et al. [144], Ge et al. [187], Dean et al. [114], Strasters et al. [503]). Note, however, that manual specification of corresponding 3D points is not an easy task, particularly in the case of medical images. This is due to the fact that commonly only 2D slices are displayed on the screen of a computer, and that the

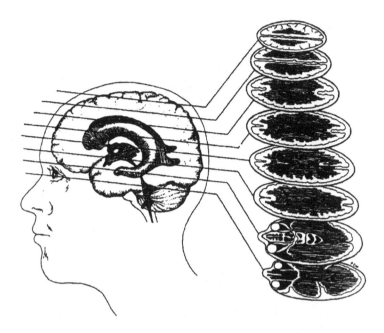

Figure 2.2.   3D anatomical structures and corresponding slices (from [59]).

difficulty of localization in 3D strongly depends on the orientation of the slices
w.r.t. the anatomical structures. Figures 2.1 and 2.2 indicate how curved 3D
structures are represented by 2D slices, from which the 3D shapes are difficult
to imagine. The problem is somewhat reduced if three orthogonal slices at a
certain position are displayed using a so-called orthoview tool, however, the
basic problem remains. As an example, we show in Figure 2.3 orthoview
images (sagittal, axial, and coronal view) of the landmark 'tip of the fourth
ventricle' (or, synonymously, tip at the cerebellum) in a 3D MR image of the
human brain. Given these images, it is actually very difficult to imagine the
3D structure of this landmark (see also later). Generally, manual selection of
anatomical point landmarks from 3D images is difficult, time-consuming, and
often lacks accuracy. Particularly, reproducibility is a problem.

Computational schemes open a possibility to improve this situation. Currently, however, there exist only a few approaches to the extraction of 3D
anatomical point landmarks. Thirion [520], for example, uses a differential
operator which consists of partial derivatives of the image up to the third order
to detect prominent points on 3D ridge lines (for 3D ridge line detection see, for
example, Monga et al. [352]). However, the computation of high order partial
derivatives is generally very sensitive to noise. Therefore, additional steps are
necessary to diminish the occurring instabilities (e.g., Monga et al. [353]). In
contrast, in this chapter we suggest low order 3D differential operators for the

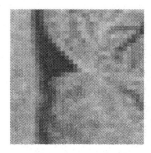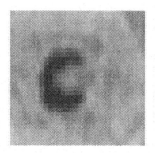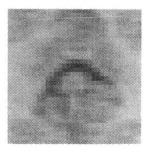

Figure 2.3. Orthoview images (sagittal, axial, coronal) at the tip of the fourth ventricle (center point in the sagittal view) in a 3D MR image of the human brain.

detection and localization of 3D anatomical point landmarks. Since only low order partial derivatives of the image are involved, these operators do not suffer from instabilities due to computing high order partial derivatives. Moreover, using only low order partial derivatives also requires less computation time. Below, we propose 3D operators that depend either only on first order partial derivatives or on first and second order partial derivatives. As a second principal class of approaches to landmark extraction we also introduce a parametric approach. While differential operators only analyze the local structure of a landmark (e.g., a $5 \times 5 \times 5$ voxels neighborhood), with parametric approaches it is possible to integrate more global information about the intensity variations in the neighborhood of a landmark. Using this additional information opens the possibility to further improve the detection and localization performance.

2.1.2 A Framework for Developing Landmark Operators

To develop computational schemes for landmark detection and localization, we find it imperative to work along a methodic framework aiming at algorithms of predictable performance, which thus can really be used in practice (Rohr and Stiehl [442]). The framework (depicted in Figure 2.4) consists of four main steps which will be detailed in the subsections below. In the first step, it is necessary to select suitable anatomical structures which represent a prominent point, and to define and characterize these structures verbally. This characterization primarily concerns geometry (e.g., characterization as a tip or a center of a region), but may also include a characterization of the corresponding intensities as well as the definition of additional attributes. The (verbal) characterization then has to be transferred to a sound mathematical description, e.g., in terms of differential geometry. Based on this description, we can now design operators for detecting and localizing landmarks. To end up with applicable operators, where one design constraint usually is computational complexity, it is often necessary to introduce well-motivated and mathematically well-founded ap-

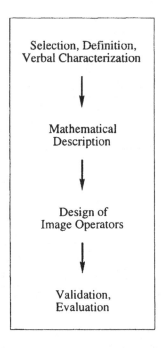

Figure 2.4.   A framework for the development of approaches to landmark extraction.

proximations. The last step of the framework is to validate and evaluate the operators using synthetic as well as real image data. This framework has clearly distinguishable modelling steps which we consider important to arrive at algorithms of predictable performance. On the basis of this framework we detail below our approach for the case of tomographic images of the human brain. Since we use generic descriptions as a basis to develop generic approaches, our schemes described below are also applicable to other regions of the human body as well as to other volume images. Prior to detailing our approach we now briefly describe the scenario in which the developed algorithms can be applied. The subject of validation and evaluation of the operators is treated separately in Chapter 3.

2.1.3   Semi-Automatic Landmark Extraction

We already mentioned that our aim is to use the extracted anatomical point landmarks as features for the registration of 3D multimodality images (see also Chapter 4). Particularly from the point of view of clinical practice we consider it important that the user has the possibility to control the results during processing (keep-the-user-in-the-loop paradigm, e.g., Gerritsen et al. [192]). Therefore, we are working on a semi-automatic procedure for the extraction of 3D anatomical point landmarks (see also Rohr et al. [443]).

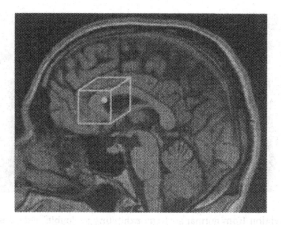

Figure 2.5.   Semi-automatic extraction of 3D anatomical point landmarks based on a region-of-interest (ROI).

Another argument for a semi-automatic approach is that a fully automatic and reliable landmark extraction scheme currently is beyond the start-of-the-art in computer vision, with the exception of special applications. In the case of using 3D differential operators, we rely on the following user-interaction scenario for the localization of a certain landmark (see also Figure 2.5): i) the user specifies a region-of-interest (ROI) together with a coarse position (e.g., the center of the ROI), ii) an automatic algorithm is applied yielding landmark candidates within the selected ROI, and then iii) the user selects the most promising candidate. To simplify the selection procedure, the landmark candidates may be ordered based on either their operator responses or their distances to the manually specified position. Note, that the positions of the landmark candidates may be refined by applying additional procedures, e.g., multi-step procedures (Frantz et al. [176],[177]). In the case of parametric approaches, we rely on the following user-interaction scenario: i) the user specifies a coarse position, ii) an automatic algorithm is applied to refine the position, and then iii) the user either accepts the refined position or defines a new coarse position starting again with step i). Note, that differential and parametric approaches can also be combined, e.g., a parametric approach can be used for refinement of the position obtained by a differential approach or can also be used for excluding false detections.

2.2   Definition and Characterization of Anatomical Point Landmarks

According to our framework depicted in Figure 2.4 the first step in developing computational approaches to landmark extraction is the selection, definition,

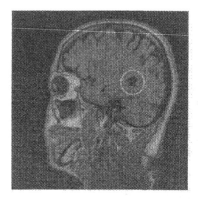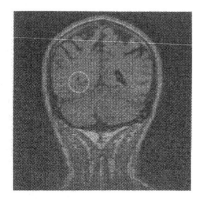

Figure 2.6.   Exception from normal anatomy exhibiting a 'double' occipital ventricular horn of the human brain: sagittal (left) and coronal view (right).

and verbal characterization of landmarks in 3D space. In our case we have focused on anatomical landmarks of the human head that are visible in either 3D MR images or 3D CT images or in both of these image modalities. To this end we have carried out a detailed analysis of anatomy on the basis of anatomical textbooks, digital atlases (VOXEL-MAN [251],[252], SAMMIE [257]), 3D plastic models of the brain and skull, as well as MR and CT images. In addition, we have reviewed existing literature (Rohr and Stiehl [441],[442]). Below, we first discuss general problems in modelling anatomical point landmarks, and then we consider the characterization of 2D and 3D landmarks in more detail.

2.2.1   Problems

In our investigation [441],[442] it soon became clear that the selection, definition, and characterization of 3D point landmarks is a very hard problem (see also Evans [147] and Hill et al. [244],[245]). The difficulties are due to the fact that the human head and brain consists of very complex anatomical structures. Also, we have to take into account the variability between different persons as well as the asymmetry between the two hemispheres of one person. Unfortunately, only sparse quantitative knowledge exists about anatomical structures of the human head. The variability between brains also includes topology differences, e.g., different topology of the sulci. An example for an untypical topology is given in Figure 2.6, which shows the occipital ventricular horn of a healthy person. Normally, there is only one tip at the horn, but this person actually has two tips, i.e., we here have a 'double horn' (see also Figure 2.11 below). Note also, that the anatomical structures can significantly be deformed due to pathologic processes (e.g., occurrence of a lesion or tumor growth). Other difficulties arise in the case of multimodality image registration since we here have to deal with the visibility and position invariance of landmarks in images

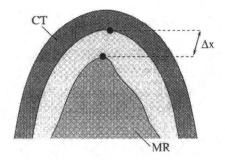

Figure 2.7.   Example for a systematic error when matching multimodality images.

from different modalities. Multimodality images generally represent different structures. For example, bone is primarily represented in CT images while soft tissue is primarily discernible in MR images. The problem of position invariance in multimodality images is illustrated in Figure 2.7. We consider to define corresponding landmarks in CT and MR images. We assume an anatomical constellation, where soft tissue is surrounded by a bony structure while there is another region between these two types of tissues (such a constellation can be found, for example, at the 'tip of convex dent below ala minor'). If we now define a landmark at the bone in the CT image and at the brain in the MR image, then we have a systematic localization error Δx that depends on the size of the transition region. Either one should compensate this systematic error prior to using these landmarks for registration or one should avoid using such landmarks. Another problem is that the localization depends, for example, on the scale of the landmarks, the degree of contrast as well as the image resolution, blur, and noise. While these dependences are generally met in computer vision, in medical image analysis we have an additional strong dependence on other imaging parameters (e.g., T_1- vs. T_2-weighted MR images). Moreover, the choice of a suitable set of 3D landmarks required for image registration depends on the imaging modality at hand (e.g., MR-MR, MR-CT, or MR-atlas matching), the clinical task (e.g., skull-base surgery), and the individual patient anatomy.

2.2.2   2D Landmarks

In our study in [441],[442] we started with the problem of defining and characterizing 2D landmarks. To this end we have considered landmarks in the midsagittal plane of MR images as depicted in Figure 2.8. The indicated landmarks have previously been used in Bookstein [50] for the registration of 2D MR images. Together with each landmark a verbal description has been given in [50]. For example, landmark Nr. 1 is defined as 'anteriormost point on genu of corpus callosum', i.e., the most frontal point of this structure (landmark

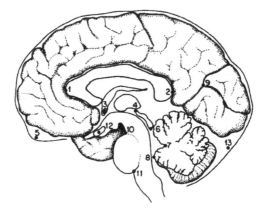

Figure 2.8.   2D Landmarks on a schematic sketch of a midsagittal MR image (from [50]).

Nr. 2 is defined analogously). Note, that this definition depends on the chosen coordinate system. Instead we could define this point as curvature extremum, which would be an invariant definition w.r.t. translations and rotations of the co-ordinate system. Some landmarks are defined as the tip of some structure (e.g., landmarks Nr. 6 and 7) or as a junction (e.g., landmark Nr. 9), which in both cases implies a point definition. Other landmarks are only coarsely described, e.g., landmark Nr. 12 as optic chiasm or landmarks Nr. 3 and 4 as anterior commissure (AC) and posterior commissure (PC), respectively. In these cases, generally several point definitions are possible, e.g., the distinguished point of the optic chiasm may be defined as the center of an elliptic area or as a tip. Note also, that landmarks Nr. 5 and 13 seem to result from an orthogonal projection of the poles onto the midsagittal plane, which, however, is a 3D definition. These points cannot be localized using the midsagittal plane alone and the position depends on the brain hemisphere from which the pole is taken. In summary, we found that in the 2D case most landmarks can geometrically be characterized as tips (peaks), which may have either a more rounded shape or may be rather sharp like a junction or cusp. Note, that both the rounded and the sharp forms can be characterized as curvature extrema since also in the latter case we have some rounding effect (due to the anatomy or due to the band-limited imaging process). Other types of landmarks are a junction of three curves, the center of an elliptic area, and an end point of a curve. In Figure 2.9 we have sketched these types of landmarks. Examples for the first four landmark types are landmarks Nr. 1, 7, 9, and 12 in Figure 2.8 (from left to right). Line ends have not be used in [50] but could be defined within sulci structures or at the pons.

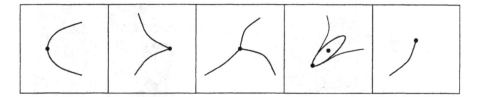

Figure 2.9. Different types of 2D point landmarks.

2.2.3 3D Landmarks

Next we investigate 3D anatomical landmarks. In comparison to the 2D case we here have a larger number of possible types of landmarks. In Figure 2.10 we have sketched the 3D geometry for some of these landmark types: tip (peak), cusp-like structure, saddle, junction of three curved surfaces, and crossing of two centerlines. Note, that these 3D landmark types (with the exception of the saddle) correspond to the first four 2D landmark types in Figure 2.9. Examples for tips (peaks) in 3D are the tips of the frontal horns of the ventricular system (cf. Figure 2.11), the poles of the cortex (landmarks Nr. 5 and 13 in Figure 2.8), or the tip of the external occipital protuberance (Figure 2.12). Saddle points can be found at the nasal bone and the zygomatic bone (Figure 2.12) as well as at the genu of corpus callosum and at the 'tip' of the fourth ventricle (landmarks Nr. 1 and 7 in Figure 2.8, see also Figure 2.11). In Figure 2.3 we have already shown orthoview images of the latter landmark. The shape of this structure is not easy to imagine since close to this landmark there are also two (tiny) tips (see the contour sketch in Figure 2.13). 3D cusp-like structures are the two junctions between pons and medulla oblongata (landmarks Nr. 10 and 11 in Figure 2.8). An example for a junction of three curved surfaces is the sulci junction landmark Nr. 9 in Figure 2.8. Besides such surface-surface crossings there also exist curve-surface crossings and curve-curve crossings. The latter definition applies to the optic chiasm (landmark Nr. 12 in Figure 2.8), which has been depicted as 3D landmark type in Figure 2.10 (most right). While this landmark has been defined as crossing of two centerlines, alternative definitions are also possible, e.g., intersection of three (orthogonal) symmetry planes.

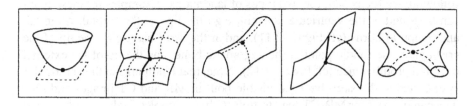

Figure 2.10. Different types of 3D point landmarks.

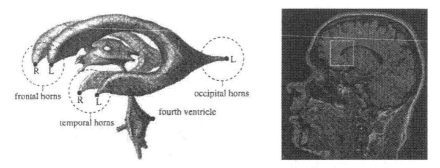

Figure 2.11.   Ventricular system of the human brain adapted from [491] with marked landmarks (left), and frontal horn of the ventricular system in a 3D MR image (right).

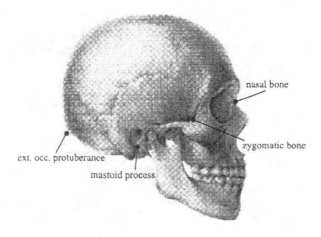

Figure 2.12.   Anatomical point landmarks at the human skull, adapted from [35].

Besides the landmark types sketched in Figure 2.10 other types can be defined, e.g., curvature extremum along a 3D curve (landmark Nr. 3 in Figure 2.8) or end point of a 3D curve.

In summary, we thus have a large number of different types of 3D anatomical point landmarks. However, it turns out that most of the 3D point landmarks can geometrically be characterized either as tips or saddle points. Therefore, in the following we focus on these two types of landmarks. Examples for these types can be found at the ventricular system, e.g., the tips of the frontal, occipital, and temporal horns (cf. Figure 2.11), and at the skull base, e.g., the tip of the crista galli, the saddle point at the zygomatic bone, and the tip of the external occipital protuberance (cf. Figure 2.12). Note, that landmarks at the ventricular system and at the skull base are visible both in MR and CT images and thus they can be used for MR-CT registration. Other examples for landmarks suited for this purpose are the junctions between pons and medulla oblongata, which

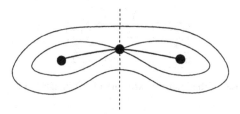

Figure 2.13. Contour sketch of the landmark 'tip of fourth ventricle' and its neighborhood (the dashed line represents the midsagittal plane), see also Fig. 2.3.

can be classified as tips, and the genu of corpus callosum, which is a saddle point.

2.3 Mathematical Description of Anatomical Point Landmarks

Above, we have defined 3D anatomical point landmarks and have characterized them verbally. In this section, we introduce mathematical descriptions of these landmarks based on *differential geometry* (e.g., Lipschutz [311], do Carmo [121], Koenderink [284]) and describe different classes of practically feasible approaches to landmark extraction.

2.3.1 General Mathematical Descriptions

We start with a classification of general structures in 2D and 3D images and motivate which descriptions are suitable to characterize point landmarks. Let us first consider a classification of the intensity surface of 2D images $g(x, y)$ which is based on the principal curvatures. The *principal curvatures* in a certain surface point can be obtained as follows: We intersect the surface with a plane containing the normal at that point, rotate this plane, and determine minimal and maximal sectional curvatures. The corresponding directions are orthogonal and are denoted *principal curvature directions*. For each point of the image the two principal curvatures λ_1 and λ_2 of the intensity surface can be computed and arranged such that $|\lambda_1| \geq |\lambda_2|$. Based on the values of the principal curvatures the classification in Table 2.1 can be established. In this table we have used the following symbols: '−' for values significantly smaller than zero, '+' for values significantly larger than zero, and '≈' for values approximately zero. Note, that we here essentially exploit the sign of the principal curvatures while the Eigenvalues of the Hessian matrix (see (2.2) below) have the same sign. Thus, we can use the Hessian matrix for classification and only need to compute second order image derivatives (see Haralick et al. [227]). From Table 2.1 we see that we can classify three

	λ_1	λ_2
blob	$- (+)$	$- (+)$
saddle	$- (+)$	$+ (-)$
line	$- (+)$	≈ 0

Table 2.1.   Classification of the intensity structure of 2D images on the basis of the principal curvatures λ_1, λ_2.

	λ_1	λ_2	λ_3
blob	$- (+)$	$- (+)$	$- (+)$
saddle	$- (+)$	$- (+)$	$+ (-)$
	$- (+)$	$+ (-)$	$- (+)$
	$+ (-)$	$- (+)$	$- (+)$
line	$- (+)$	$- (+)$	≈ 0
	$- (+)$	$+ (-)$	≈ 0
plane	$- (+)$	≈ 0	≈ 0

Table 2.2.   Classification of the intensity structure of 3D images on the basis of the principal curvatures $\lambda_1, \lambda_2, \lambda_3$.

different structures: blobs, saddles, and lines. This approach can be extended for the intensity surface of 3D images $g(x, y, z)$. Now we have three principal curvatures arranged by $|\lambda_1| \geq |\lambda_2| \geq |\lambda_3|$, but note that we now consider a 3D hypersurface in 4D which is difficult to visualize in comparison to the 2D case. Based on the principal curvatures (or the Eigenvalues of the Hessian matrix) we can classify blobs, saddles, lines, and planes as summarized in Table 2.2 (see also Rohr et al. [443]). For related classifications for 3D images primarily for the purpose of vessel extraction see, e.g., Sato et al. [460], Lorenz et al. [315], and Frangi et al. [174]. In our case, we are interested in the definition of point landmarks. One possibility is to use the classified lines and planes and then compute intersections of these structures to arrive at points. In this case we identify line-plane intersections with point landmarks. Another possibility it to use the centerpoint of a blob or a saddle. However, all these structures are defined on the basis of the intensity structure and they generally do not correspond to the most occurring types of 3D anatomical point landmarks, namely tips and saddle points as sketched in Figure 2.10.

Actually, the sketches of the 3D landmark types in Figure 2.10 represent the contours of structures in 3D images but not directly the intensity structure. Thus a more related description of these 3D landmark types relies on curvature properties of the contours, which are surfaces in 3D space. However, this requires to first extract the contours from 3D images. The usual approach in computer vision to extract contours is to exploit the image gradient. Canny [79], for example, computes contours (edges) in 2D images by searching for points with maximal gradient magnitude in the direction of the gradient. Actually, the

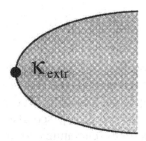

Figure 2.14.   Curvature extremum along 2D contour.

same definition can be applied in the 3D case. Alternatively, we could use a 3D extension of the Laplacian operator

$$\Delta g = g_{xx} + g_{yy} + g_{zz}, \tag{2.1}$$

where the partial derivatives of the image w.r.t. the coordinate axes have been denoted by subscripts, e.g., $g_x = \partial g/\partial x, g_{xx} = \partial^2 g/(\partial x)^2$. Here, edges are defined as zero-crossings of this operator. However, the Laplacian has disadvantages particularly at strongly curved image structures (e.g., [117], [427]). Therefore, we prefer the Canny criterion [79] which is detailed below. We first discuss the 2D case. Suppose we have a curved structure as depicted in Figure 2.14 and we want to compute the contour (edge) of this structure and then the curvature extremum along this curve. This gives a uniquely defined point. The criterion 'maximal gradient in gradient direction' means that the second directional derivative in this direction has to be zero. With the image gradient and the Hessian matrix,

$$\nabla g = \begin{pmatrix} g_x \\ g_y \end{pmatrix}, \qquad\qquad \mathbf{H}_g = \begin{pmatrix} g_{xx} & g_{xy} \\ g_{xy} & g_{yy} \end{pmatrix}, \tag{2.2}$$

and the normalized gradient $\mathbf{n} = \nabla g/|\nabla g|$, we have the criterion

$$\frac{\partial^2 g}{(\partial \mathbf{n})^2} = \frac{(\nabla g)^T \mathbf{H}_g \, \nabla g}{|\nabla g|^2} = 0. \tag{2.3}$$

Denoting the contour curve by Γ we can write this criterion as

$$\Gamma = g_x^2 g_{xx} + 2 g_x g_y g_{xy} + g_y^2 g_{yy} = 0. \tag{2.4}$$

We see that (2.4) incorporates partial derivatives of the image up to the second order. To compute the curvature along this curve, we need to compute first and second order partial derivatives of Γ. To determine the curvature extremum along this curve,

$$\kappa \rightarrow extr, \qquad (2.5)$$

we thus need partial derivatives of Γ up to the third order. Since Γ is already defined by partial derivatives up to the second order, we therefore need partial derivatives of the image up to the fifth order to compute the curvature extremum along the contour curve (Rieger [416]; see also Rohr [430]). Additionally, computing the expression for the curvature extremum symbolically, it turns out that it is rather extensive and consists of several hundred terms. On the one hand, in computer vision is it currently not possible to reliably compute partial derivatives of such high order (due to discretization and noise effects). On the other hand, since the expression is very extensive even small estimation errors of the partial derivatives would sum up yielding significant instabilities. For 3D images the resulting expression is even more complex (see Rieger [418] for a recent study of generic properties of edge surfaces). In this case, the image gradient and the Hessian matrix are given by

$$\nabla g = \begin{pmatrix} g_x \\ g_y \\ g_z \end{pmatrix}, \qquad \mathbf{H}_g = \begin{pmatrix} g_{xx} & g_{xy} & g_{xz} \\ g_{xy} & g_{yy} & g_{yz} \\ g_{xz} & g_{yz} & g_{zz} \end{pmatrix}, \qquad (2.6)$$

and the contour (surface) is defined analogously to the 2D case in (2.3),(2.4):

$$\begin{aligned} \Gamma &= (\nabla g)^T \mathbf{H}_g \nabla g \qquad\qquad (2.7)\\ &= g_x^2 g_{xx} + g_y^2 g_{yy} + g_z^2 g_{zz} + 2(g_x g_y g_{xy} + g_x g_z g_{xz} + g_y g_z g_{yz}) = 0. \end{aligned}$$

Thus, we conclude that this approach is not practically feasible for landmark extraction. Note, that an approach based on the Laplacian operator in (2.1) also incorporates the same (maximal) order of partial derivatives and therefore is also not useful in practical applications.

2.3.2   Applicable Approaches to Landmark Extraction

To end up with practically feasible algorithms we have to introduce some approximation. Note, however, that the introduction of an approximation generally leads to systematic localization errors. In this section, we describe different classes of applicable approaches to landmark extraction.

   One possibility to develop applicable operators is based on approximating the contour of the landmarks, i.e. the surface of organs, by *isointensity surfaces* (*isocontours*). Isointensity surfaces consist of points within a 3D intensity image which have the same intensity, i.e.,

$$g(x, y, z) = const., \qquad (2.8)$$

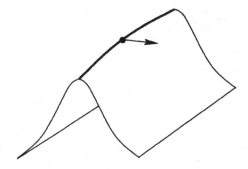

Figure 2.15.   Sketch of a ridge curve.

or, equivalently,

$$g(x, y, z) - const. = 0. \tag{2.9}$$

In comparison to the previously discussed contour surfaces based on the Canny criterion or the Laplacian operator, we see that no partial derivatives are involved in this definition. Thus, to determine prominent points on isocontour surfaces based on curvature properties, we only need partial derivatives up to the third order of the image. Additionally, if we implement the search for prominent points by utilizing a maximum (or minimum) search instead of computing zero-crossings, then we save one order of derivatives, and in total we only require partial derivatives up to the second order. Such an approach is detailed below in Section 2.4, where we exploit the *mean* and *Gaussian curvature* of isocontour surfaces. We will also see that the resulting operators are not very extensive.

An alternative approach on the basis of isocontour surfaces relies on 3D *ridge curves* (ridge lines, crest lines). Ridge curves are defined by extremal curvature in principal curvature directions, e.g., Monga et al. [352], Eberly et al. [137],[136]; see also Figure 2.15. By this approach we obtain curves in 3D space and we only need to impose one additional extremality criterion to arrive at prominent points. Such a scheme has been introduced by Thirion [520] using partial derivatives up to the third order and by Beil et al. [30] using partial derivatives up to the second order.

Another possibility instead of considering isocontour surfaces is to generalize existing *differential corner operators* from 2D to 3D (Rohr [434]; see Section 2.5 below). Corner operators have previously been applied in computer vision to extract prominent points from 2D images. These operators generally require partial derivatives up to the second order while some of them only require first order partial derivatives. Thus, also here we arrive at practically feasible point landmark operators. Actually, it can be shown that partially there exists a relation between these 3D operators and those based on isocontour properties. A 3D extension of the Moravec interest operator [354] has been

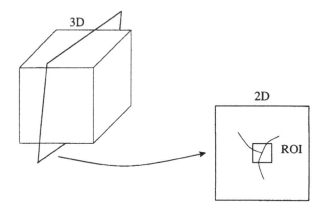

Figure 2.16. Alternative approach to 3D landmark localization: Extraction of a slice from a 3D image and application of 2D operators.

described in Yeung et al. [572]. This operator is not a differential operator, but exploits the image variance along certain discrete directions.

Besides the above mentioned classes of 3D differential operators, there is a principally different approach, which does not require any 3D operators (see the sketch in Figure 2.16). With this approach we first extract a certain slice from the 3D image (e.g., one can automatically extract the midsagittal plane), and then apply *2D operators* only to this slice. Note, that this slice may have an arbitrary orientation within the 3D image. An advantage is that we only need 2D operators, however, when using an automatic approach for slice selection we are restricted to certain characteristic planes within the 3D dataset.

Differential operators are generally very efficient, since only the local image structure is analyzed. A different class of approaches is based on *parametric models* of landmarks. This approach is more time-consuming, but we can integrate more global and specific information, which opens the possibility to improve the detection and localization performance (see Section 2.6).

2.4 3D Differential Operators Based on Curvature Properties of Isocontours

In this section, we describe an approach to landmark extraction which is based on curvature properties of *isointensity contours* (*isocontours*). Our focus is on tips and saddle points which are the most frequently occurring types of 3D anatomical point landmarks. The underlying assumption is that the surface of a landmark is well approximated by an isocontour. Isocontours have previously been exploited for detecting 3D crest or ridge curves (e.g., Monga et al. [352], Eberly et al. [137],[136], Florack et al. [154],[155], Le Goualher et al. [303],

Maintz et al. [320], Monga and Benayoun [351], Thirion and Gourdon [523], Dean et [114]) or certain points on these curves (e.g., Cutting et al. [109], Thirion [520],[521]). In our case, we use 3D differential operators for point landmark detection which are based on the *mean* or *Gaussian curvature* of isocontours (Rohr et al. [443], Beil et al. [30]). The mean and Gaussian curvature, denoted by H and K respectively, are defined on the basis of the principal curvatures κ_1, κ_2 as

$$H = \frac{1}{2}(\kappa_1 + \kappa_2), \qquad K = \kappa_1 \cdot \kappa_2. \tag{2.10}$$

H and K are differential invariants. The mean curvature is invariant under rigid transformations, while the Gaussian curvature is invariant under rigid and isometric transformations. While rigid transformations preserve distances between any two points on an object, isometric transformations preserve lengths along surfaces and angles between curves on surfaces (e.g., [268]). Suppose to bend a piece of paper. In this case, the mean curvature changes its value while the Gaussian curvature is preserved.

What we need in our approach are expressions for the mean and Gaussian curvature of isocontours defined in (2.9) above. The isocontours, however, are given in implicit form and the computation of curvature properties is more difficult than for surfaces given in parametric form. To compute the curvatures of implicitly given surfaces, we can apply the *implicit function theorem* (e.g., [71],[430],[523]). We first consider the 2D case, i.e., implicitly defined (planar) curves

$$F(x, y) = g(x, y) - const. = 0. \tag{2.11}$$

Now we parameterize $y = y(x)$ in a small neighborhood of a point (x_0, y_0) provided that $F_y(x_0, y_0) \neq 0$, i.e. we have

$$F(x, y(x)) = 0. \tag{2.12}$$

Computing the partial derivatives gives

$$F_x + F_y\, y_x = 0, \tag{2.13}$$

where y_x is the partial derivative of y w.r.t. x, and thus we have

$$y_x = -\frac{F_x}{F_y}. \tag{2.14}$$

Further differentiation leads to

$$y_{xx} = -\frac{F_x^2 F_{yy} - 2F_x F_y F_{xy} + F_y^2 F_{xx}}{F_y^3}. \tag{2.15}$$

Using (2.11) we have $F_x = g_x, F_{xx} = g_{xx}$, etc., and finally we obtain for the curvature of an implicitly defined curve

$$\kappa \;\; = \;\; \frac{y_{xx}}{(1+y_x^2)^{3/2}}$$

$$= \;\; -\frac{g_x^2 g_{yy} - 2g_x g_y g_{xy} + g_y^2 g_{xx}}{(g_x^2 + g_y^2)^{3/2}} \tag{2.16}$$

Analogously, the 3D case can be treated (e.g., Thirion and Gourdon [523]). In this case we have implicitly defined surfaces in 3D images

$$F(x, y, z) = g(x, y, z) - const. = 0, \tag{2.17}$$

and we can use a parameterization $z(x, y)$ in a small neighborhood of a point (x_0, y_0, z_0) provided that $F_z(x_0, y_0, z_0) \neq 0$, i.e. we have

$$F(x, y, z(x, y)) = 0. \tag{2.18}$$

Based on this parameterization we can compute the two principal curvatures κ_1, κ_2 as well as the mean and Gaussian curvature H and K, respectively, which are related by

$$\kappa_{1,2} = H \pm \sqrt{H^2 - K}. \tag{2.19}$$

For the mean and Gaussian curvature we obtain the following expressions

$$H \;\; = \;\; \Big(g_x^2(g_{yy} + g_{zz}) + g_y^2(g_{xx} + g_{zz}) + g_z^2(g_{xx} + g_{yy})$$
$$-2(g_x g_y g_{xy} + g_x g_z g_{xz} + g_y g_z g_{yz}) \Big) / 2(g_x^2 + g_y^2 + g_z^2)^{3/2} \tag{2.20}$$

and

$$K \;\; = \;\; \Big(g_x^2(g_{yy}g_{zz} - g_{yz}^2) + g_y^2(g_{xx}g_{zz} - g_{xz}^2) + g_z^2(g_{xx}g_{yy} - g_{xy}^2)$$
$$+2(g_y g_z(g_{xz}g_{xy} - g_{xx}g_{yz}) + g_x g_z(g_{yz}g_{xy} - g_{yy}g_{xz})$$
$$+g_x g_y(g_{xz}g_{yz} - g_{zz}g_{xy})) \Big) / (g_x^2 + g_y^2 + g_z^2)^2. \tag{2.21}$$

We see that these expressions are not very extensive. The involved partial derivatives up to the second order can directly be computed from the 3D image using, e.g., Gaussian derivative filters. Based on the principal curvatures $|\kappa_1| \geq |\kappa_2|$, we can classify the surface points on isocontours as given in Table 2.3 (see a standard textbook on differential geometry, e.g., [311],[121]). We have elliptic, hyperbolic and parabolic points as sketched in Figure 2.17 (assuming that not both principal curvatures vanish). Tips are elliptic points and saddle points are hyperbolic points. A special case of elliptic points are

	κ_1	κ_2
tip (elliptic)	$-\ (+)$	$-\ (+)$
saddle (hyperbolic)	$-\ (+)$	$+\ (-)$
parabolic	$-\ (+)$	≈ 0

Table 2.3. Classification of isocontour surface points in 3D images on the basis of the principal curvatures κ_1, κ_2.

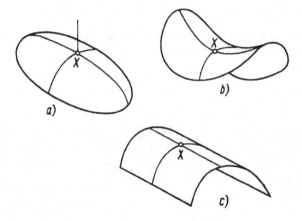

Figure 2.17. Classification of surface points: (a) elliptic, (b) hyperbolic, and (c) parabolic point (from [473]).

umbilic points, where both principal curvatures have same values, i.e., $\kappa_1 = \kappa_2$. This classification is analogous to the classification of 2D intensity surfaces in Table 2.1 (see Section 2.3.1 above). However, here we deal with the contours of 3D objects and thus this classification is directly related to our geometric characterization of brain landmarks from Section 2.2 above.

The mean and Gaussian curvature are scalar quantities and we can find prominent points by searching extremal values of them. Let's see how this works for tip and saddle structures. To this end we have first modelled the isocontour of a (rather rounded) tip in 3D by a bivariate polynomial

$$z(x, y) = -\frac{1}{2}(x^2 + y^2) \qquad (2.22)$$

as shown in Figure 2.18 on the left. Using the expressions for H and K in (2.20),(2.21) we have computed the operator responses for this tip model. The result is shown in Figure 2.18 (middle and right). Note, that we have displayed the negative mean curvature to allow for a better assessment of the result. It can be seen that the strongest operator response is obtained at the center of the tip which is what we expect. The response of the Gaussian curvature is sharper in comparison to that of the mean curvature, thus the discrimination power of

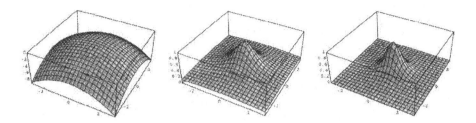

Figure 2.18.   Polynomial model of a rounded tip (left) and result of the negative mean curvature (middle) and the Gaussian curvature (right).

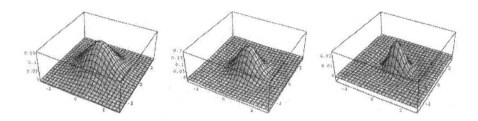

Figure 2.19.   Gaussian model of a tip (left) and result of the negative mean curvature (middle) and the Gaussian curvature (right).

the Gaussian curvature seems to be better, i.e., the prominent point is better distinguished from its neighborhood. Qualitatively the same result is obtained if we model a tip by a bivariate Gaussian function

$$z(x,y) = \frac{1}{2\pi}e^{-\frac{x^2+y^2}{2}} \tag{2.23}$$

as shown in Figure 2.19. Next we model the isocontours of a saddle point by a bivariate polynomial

$$z(x,y) = -\frac{1}{2}(x^2 - y^2). \tag{2.24}$$

The model of the saddle and the operator responses of H and K are shown in Figure 2.20. Note, that in both cases we have displayed negative values of the operator values. For the mean curvature we see that we obtain a rather complicated operator response where the largest operator response is not at the saddle point. Thus, the mean curvature is unsuited for localizing saddle points. Instead, the Gaussian curvature gives the strongest operator response at the saddle point and can well be used to localize this structure. In summary, the use of the Gaussian curvature has two advantages over the mean curva-

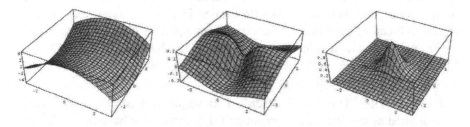

Figure 2.20.   Polynomial model of a saddle (left) and result of the negative mean curvature (middle) and the negative Gaussian curvature (right).

ture: It is invariant w.r.t. a more general class of transformations (isometric transformations) and it can be used for localizing tips as well as saddle points.

So far, we have considered the case of a single isocontour surface, however, in 3D images there are infinitely many isocontours (if we assume a continuous image function instead of discrete samples). To select one isocontour two different schemes can be applied, which both assume that the landmark's surface is well represented by image edges. With the first scheme we first extract 3D edge points, then compute the mean and Gaussian curvature only for these points, and finally determine local extrema of the curvature result. With the second scheme, we multiply the expressions for the mean and Gaussian curvature with some power of the gradient magnitude, and search local extrema of the thus modified operators. In this case, the most efficient operators are obtained when multiplying the mean and Gaussian curvature in (2.20),(2.21) with the third and fourth power of the gradient magnitude, resp, i.e., $H^* = H \cdot 2|\nabla g|^3$ and $K^* = K \cdot |\nabla g|^4$, where $|\nabla g| = \sqrt{g_x^2 + g_y^2 + g_z^2}$. Then we have

$$
\begin{aligned}
H^* \;=\;& g_x^2(g_{yy} + g_{zz}) + g_y^2(g_{xx} + g_{zz}) + g_z^2(g_{xx} + g_{yy}) \\
& -2(g_x g_y g_{xy} + g_x g_z g_{xz} + g_y g_z g_{yz})
\end{aligned}
\tag{2.25}
$$

and

$$
\begin{aligned}
K^* \;=\;& g_x^2(g_{yy}g_{zz} - g_{yz}^2) + g_y^2(g_{xx}g_{zz} - g_{xz}^2) + g_z^2(g_{xx}g_{yy} - g_{xy}^2) \\
& + 2(g_y g_z(g_{xz}g_{xy} - g_{xx}g_{yz}) + g_x g_z(g_{yz}g_{xy} - g_{yy}g_{xz}) \\
& + g_x g_y(g_{xz}g_{yz} - g_{zz}g_{xy})).
\end{aligned}
\tag{2.26}
$$

Experimentally we found, that the second scheme yields better results and that the operator K^* is superior to H^* (Beil et al. [30], Hartkens et al. [233]–[235]; see also Section 3.3 below). Note, that tips and saddle points can be distinguished on the basis of the sign of K^* and without the necessity of computing the principal curvatures explicitly. For tips we have $K = \kappa_1 \kappa_2 > 0$ and thus also $K^* > 0$, and for saddles we have $K < 0$ and thus also $K^* < 0$

(cf. Table 2.3). Figure 2.21 shows the operator response of K^* for the right frontal ventricular horn in a 3D MR dataset in sagittal, axial, and coronal sections. It can be seen that we obtain a strong operator response at the tip of the frontal horn which enables semi-automatic localization of this landmark. More detailed studies on the performance of the operators H^* and K^* as well as others are described in Section 3.3 below.

Previously, the 3D operators described above (as well as related ones) have been applied as measures for segmenting ridge curves, but have not been used for detecting 3D anatomical point landmarks (e.g., Florack et al. [154], Le Goualher et al. [303], Monga and Benayoun [351], Thirion and Gourdon [523], Maintz et al. [320]). Thirion [520],[521] has proposed a ridge curve based approach, where prominent points are defined as intersection set of different extremality criteria, which requires substantial implementation. Instead, with our approach we are searching extremal values of scalar quantities which can efficiently and easily be implemented. Another advantage is that our approach can localize more general types of tips in comparison to the approach in [520], [521]. Imagine the tip of an ellipsoid. If all semi-axes of the ellipsoid are equal (special case of a sphere), then there is no change in curvature along the surface and thus no prominent point can be detected. Now, assume that two semi-axes are equal and that the other semi-axis (which is in normal direction at the tip) is larger than these two. Then the structure is still rotational symmetric w.r.t. the largest axis, but the curvature on the surface changes and thus our approach yields a prominent point. However, due to the rotational symmetry, there is no ridge curve in this case and thus the approach in [520],[521] will not locate the tip.

2.5   3D Generalization of Differential Corner Operators

We now introduce 3D differential operators for point landmark detection which are generalizations of existing 2D corner operators (Rohr [446]). An advantage of these operators is that only low order partial derivatives of an image are required. Therefore, these operators are computationally efficient and they do not suffer from instabilities of computing high order partial derivatives. In this section, we propose 3D operators that depend either only on first order partial derivatives or on first and second order partial derivatives. In the 2D case a large number of corner operators has been proposed in the literature. Recent approaches are based on, e.g., orientation selective filters (e.g., [486],[422], [574]), covariance propagation (e.g., [263]), scale space analysis (e.g., [309], [152],[350],[495]), simple comparisons of grey values (e.g., [490]), moments (e.g., [454]), or mathematical morphology (e.g., [296]). For approaches based

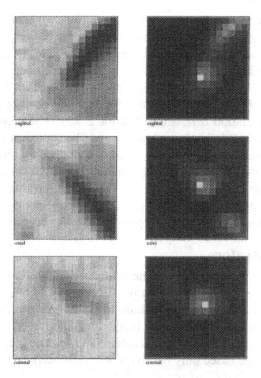

Figure 2.21. Right frontal horn within a 3D MR dataset (left) and result of computing the gradient-weighted 3D Gaussian curvature K^* (right) in sagittal, axial, and coronal sections.

on parametric models see Section 2.6 below. Differential corner operators have usually been designed to detect grey-value corners while different definitions have been applied. The general criterion is to find *'points of high intensity variations'*, i.e., points where the intensity surface is strongly curved, and actually in many applications these operators have been used to extract *general* prominent points. Based on this criterion we expect that the 3D extensions also detect general characteristic 3D points of high intensity variations. This includes tips and saddle points, but also other prominent points such as line-plane intersections or line ends. Below, we show that some of the resulting 3D operators can be related to the 3D operators based on isocontour properties as introduced in Section 2.4 above.

For an analytic study of ten 2D differential corner detectors see Rohr [430]. In this study an analytic corner model has been used to analyze the performance of the different operators (see also Section 3.2.1 below). This study reveals that four corner detection schemes out of those ten seem to be most promising to use: They yield a unique position and no post-processing steps are necessary. Note, however, that this study is only based on a prototype corner model but not on other models. In the following, we briefly review these four operators (Section 2.5.1) and then propose extensions of them for 3D images (Section 2.5.2). Also, we describe how the 3D operators can be generalized to arbitrary dimension (Section 2.5.3). Experimental results will be presented for 2D as well as 3D MR and CT images of the human brain (Section 2.5.4). After that, we show that for a certain class of these operators a statistical interpretation is possible (Section 2.5.5). These operators require only first order partial derivatives of an image. The statistical interpretation is based on the Cramér-Rao bound. We found that all operators belonging to this class find points of minimal localization uncertainty. In Section 2.5.6 we show that these operators can also be derived on the basis of invariance principles. It turns out, that the operators form a complete set of principal invariants. Finally, in Section 2.5.7 we consider multi-step procedures for landmark extraction.

2.5.1   2D Operators

In this section, we briefly describe the four differential 2D corner operators of Kitchen and Rosenfeld [280], Förstner [168], Rohr [424], and Blom et al. [47], which subsequently will be extended to 3D. We use the gradient ∇g and the Hessian matrix $\mathbf{H}_g$ of the 2D image function $g(x, y)$ as given in (2.2) above. We distinguish between operators based on first and second order partial derivatives and those based only on first order partial derivatives.

2.5.1.1   Operators Based on First and Second Order Partial Derivatives

Kitchen and Rosenfeld (1982).   To detect grey-value corners Kitchen and Rosenfeld [280] proposed a differential operator that consists of first and second order partial derivatives of the image $g(x, y)$:

$$
\begin{aligned}
KR(x, y) &= \frac{(\nabla g^\perp)^T \mathbf{H}_g \, \nabla g^\perp}{|\nabla g|^2} \\
&= \frac{g_x^2 g_{yy} - 2 g_x g_y g_{xy} + g_y^2 g_{xx}}{g_x^2 + g_y^2} \quad \to \quad extr, \qquad (2.27)
\end{aligned}
$$

where $\nabla g^\perp = (-g_y, g_x)^T$ is orthogonal to ∇g, and $(\nabla g^\perp)^T$ denotes the transposed vector. The operator represents the curvature κ of a plane curve (isophote, level curve, isocontour) multiplied by the gradient magnitude $|\nabla g| = \sqrt{g_x^2 + g_y^2}$:

$$
KR(x, y) = -\kappa \cdot |\nabla g|, \qquad (2.28)
$$

where

$$
\kappa = -\frac{(\nabla g^\perp)^T \mathbf{H}_g \, \nabla g^\perp}{|\nabla g|^3} \qquad (2.29)
$$

as derived in Section 2.4 above, see (2.16). Note, that the sign of the curvature depends on the chosen orientation of the curve. Corners are identified with local extrema of the operator values.

This operator has also been applied to 2D medical image data as point detector (e.g., Le Briquer et al. [66]), in 2D and 3D as a measure of ridgeness (e.g., van den Elsen [142], Maintz et al. [320]), and in 3D to separate certain elongated anatomical structures (sulci and gyri of the human brain; see Le Goualher et al. [303]). Gauch and Pizer [185] have directly used the level curvature κ to detect ridges and valleys in 2D medical images.

Blom et al. (1992).   Closely related to the cornerness measure of Kitchen and Rosenfeld [280] in (2.27) is the operator of Blom et al. [47]

$$
\begin{aligned}
BRK(x,y) &= -(\nabla g^\perp)^T \mathbf{H}_g \, \nabla g^\perp \\
&= -(g_x^2 g_{yy} - 2g_x g_y g_{xy} + g_y^2 g_{xx}) \rightarrow extr. \quad (2.30)
\end{aligned}
$$

This measure is the (negative) numerator of $KR(x,y)$ in (2.27) and has also been used in Brunnström et al. [74]. Note, that we use the terms operator and measure synonymously. With the isophote curvature κ in (2.29) we can write

$$
BRK(x,y) = \kappa \cdot |\nabla g|^3
$$

which shows that points with large gradients are emphasized in comparison to (2.28).

2.5.1.2   Operators Based on First Order Partial Derivatives

Förstner (1986).   The corner detector of Förstner [168] (see also [173]) is based on the matrix $\mathbf{C}_g$ which represents the averaged dyadic product of the grey-value gradient:

$$
\mathbf{C}_g = \overline{\nabla g \, (\nabla g)^T} = \begin{pmatrix} \overline{g_x^2} & \overline{g_x g_y} \\ \overline{g_x g_y} & \overline{g_y^2} \end{pmatrix}, \quad (2.31)
$$

where the overline means average in a local neighborhood, i.e., in the discrete case we have, for example, $\overline{g_x^2} = \frac{1}{m} \sum_{i=1}^m g_{x_i}^2$, where m is the number of pixels in the neighborhood. Alternatively, we can weight the terms in the sum by a bivariate Gaussian function. The matrix in (2.31) is also known as *orientation tensor* or *structure tensor* (e.g., [282],[41],[260]). The corner detector in [168], [173] minimizes the trace of the inverse of $\mathbf{C}_g$:

$$
F(x,y) = tr\mathbf{C}_g^{-1} \rightarrow min, \quad (2.32)
$$

which is equivalent to maximizing the ratio between the determinant and the trace of $\mathbf{C}_g$:

$$F(x, y) = \frac{det\mathbf{C}_g}{tr\mathbf{C}_g}$$

$$= \frac{\overline{g_x^2}\,\overline{g_y^2} - (\overline{g_x g_y})^2}{\overline{g_x^2} + \overline{g_y^2}} \rightarrow max. \qquad (2.33)$$

Actually, the expression in (2.33) is equivalent to minimizing the inverse of it as done by Harris (Plessey corner detector; see Noble [383]). Note, that only first order partial derivatives are needed to implement this operator.

Rohr (1987). The differential operator of Rohr [424] (see also [426]) is also based on the matrix $\mathbf{C}_g$ given in (2.31). Here, points of high intensity variations are identified with local maxima of the determinant of $\mathbf{C}_g$:

$$R(x, y) = det\mathbf{C}_g$$

$$= \overline{g_x^2}\,\overline{g_y^2} - (\overline{g_x g_y})^2 \rightarrow max. \qquad (2.34)$$

In [424],[426] an approximation of $\mathbf{C}_g$ has been implemented which results from developing the image gradient up to a first order expansion:

$$\mathbf{C}_g \approx \nabla g\,(\nabla g)^T + c\mathbf{H}_g^2, \qquad (2.35)$$

where $\mathbf{H}_g$ is the Hessian matrix and where c is a measure for the size of the area over which the gradient components are averaged. Alternatively to (2.35), one can directly use $\mathbf{C}_g$ as given in (2.31). This has the advantage that we only have to compute first order partial derivatives of the image function.

2.5.1.3   Excluding Insignificant Points

To suppress insignificant points resulting from the application of the operators of Kitchen and Rosenfeld [280] and Blom et al. [47] a threshold on the operator values can be used.

With the approaches of Förstner [168],[173] and Rohr [424],[426] two threshold operations are performed to exclude insignificant points. First, local maxima in homogeneous regions due to noise are suppressed by comparing the operator responses with a threshold. Second, pure edge points with large operator values are removed using the measure

$$\frac{det\mathbf{C}_g}{(\frac{1}{2}tr\mathbf{C}_g)^2}, \qquad (2.36)$$

which represents the (squared) ratio between the geometric and arithmetic mean of the two Eigenvalues of $\mathbf{C}_g$. Because of the rotational invariance of the determinant and the trace of a matrix, this measure as well as the measures in (2.33) and (2.34) have the advantage that we don't have to compute the Eigenvalues of $\mathbf{C}_g$ explicitly.

2.5.2 3D Operators

We now derive 3D generalizations of the four 2D operators described above. We use the gradient ∇g and the Hessian matrix $\mathbf{H}_g$ of the 3D image function $g(x, y, z)$ as given in (2.6) above.

2.5.2.1 Operators Based on First and Second Order Partial Derivatives

The operators derived in this section are extensions of the 2D operators of Kitchen and Rosenfeld [280] and Blom et al. [47].

First 3D Operator. The 2D measure in Kitchen and Rosenfeld [280] is the curvature of the isophote (isocontour) through a considered image point. The isophote can be represented by the implicit equation

$$g(x, y) - const. = 0, \tag{2.37}$$

which describes a curve in the plane. For this curve the curvature can be obtained by implicit differentiation of (2.37) which leads to the measure given in (2.27), see also Section 2.4 above.

Extending (2.37) to 3D we have

$$g(x, y, z) - const. = 0. \tag{2.38}$$

This implicit equation, however, describes surfaces in 3D space (isocontour surfaces). Since surfaces are characterized by two principal curvatures a straightforward extension of the derivation in 2D to 3D is not obvious.

On the other hand, since in 3D we know the gradient ∇g and the Hessian matrix $\mathbf{H}_g$ as given in (2.6) one could think about a purely formal extension of (2.27) to 3D. However, we need the vector $\nabla g^\perp$ orthogonal to ∇g and this vector is not uniquely defined, but there exist an infinite number of directions orthogonal to the gradient. Therefore, an extension to 3D does not lie at hand. To end up with a unique measure a certain direction has to be chosen. To obtain a unique ridgeness measure in 3D van den Elsen [142], for example, uses the direction in which the second partial derivative is minimal under the constraint that this direction is perpendicular to the gradient. To compute this direction a constraint optimization problem is formulated which has to be solved for every image point.

In the following, we propose a more direct 3D extension of the measure in Kitchen and Rosenfeld [280], which results in a unique operator for which an explicit formula can be given. The measure can be implemented in 3D as easily as in 2D. Our extension exploits a certain relation between different well-known differential operators.

We start out from the fact that the 2D measure of Kitchen and Rosenfeld in (2.27) can be expressed as the second derivative of the image function in the direction $\mathbf{n}^\perp = \nabla g^\perp / |\nabla g|$, $\nabla g^\perp = (-g_y, g_x)^T$, perpendicular to the grey-value gradient.

$$KR(x,y) = \frac{\partial^2 g}{(\partial \mathbf{n}^\perp)^2} = \frac{(\nabla g^\perp)^T \mathbf{H}_g \nabla g^\perp}{|\nabla g|^2}$$

$$= \frac{g_x^2 g_{yy} - 2g_x g_y g_{xy} + g_y^2 g_{xx}}{g_x^2 + g_y^2} \qquad (2.39)$$

On the other hand, the second derivative of the image function in the gradient direction $\mathbf{n} = \nabla g / |\nabla g|$, where $\nabla g = (g_x, g_y)^T$, is given by

$$\frac{\partial^2 g}{(\partial \mathbf{n})^2} = \frac{(\nabla g)^T \mathbf{H}_g \nabla g}{|\nabla g|^2}$$

$$= \frac{g_x^2 g_{xx} + 2g_x g_y g_{xy} + g_y^2 g_{yy}}{g_x^2 + g_y^2} \qquad (2.40)$$

and has usually been used to detect grey-value edges (e.g., Canny [79]). If, in addition, we denote the Laplacian of $g(x,y)$ by

$$\Delta g = g_{xx} + g_{yy}, \qquad (2.41)$$

then the following relation in 2D can be stated (see, for example, Torre and Poggio [531])

$$\Delta g = \frac{\partial^2 g}{(\partial \mathbf{n})^2} + \frac{\partial^2 g}{(\partial \mathbf{n}^\perp)^2} \qquad (2.42)$$

This means if we know Δg and $\partial^2 g / (\partial \mathbf{n})^2$, then we can compute the 2D measure of Kitchen and Rosenfeld [280] by

$$KR(x,y) = \Delta g - \frac{\partial^2 g}{(\partial \mathbf{n})^2}. \qquad (2.43)$$

We now use a generalization of this relation to 3D to obtain a unique 3D extension of $KR(x,y)$. In 3D we have

$$\Delta g = g_{xx} + g_{yy} + g_{zz} \qquad (2.44)$$

and with the gradient and the Hessian matrix in 3D as given in (2.6) we have

$$\frac{\partial^2 g}{(\partial \mathbf{n})^2} = \frac{(\nabla g)^T \mathbf{H}_g \nabla g}{|\nabla g|^2} \qquad (2.45)$$

$$= \frac{g_x^2 g_{xx} + g_y^2 g_{yy} + g_z^2 g_{zz} + 2(g_x g_y g_{xy} + g_x g_z g_{xz} + g_y g_z g_{yz})}{g_x^2 + g_y^2 + g_z^2}.$$

Using (2.43) for the 3D case we can straightforwardly derive the new 3D operator as

$$Op1(x, y, z) = \Delta g - \frac{\partial^2 g}{(\partial \mathbf{n})^2} \tag{2.46}$$

$$= \left(g_x^2(g_{yy} + g_{zz}) + g_y^2(g_{xx} + g_{zz}) + g_z^2(g_{xx} + g_{yy})\right.$$
$$\left. - 2(g_x g_y g_{xy} + g_x g_z g_{xz} + g_y g_z g_{yz})\right) / (g_x^2 + g_y^2 + g_z^2).$$

Note, that the operator directly follows from the 3D generalization of (2.43), i.e., for our derivation there is no need to choose a certain direction of a vector perpendicular to the 3D gradient. Actually, the measure in (2.46) represents the 3D mean curvature of isointensity contours multiplied with the gradient magnitude (up to a factor 2; see also [154],[523],[320], as well as Section 2.4 above). Thus, we have also a direct geometric interpretation of this measure. Note, if we set all partial derivatives w.r.t. z to zero then the original 2D measure in (2.27) turns out as a special case.

The operator in (2.46) can also be written as

$$Op1(x, y, z) =$$
$$= \frac{(\nabla g_1^\perp)^T \mathbf{H}_{g1} \, \nabla g_1^\perp + (\nabla g_2^\perp)^T \mathbf{H}_{g2} \, \nabla g_2^\perp + (\nabla g_3^\perp)^T \mathbf{H}_{g3} \, \nabla g_3^\perp}{|\nabla g|^2}$$

$$= \sum_{i=1}^{3} \frac{(\nabla g_i^\perp)^T \mathbf{H}_{gi} \, \nabla g_i^\perp}{|\nabla g|^2} \tag{2.47}$$

using

$$\nabla g_1^\perp = \begin{pmatrix} -g_y \\ g_x \end{pmatrix}, \quad \nabla g_2^\perp = \begin{pmatrix} -g_z \\ g_x \end{pmatrix}, \quad \nabla g_3^\perp = \begin{pmatrix} -g_z \\ g_y \end{pmatrix} \tag{2.48}$$

and

$$\mathbf{H}_{g1} = \begin{pmatrix} g_{xx} & g_{xy} \\ g_{xy} & g_{yy} \end{pmatrix}, \mathbf{H}_{g2} = \begin{pmatrix} g_{xx} & g_{xz} \\ g_{xz} & g_{zz} \end{pmatrix}, \mathbf{H}_{g3} = \begin{pmatrix} g_{yy} & g_{yz} \\ g_{yz} & g_{zz} \end{pmatrix} \tag{2.49}$$

as well as $\nabla g = (g_x, g_y, g_z)^T$. With (2.47) the measure can be regarded as a superposition of differential measures which are closely related to the original 2D measure in (2.27), e.g., $(\nabla g_1^\perp)^T \mathbf{H}_{g1} \, \nabla g_1^\perp$ is exactly the numerator of the measure in (2.27). Alternatively, we can use

$$\nabla g^{\perp *} = \begin{pmatrix} -g_y \\ g_x \\ -g_z \\ g_x \\ -g_z \\ g_y \end{pmatrix}, \qquad \mathbf{H}_g^* = \begin{pmatrix} \mathbf{H}_{g1} & 0 & 0 \\ 0 & \mathbf{H}_{g2} & 0 \\ 0 & 0 & \mathbf{H}_{g3} \end{pmatrix}, \tag{2.50}$$

where $\mathbf{0}$ is a 2×2 zero matrix, to write

$$Op1(x, y, z) = \frac{(\nabla g^{\perp *})^T \mathbf{H}_g^* \nabla g^{\perp *}}{|\nabla g|^2} \tag{2.51}$$

With the last formulation we have an even more direct formal relation to the original 2D measure of Kitchen and Rosenfeld [280]. Having defined the new 3D measure we can now identify 3D point landmarks with local extrema of the operator values:

$$Op1(x, y, z) \;\rightarrow\; extr. \tag{2.52}$$

Second 3D Operator.   With $Op1$ as the 3D extension of the 2D measure of Kitchen and Rosenfeld [280] we can easily define a second 3D operator which is related to the 2D measure of Blom et al. [47]. Analogously to [47] we take the numerator of $Op1$ (omitting the negative sign as used in [47]) to obtain

$$\begin{aligned}
Op2(x, y, z) &= g_x^2(g_{yy} + g_{zz}) + g_y^2(g_{xx} + g_{zz}) + g_z^2(g_{xx} + g_{yy}) \\
&\quad - 2(g_x g_y g_{xy} + g_x g_z g_{xz} + g_y g_z g_{yz}) \\
&= \sum_{i=1}^{3} (\nabla g_i^{\perp})^T \mathbf{H}_{gi} \nabla g_i^{\perp} \\
&= (\nabla g^{\perp *})^T \mathbf{H}_g^* \nabla g^{\perp *} \;\rightarrow\; extr.
\end{aligned} \tag{2.53}$$

One can interpret this measure in such a way that points with large gradients are emphasized in comparison to $Op1$. Up to a factor 2 the measure represents the 3D mean curvature of isointensity contours multiplied with the third power of the gradient magnitude. Actually, this operator is identical to the operator H^* described in Section 2.4 above.

2.5.2.2   Operators Based on First Order Partial Derivatives

The operators derived in this section are extensions of the 2D measures of Förstner [168] and Rohr [424].

Third 3D Operator.   The 2D measure of Förstner [168] is based on the matrix $\mathbf{C}_g$ given in (2.31). In 3D, this matrix is obtained as the averaged dyadic product of the 3D grey-value gradient $\nabla g = (g_x, g_y, g_z)^T$:

$$\mathbf{C}_g = \overline{\nabla g \, (\nabla g)^T} = \begin{pmatrix} \overline{g_x^2} & \overline{g_x g_y} & \overline{g_x g_z} \\ \overline{g_x g_y} & \overline{g_y^2} & \overline{g_y g_z} \\ \overline{g_x g_z} & \overline{g_y g_z} & \overline{g_z^2} \end{pmatrix} \tag{2.54}$$

Using (2.54) we can define a 3D operator analogously to the 2D case as the ratio between the determinant and the trace of $\mathbf{C}_g$:

$$Op3(x, y, z) = \frac{det\mathbf{C}_g}{tr\mathbf{C}_g} \rightarrow max. \tag{2.55}$$

Alternatively, we could start from the inverse of $\mathbf{C}_g$ and define

$$Op3'(x, y, z) = tr\mathbf{C}_g^{-1} \rightarrow min, \tag{2.56}$$

which is more directly related to the original 2D measure in [168]. Note, that in the 2D case $det\mathbf{C}_g/tr\mathbf{C}_g$ is equivalent to $tr\mathbf{C}_g^{-1}$ which can easily be seen as follows. Suppose that λ_1 and λ_2 are the Eigenvalues of $\mathbf{C}_g$. Then we have $tr\mathbf{C}_g^{-1} = 1/\lambda_1 + 1/\lambda_2 = (\lambda_1 + \lambda_2)/(\lambda_1\lambda_2)$ which is equivalent to $tr\mathbf{C}_g/det\mathbf{C}_g$. Since additionally maximization of an expression is equivalent to minimizing the inverse of it, we have the above stated equivalence. In the 3D case, however, $det\mathbf{C}_g/tr\mathbf{C}_g$ is not equivalent to $tr\mathbf{C}_g^{-1}$. Therefore, we here obtain an additional operator. Note, that the operators in (2.55) and (2.56) in general do not yield equivalent points. Considering the computational complexity, we see that for both operators we only have to compute the three first order partial derivatives of the 3D image (g_x, g_y, g_z), average them, and then find local extrema of the measures in (2.55) or (2.56). In contrast to this, Thirion [520], for example, computes 20 partial derivatives up to order three to find his 'extremal points'.

Fourth 3D Operator. Analogously to Rohr [424] we define a fourth 3D operator as the determinant of the 3×3 matrix $\mathbf{C}_g$ in (2.54):

$$Op4(x, y, z) = det\mathbf{C}_g \rightarrow max. \tag{2.57}$$

Alternatively to employing $\mathbf{C}_g$ in (2.54) one could use an approximation to this matrix:

$$\mathbf{C}_g \approx \nabla g \, (\nabla g)^T + c\mathbf{H}_g^2, \tag{2.58}$$

where $\mathbf{H}_g$ is the Hessian matrix in 3D. In this case, we would need first as well as second order partial derivatives of the image function instead of using only first order partial derivatives.

2.5.2.3 Excluding Insignificant Points

Insignificant points resulting from the application of $Op1$, $Op2$, $Op3$, and $Op4$ can be excluded analogously to the 2D case. First, the measures can be compared with a threshold. Second, for $Op3$ and $Op4$ we can use an extension of the 2D measure $det\mathbf{C}_g/(\frac{1}{2}tr\mathbf{C}_g)^2$ in (2.36). Since this measure represents the ratio between the geometric and arithmetic mean of the Eigenvalues of $\mathbf{C}_g$ a generalization to 3D is straightforward and leads to

$$OpR(x,y,z) = \frac{det\mathbf{C}_g}{\left(\frac{1}{3}tr\mathbf{C}_g\right)^3} \qquad (2.59)$$

(compare also with the n-dimensional case in (2.68) below). In 2D as well as in 3D this measure yields values between 0 and 1 and characterizes the similarity of the Eigenvalues of $\mathbf{C}_g$. For example, we obtain a value of 1 when all Eigenvalues are equal and we obtain low values when there is a large difference between the Eigenvalues. As in 2D the Eigenvalues of $\mathbf{C}_g$ have not to be computed explicitly.

2.5.3 nD Operators

Below, we generalize the four 3D operators considered above to arbitrary dimension n, i.e. for use in nD images. An example for 4D images are time-varying 3D tomographic images. In this case, a 4D operator could be applied to yield characteristic points in the space-time continuum. The involved gradient and the Hessian matrix of the n-dimensional image function $g(x_1, ..., x_n)$ can be written as

$$\nabla g = \begin{pmatrix} g_{x_1} \\ \vdots \\ g_{x_n} \end{pmatrix}, \qquad \mathbf{H}_g = \begin{pmatrix} g_{x_1 x_1} & \cdots & g_{x_1 x_n} \\ \vdots & \ddots & \vdots \\ g_{x_n x_1} & \cdots & g_{x_n x_n} \end{pmatrix}. \qquad (2.60)$$

2.5.3.1   Operators Based on First and Second Order Partial Derivatives

First n-Dimensional Operator.   An extension of $Op1$ to n dimensions is straightforward, since we already introduced suitable representations for the 3D case in (2.47) and (2.51). Thus, we can write:

$$
\begin{aligned}
Op1(x_1, ..., x_n) &= \sum_{i=1}^{\binom{n}{2}} \frac{(\nabla g_i^{\perp})^T \mathbf{H}_{gi} \nabla g_i^{\perp}}{|\nabla g|^2} \\
&= \frac{(\nabla g^{\perp *})^T \mathbf{H}_g^* \nabla g^{\perp *}}{|\nabla g|^2} \rightarrow extr, \qquad (2.61)
\end{aligned}
$$

with $\nabla g_i^{\perp}$, $\mathbf{H}_{gi}$, $\nabla g^{\perp *}$, and $\mathbf{H}_g^*$ defined analogously as in (2.48), (2.49), and (2.50).

2.5.3.2 Second n-Dimensional Operator

As a second n-dimensional operator the numerator of $Op1(x_1, ..., x_n)$ is taken to obtain:

$$
\begin{aligned}
Op2(x_1, ..., x_n) &= \sum_{i=1}^{\binom{n}{2}} (\nabla g_i^{\perp})^T \mathbf{H}_{gi} \, \nabla g_i^{\perp} \\
&= (\nabla g^{\perp *})^T \mathbf{H}_g^* \, \nabla g^{\perp *} \quad \rightarrow \quad extr.
\end{aligned}
\tag{2.62}
$$

2.5.3.3 Operators Based on First Order Partial Derivatives

Third n-Dimensional Operator. A generalization of $Op3$ is defined using the $n \times n$ matrix $\mathbf{C}_g$:

$$
\mathbf{C}_g = \overline{\nabla g \, (\nabla g)^T} = \begin{pmatrix} \overline{g_{x_1}^2} & \cdots & \overline{g_{x_1} g_{x_n}} \\ \vdots & \ddots & \vdots \\ \overline{g_{x_1} g_{x_n}} & \cdots & \overline{g_{x_n}^2} \end{pmatrix}
\tag{2.63}
$$

as

$$
Op3(x_1, ..., x_n) = \frac{\det \mathbf{C}_g}{\operatorname{tr} \mathbf{C}_g} \quad \rightarrow \quad max.
\tag{2.64}
$$

Alternatively, we have

$$
Op3'(x_1, ..., x_n) = \operatorname{tr} \mathbf{C}_g^{-1} \quad \rightarrow \quad min.
\tag{2.65}
$$

Fourth n-Dimensional Operator. Using $\mathbf{C}_g$ in (2.63) an extension of $Op4$ can analogously be defined as:

$$
Op4(x_1, ..., x_n) = \det \mathbf{C}_g \quad \rightarrow \quad max.
\tag{2.66}
$$

Excluding Insignificant Points. Analogously to the 2D and 3D case, insignificant points can be excluded by comparing the measures $Op1$, $Op2$, $Op3$, and $Op4$ with a threshold. For $Op3$ and $Op4$ an additional measure OpR can be applied to exclude pure 'edge points'. As in the 2D and 3D case, we can use the ratio between the geometric and arithmetic mean of the Eigenvalues λ_i of $\mathbf{C}_g$. For n-dimensional images this ratio is

$$
\left(\prod_{i=1}^{n} \lambda_i \right)^{\frac{1}{n}} \Bigg/ \frac{1}{n} \sum_{i=1}^{n} \lambda_i
\tag{2.67}
$$

Taking the ratio to the power of n we finally obtain

$$OpR(x_1, ..., x_n) = \frac{\prod\limits_{i=1}^{n} \lambda_i}{\left(\dfrac{1}{n}\sum\limits_{i=1}^{n} \lambda_i\right)^n} = \frac{det\mathbf{C}_g}{\left(\dfrac{1}{n}tr\mathbf{C}_g\right)^n} \qquad (2.68)$$

2.5.4   Experimental Results

We now present experimental results from applying the described operators to medical image data. We investigate 2D and 3D MR as well as CT images.

2.5.4.1   2D Images

We first show some results for 2D images using the 2D operator of Förstner [168] in (2.33). Previously, this operator has been applied to images of different domains, but to our knowledge has not yet been used for medical images. In the analytic 2D study in Rohr [430] this operator turned out to have very good localization properties in comparison to other approaches. In our implementation, we determine local maxima of the measure in (2.33) and, to remove insignificant points, we use thresholds on the measure itself and on the measure in (2.36), i.e., $det\mathbf{C}_g/tr\mathbf{C}_g \geq s_1$ and $det\mathbf{C}_g/(\frac{1}{2}tr\mathbf{C}_g)^2 \geq s_2$. For all 2D images we have used the thresholds $s_1 = 15$ or $s_1 = 20$ (for low- or high-contrast images, respectively) and $s_2 = 0.25$. Assuming similar Eigenvalues of $\mathbf{C}_g$ (which should be the case for prominent points) this means that each Eigenvalue λ_i has to exceed 30 or 40, respectively. The second threshold removes such points where the ratio of the Eigenvalues is larger than about 14. For computing the partial derivatives of the image we have here used the operators of Beaudet [28], but Gaussian derivative filters could also be used, for example.

The result for a midsagittal MR slice of the human brain is shown in Figure 2.22. The total number of detected point landmarks is 75. It can be seen that a large number of important anatomical point landmarks has successfully been detected. Actually, a larger number of these landmarks agree, for example, with the manually selected landmarks in Bookstein [50], e.g., the anteriormost and posteriormost points of the corpus callosum, the posterior commissure, the tip of the inferior colliculus, the tip of the cerebellum, and the cusps at the pons (see the sketch in Figure 2.8 as well as Section 2.2.2 above). However, we also obtain some misdetections which do not correspond to prominent points of anatomy, for example, detections at the outer contour of the head. Using an axial MR slice of a different dataset yields the points depicted in Figure 2.23. Besides some misdetections at the outer contour of the head, the tips of the ventricular system (cf. Figure 2.11 above) as well as prominent points at the

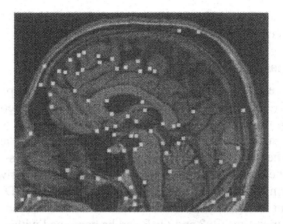

Figure 2.22. Detected point landmarks in a 2D sagittal MR image of a human brain using the 2D operator of Förstner in (2.33).

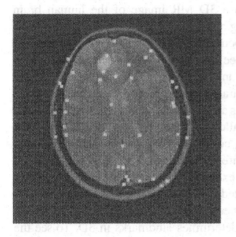

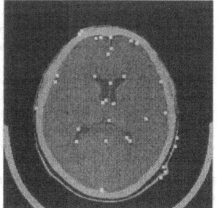

Figure 2.23. Same as Fig. 2.22 but for a 2D axial MR image of a different human brain.

Figure 2.24. Same as Fig. 2.22 but for a 2D axial CT image of a human brain.

symmetry line of the brain, for example, have well been detected. The application to a 2D CT image is shown in Figure 2.24. Also for this kind of image modality significant structures have been detected, for example, the tips of the ventricular system. However, again some misdetections appear, mainly at the outer contour of the head.

Recently, we have evaluated the 2D operators as described above w.r.t. their detection capabilities on the basis of a larger number of 2D tomographic images of the human brain (Hartkens et al. [232]). In this study the operator of Förstner [168] yielded the best result followed by the operator of Rohr [424]. With the operators of Blom et al. [47] and Kitchen and Rosenfeld [280] we obtained worse results (see also Section 3.3 below).

2.5.4.2   3D Images

Next, we show results for 3D images. We first apply the 3D operator $Op3 = det\mathbf{C}_g/tr\mathbf{C}_g$ in (2.55). Here, thresholds are applied on the cornerness measure itself and on the measure $OpR(x, y, z) = det\mathbf{C}_g/(\frac{1}{3}tr\mathbf{C}_g)^3$ in (2.59). For all 3D images we have used the thresholds $s_1 = 75$ or $s_1 = 133$ and $s_2 = 0.1$. Note, that for the operator $Op3$ we only have to compute first order partial derivatives of the image function. In our case, the partial derivatives of the image have been determined using a 3D extension of the 2D operators of Beaudet [28], but 3D Gaussian derivative filters could also be used, for example. Note, that both measures $Op3$ and OpR can be computed without the need of determining the Eigenvalues of $\mathbf{C}_g$ explicitly because these measures are based on the determinant and the trace of $\mathbf{C}_g$ which are both rotationally invariant.

Our approach has been applied to a 3D MR image of the human brain which consists of 68 slices each having a resolution of 165×210 voxels. The total number of detected points is about 1000. The result for a number of slices is shown in Figure 2.25. We see that significant structures have been detected. For example, in slices 7, 20, and 48 the tips of the ventricular system (cf. Figure 2.11 above) and certain characteristic points on the sulci have been found. Additionally detected landmarks are, for example, in slice 36 the anterior commissure and the genu of corpus callosum, in slice 37 the tips between the midbrain and the pons, the posterior commissure, and the splenium of the corpus callosum, and in slice 38 the inferior colliculus (see also Section 2.2.2 and Figure 2.8 above). Note that, for example, the posterior commissure and the inferior colliculus have been detected in different slices, whereas in the 2D case these two point landmarks have been detected in one slice. This means that the applied 3D operator actually determines landmarks in 3D. To see the fundamental differences between the 2D and 3D case more clearly we show in Figure 2.26 the result of the 3D corner operator for the adjacent slices 36, 37, and 38 in comparison to the result of applying the corresponding 2D operator separately to each of the slices. Generally, we see that in the 3D case we have a smaller number of misdetections at the outer contour of the head than in the 2D case (see also Figures 2.22 and 2.23 above). It seems that the 3D operator actually takes into account the information of the structure of the 3D contour (surface) which is relatively smooth. Hence, small perturbations of the contour (curves) within single 2D slices of the 3D data generally do not lead to misdetetions in 3D. A similar argument holds for the triangular shape at the bottom of the slices 36, 37, and 38, which has not been detected in the 3D dataset, while in the 2D case the three sharp corners of this structure have well been detected. In 3D, however, this structure has hardly any variations in the

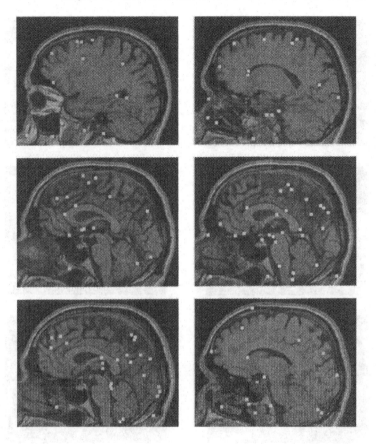

Figure 2.25. Detected point landmarks for a 3D MR image of a human brain using the 3D operator $Op3$ (slices 7, 20, 36, 37, 38, and 48).

direction perpendicular to the slices. Thus, this structure has no prominent 3D point and this fact is justified by the operator result. However, in addition to well-detected 3D point landmarks we also obtain some points which we cannot relate to points of anatomical relevance, e.g., in slices 37 and 38 in the upper and right part of the brain. Here, the reason may be the gap between the two hemispheres of the brain which is partly visible as dark areas in these slices.

In addition to displaying the detection result in a slice-by-slice manner, we have also provided orthoview images of some of the landmarks. These images show the three orthogonal planes (sagittal, axial, coronal) within the 3D image at the detected point. In Figure 2.27 the orthoview images of the genu of corpus callosum detected in slice 36 of Figure 2.25 can be seen. Figure 2.28 shows orthoview images of the posterior commissure detected in slice 37 of Figure 2.25. Note that, although this visualization technique gives

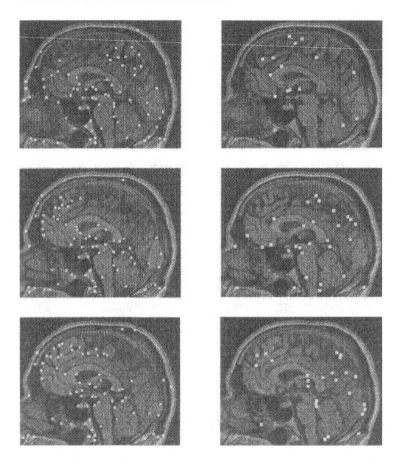

Figure 2.26.   Comparison between 3D operator *Op*3 (right) and corresponding 2D operator (left) for adjacent slices 36, 37, and 38 of a 3D MR image.

some additional insight, the detection result is generally not easy to assess by visual inspection.

The 3D operator *Op*3 has also been applied to a 3D CT image of the human brain. The original dataset consisted of 16 slices each having a resolution of 256 × 256 voxels. To obtain a dataset which has a comparable resolution in all three coordinate directions we have interpolated the original dataset which resulted in about 60 slices. For this image the result of *Op*3 is shown in Figure 2.29. The total number of detected points is about 100 and reflects the fact that in CT images the number of visible brain structures and thus the number of prominent points is much lower than in MR data. In Figure 2.29 we see that prominent points at the ventricular system of the brain are well detected. We also obtain some relevant landmarks along the symmetry line of

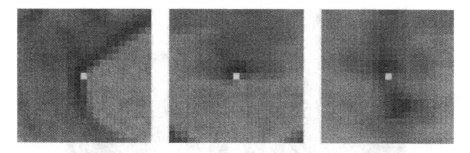

Figure 2.27.   Orthoview images (sagittal, axial, coronal) of the genu of corpus callosum in slice 36 of Fig. 2.25.

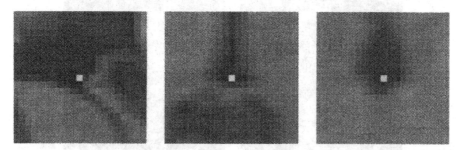

Figure 2.28.   Orthoview images (sagittal, axial, coronal) of the posterior commissure in slice 37 of Fig. 2.25.

the brain. However, it seems that the result for the 3D MR image in Figure 2.25 is better than the result for the 3D CT image. A reason for this is probably that the quality of the MR image is significantly better than that of the CT image.

We also present some experiments with the 3D operator $Op1$ in (2.46). This operator is based on first as well as second order partial derivatives. The result of $Op1$ for the 3D MR dataset used above is shown in Figure 2.30. The threshold for this operator has been set in such a way that we obtain about the same number of detected landmarks within the brain as with $Op3$. Partially, the same landmarks have been detected as with $Op3$ (compare with Figure 2.25), for example, the tips of the ventricular system or the genu of corpus callosum. Note, however, that one has to be careful with such a comparison based on single slices because already relatively small differences may lead to a detection result in an adjacent slice. Therefore, for a sound comparison all detections within the 3D dataset should be taken into account. To diminish the problem of analyzing and comparing the results, we have displayed three adjacent slices from the middle part of the brain (slices 36, 37, and 38 in Figures 2.25 and 2.30). W.r.t. this brain region a comparison of the results is less problematic. Generally, the application of $Op1$ leads to more unwanted points at the outer contour of the

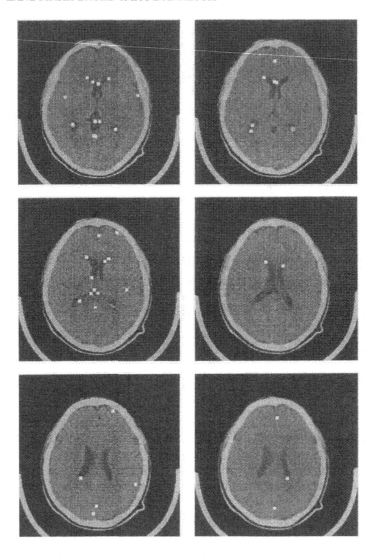

Figure 2.29. Detected point landmarks for a 3D CT image of a human brain using the 3D operator *Op*3 (slices 12, 16, 20, 25, 32, and 33).

head than the operator *Op*3. Actually this seems to be an intrinsic property of *Op*1 and does not result from the fact that only one threshold is used in comparison to two for *Op*3 (see also Section 3.3 below).

We also provide orthoview images of the landmarks at the genu of corpus callosum and the posterior commissure (see Figures 2.31,2.32). For the genu of corpus callosum it seems that we obtain a larger localization error with

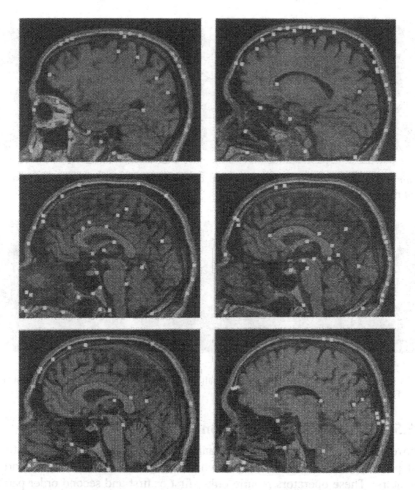

Figure 2.30. Detected point landmarks for a 3D MR image of a human brain using the 3D operator $Op1$ (slices 7, 21, 36, 37, 38, and 47).

$Op1$ than with $Op3$ (Figures 2.27,2.31). For the posterior commissure the two operators yield nearly the same position (Figures 2.28,2.32).

The application of $Op1$ for the 3D CT dataset gives the result shown in Figure 2.33. With this image the effect of the misdetections at the outer contour of the head can be seen more clearly, in particular, when comparing this result with the result of $Op3$ in Figure 2.29. On the other hand, significant 3D landmarks within the brain have well been detected, e.g., the tips of the ventricular system. For a more comprehensive and detailed study of the performance of the described 3D operators as well as others, see Section 3.3 below.

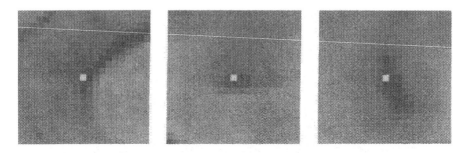

Figure 2.31.   Orthoview images (sagittal, axial, coronal) of the genu of corpus callosum in slice 37 of Fig. 2.30.

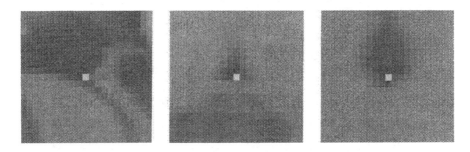

Figure 2.32.   Orthoview images (sagittal, axial, coronal) of the posterior commissure in slice 37 of Fig. 2.30.

2.5.5   Statistical Interpretation

Above we have introduced 3D differential operators for the detection of anatomical point landmarks in 3D images which are generalizations of 2D corner operators. These operators require either first or first and second order partial derivatives and have been motivated by the criterion of finding *points with high intensity variations*. Whereas this criterion is rather general and unspecific, in this section we provide a statistical interpretation of a certain class of the 3D operators (Rohr [436],[437]). This class of operators require only first order partial image derivatives. The operators are 3D generalizations of the 2D corner detectors of Förstner [168] and Rohr [424]:

$$Op3 = \frac{det\mathbf{C}_g}{tr\,\mathbf{C}_g}, \qquad Op3' = \frac{1}{tr\,\mathbf{C}_g^{-1}}, \qquad Op4 = det\mathbf{C}_g, \qquad (2.69)$$

where

$$\mathbf{C}_g = \overline{\nabla g \,(\nabla g)^T} \qquad (2.70)$$

is a symmetric 3×3 matrix which represents the averaged dyadic product of the 3D intensity gradient (see also Section 2.5.2 above). If $\mathbf{C}_g$ has full rank,

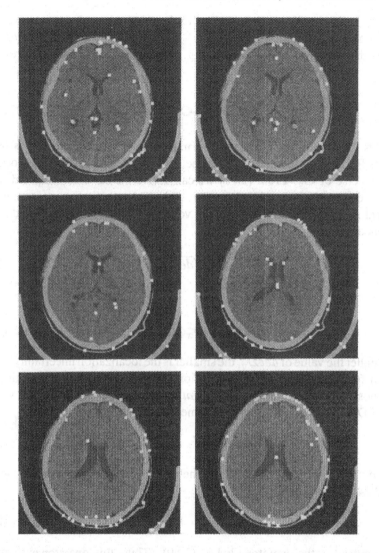

Figure 2.33. Detected point landmarks for a 3D CT image of a human brain using the 3D operator $Op1$ (slices 12, 16, 18, 24, 28, and 29).

then C_g is positive definite and all Eigenvalues of C_g as well as those of its inverse are larger than zero. Therefore, the responses of the operators in (2.69) are always larger (or equal) to zero, and landmark points can be found by computing local maxima of the expressions in (2.69).

In the following, let σ_n^2 denote the variance of additive white Gaussian image noise that is independent of the signal and let m be the number of voxels in a local 3D window. Then, we can relate the matrix C_g, which captures the intensity variations inside the window, to the minimal localization uncertainty of the center of the window $\mathbf{x} = (x, y, z)$. The minimal localization uncertainty is given by the *Cramér-Rao bound* (e.g., van Trees [533]) and is represented by the covariance matrix

$$\Sigma_g = \frac{\sigma_n^2}{m} \mathbf{C}_g^{-1}, \tag{2.71}$$

which is the inverse of the Fisher information matrix (for more details on the Cramér-Rao bound see Section 3.2.2 below). We see, that Σ_g is proportional to the inverse of $\mathbf{C}_g$. From (2.71) we can derive the 3D error ellipsoid of the position estimate with semi-axes σ_x, σ_y, and σ_z. A quantitative measure for the minimal localization uncertainty is the volume of the 3D error ellipsoid which is defined as

$$V = \frac{4}{3} \pi \sqrt{det\Sigma_g}, \tag{2.72}$$

where

$$det\Sigma_g = \sigma_x^2 \sigma_y^2 \sigma_z^2. \tag{2.73}$$

The smaller the value of $det\Sigma_g$, the smaller is the localization uncertainty. Thus, we can formulate the following criterion for localizing 3D point landmarks: Find those points with *minimal localization uncertainty*, i.e., minimal volume of the 3D error ellipsoid. This requirement can be stated as

$$det\Sigma_g \rightarrow min. \tag{2.74}$$

Since $det\Sigma_g = 1/det\Sigma_g^{-1}$ and Σ_g is the inverse of $\mathbf{C}_g$ (up to a factor), we see that (2.74) is equivalent to

$$det\mathbf{C}_g \rightarrow max, \tag{2.75}$$

which indeed is the operator $Op4$ in (2.69). Thus, this operator extracts 3D points with *minimal localization uncertainty*, i.e., *highest possible localization precision*. Analogously, with (2.69) and (2.71) we see that the operator $Op3'$ minimizes $tr\Sigma_g$ which is the sum of the squared semi-axes of the 3D error ellipsoid (for the 2D case see also Förstner [168])

$$tr\Sigma_g = \sigma_x^2 + \sigma_y^2 + \sigma_z^2. \tag{2.76}$$

If the semi-axes are small, then generally also the error ellipsoid is small and vice versa. Therefore, this operator can be seen as a measure for the size of the ellipsoid.

Finally, with $det\mathbf{\Sigma}_g tr\mathbf{\Sigma}_g^{-1} = 1/2((tr\mathbf{\Sigma}_g)^2 - tr\mathbf{\Sigma}_g^2)$ (see also Section 2.5.6 below) and $det\mathbf{\Sigma}_g = 1/det\mathbf{\Sigma}_g^{-1}$, $Op3$ turns out to be equivalent to

$$\frac{1}{2}((tr\mathbf{\Sigma}_g)^2 - tr\mathbf{\Sigma}_g^2) = \sigma_x^2\sigma_y^2 + \sigma_x^2\sigma_z^2 + \sigma_y^2\sigma_z^2, \tag{2.77}$$

which can further be written as

$$\frac{1}{\pi^2}((\pi\sigma_x\sigma_y)^2 + (\pi\sigma_x\sigma_z)^2 + (\pi\sigma_y\sigma_z)^2). \tag{2.78}$$

Now we can see, that the three terms in the parentheses represent the areas of three (2D) ellipses with corresponding semi-axes, and the total expression is the sum of the squared areas of the ellipses. Actually, these ellipses are the three orthogonal sections of the 3D error ellipsoid the orientation of which are determined through the directions of the Eigenvectors of $\mathbf{\Sigma}_g$. Thus, also $Op3$ represents a measure for the size of the 3D error ellipsoid.

In summary, all three operators $Op3$, $Op3'$, and $Op4$ can be interpreted as measures for the size of the minimal 3D error ellipsoid, using either the sum of (squared) sectional ellipse areas, the sum of the (squared) lengths of the semi-axes, or the (squared) volume of the ellipsoid, respectively. In Figure 2.34 we have visualized the different measures. Examples for estimating the 3D error ellipsoids directly from image data are provided in Figures 4.31,4.32 in Section 4.6.4 below. There, we use the estimated ellipsoids as additional information for image registration.

2.5.6 Interpretation as Principal Invariants

Having provided a statistical interpretation of the 3D differential operators $Op3$, $Op3'$, and $Op4$ we show in this section that these operators can also be derived on the basis of invariance principles (Rohr [437]). Invariance (absolute or relative invariance) is an important property which indicates preservation under certain types of transformations (e.g., rotations). Our analysis is based on the covariance matrix $\mathbf{\Sigma}_g$ as introduced above in Section 2.5.5 and which represents the minimal positional uncertainty according to the Cramér-Rao bound. We consider the *principal invariants* of this matrix.

2.5.6.1 Principal invariants of a matrix

Generally, the principal invariants of a $d \times d$ matrix $\mathbf{B} = (b_{ij})$ are the coefficients $\iota_1, ..., \iota_d$, also denoted $\iota_1(\mathbf{B}), ..., \iota_d(\mathbf{B})$ if we wish to make the dependence on $\mathbf{B}$ explicit. These coefficients appear in the characteristic polynomial of $\mathbf{B}$

$$det(\mathbf{B} - \lambda\mathbf{I}) = \tag{2.79}$$
$$(-1)^d\lambda^d + (-1)^{d-1}\iota_1(\mathbf{B})\lambda^{d-1} + \cdots - \iota_{d-1}(\mathbf{B})\lambda + \iota_d(\mathbf{B}),$$

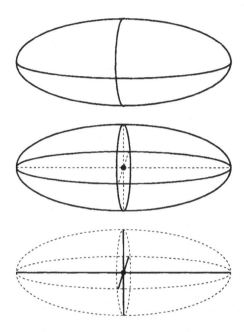

Figure 2.34.   Different measures for the size of the minimal error ellipsoid corresponding to the 3D operators *Op4*, *Op3*, and *Op3′*: volume (top), area of the three principal sections (middle), and lengths of the principal axes (bottom).

where $\mathbf{I}$ is a $d \times d$ unit matrix, such that $\iota_1(\mathbf{B}) = tr\mathbf{B}$, $\iota_{d-1}(\mathbf{B}) = tr(cof\ \mathbf{B})$ $(= det\mathbf{B}\ tr\mathbf{B}^{-1}$ if $\mathbf{B}$ is invertible), and $\iota_d(\mathbf{B}) = det\mathbf{B}$ ([96]). The complete set of the principal invariants can be abbreviated by $\iota_{\mathbf{B}} = (\iota_1(\mathbf{B}), ..., \iota_d(\mathbf{B}))$. The $\iota_i(\mathbf{B})$ are invariant under similarity transformations (translation, rotation, scaling) and they are independent of each other.

In the case of a 3×3 matrix we have the coefficients $\iota_{\mathbf{B}} = (\iota_1(\mathbf{B}), \iota_2(\mathbf{B}), \iota_3(\mathbf{B}))$ which appear in the characteristic polynomial

$$det(\mathbf{B} - \lambda\mathbf{I}) = -\lambda^3 + \iota_1(\mathbf{B})\lambda^2 - \iota_2(\mathbf{B})\lambda + \iota_3(\mathbf{B}). \qquad (2.80)$$

If we denote the Eigenvalues of $\mathbf{B}$ by $\lambda_1, \lambda_2, \lambda_3$ then the following relations can be deduced

$$\begin{aligned}
\iota_1(\mathbf{B}) &= tr\mathbf{B} = \lambda_1 + \lambda_2 + \lambda_3, \\
\iota_2(\mathbf{B}) &= \frac{1}{2}((tr\mathbf{B})^2 - tr\mathbf{B}^2) = \lambda_1\lambda_2 + \lambda_2\lambda_3 + \lambda_1\lambda_3, \qquad (2.81) \\
\iota_3(\mathbf{B}) &= det\mathbf{B} = \lambda_1\lambda_2\lambda_3.
\end{aligned}$$

Other examples of invariants are $tr\mathbf{B}^2$ or $tr\mathbf{B}^3$, however, these invariants are not principal invariants. In the 2D case, i.e., for a 2×2 matrix, we have $det(\mathbf{B} - \lambda\mathbf{I}) = \lambda^2 - \iota_1(\mathbf{B})\lambda + \iota_2(\mathbf{B})$ with the two principal invariants $\iota_1(\mathbf{B}) = tr\mathbf{B}$ and $\iota_2(\mathbf{B}) = det\mathbf{B}$.

2.5.6.2 Interpretation of the 3D Operators $Op3$, $Op3'$, and $Op4$

The covariance matrix $\boldsymbol{\Sigma}_g$ given in (2.71) transforms under similarity transformations $\tilde{\mathbf{x}} = \mathbf{A}\mathbf{x}$ as $\tilde{\boldsymbol{\Sigma}}_g = \mathbf{A}\boldsymbol{\Sigma}_g\mathbf{A}^T$. In the 3D case, according to (2.81), the three principal invariants are

$$\iota_1(\boldsymbol{\Sigma}_g) = tr\boldsymbol{\Sigma}_g, \quad \iota_2(\boldsymbol{\Sigma}_g) = \frac{1}{2}((tr\boldsymbol{\Sigma}_g)^2 - tr\boldsymbol{\Sigma}_g^2), \quad \iota_3(\boldsymbol{\Sigma}_g) = det\boldsymbol{\Sigma}_g. \quad (2.82)$$

Regarding the first principal invariant and knowing from (2.71) that $\mathbf{C}_g$ is the inverse of $\boldsymbol{\Sigma}_g$ (up to a factor) it follows that $\iota_1(\boldsymbol{\Sigma}_g)$ is equivalent to $Op3' = 1/tr\mathbf{C}_g^{-1}$ in (2.69). Note, that for localizing landmarks, we compute local maxima of the operator values. Thus, constant factors of the operators are not relevant. Also note, that maximizing an expression is equivalent to minimizing the inverse of it. Considering $\iota_2(\boldsymbol{\Sigma}_g)$ in order to derive a relation to our 3D operators, we first rewrite the second principal invariant as $\iota_2(\boldsymbol{\Sigma}_g) = det\boldsymbol{\Sigma}_g tr\boldsymbol{\Sigma}_g^{-1}$. Since $det\boldsymbol{\Sigma}_g = 1/det\boldsymbol{\Sigma}_g^{-1}$ we have $\iota_2(\boldsymbol{\Sigma}_g) = tr\boldsymbol{\Sigma}_g^{-1}/det\boldsymbol{\Sigma}_g^{-1}$. Thus, $\iota_2(\boldsymbol{\Sigma}_g)$ is equivalent to $Op3 = det\mathbf{C}_g/tr\mathbf{C}_g$. Finally, again since $det\boldsymbol{\Sigma}_g = 1/det\boldsymbol{\Sigma}_g^{-1}$ and due to (2.71), it follows that the third principal invariant $\iota_3(\boldsymbol{\Sigma}_g)$ is equivalent to $Op4 = det\mathbf{C}_g$. In summary, the 3D operators $Op3$, $Op3'$, and $Op4$ in (2.69) are equivalent to the principal invariants of the covariance matrix $\boldsymbol{\Sigma}_g$. The operators represent the complete set of principal invariants of this matrix. With $\propto$ denoting proportional or inverse proportional, we can write

$$\iota_1(\boldsymbol{\Sigma}_g) \propto \frac{1}{tr\mathbf{C}_g^{-1}}, \quad \iota_2(\boldsymbol{\Sigma}_g) \propto \frac{det\mathbf{C}_g}{tr\mathbf{C}_g}, \quad \iota_3(\boldsymbol{\Sigma}_g) \propto det\mathbf{C}_g. \quad (2.83)$$

Note, that $\iota_1(\boldsymbol{\Sigma}_g)$ can also be expressed exclusively in terms of the matrix $\mathbf{C}_g$ as $\iota_1(\boldsymbol{\Sigma}_g) \propto 2\,det\mathbf{C}_g/((tr\mathbf{C}_g)^2 - tr\mathbf{C}_g^2)$.

If instead, we take the matrix $\mathbf{C}_g$ as the basis of our analysis and consider the principal invariants of this matrix, then we obtain

$$\iota_1(\mathbf{C}_g) = tr\mathbf{C}_g, \quad \iota_2(\mathbf{C}_g) = \frac{1}{2}((tr\mathbf{C}_g)^2 - tr\mathbf{C}_g^2), \quad \iota_3(\mathbf{C}_g) = det\mathbf{C}_g. \quad (2.84)$$

We immediately see, that $\iota_3(\mathbf{C}_g)$ is equivalent to $\iota_3(\boldsymbol{\Sigma}_g)$, while the other two invariants are different from the invariants of $\boldsymbol{\Sigma}_g$. Thus, we have two additional invariants and in total there are five different principal invariants. All invariants are given in terms of the matrix $\mathbf{C}_g$ which is easier to implement in comparison to using the matrix $\boldsymbol{\Sigma}_g$. However, since $\boldsymbol{\Sigma}_g$ is the basis for the statistical interpretation in terms of the minimal uncertainty of the position estimate, we favor those operators which are based on this matrix, i.e., $\iota_1(\Sigma_g)$, $\iota_2(\Sigma_g)$, and $\iota_3(\Sigma_g)$.

In the 2D case, we have the principal invariants $\iota_1(\Sigma_g) = tr\Sigma_g$ and $\iota_2(\Sigma_g) = det\Sigma_g$ which are indeed equivalent to the 2D corner detectors of Förstner [168] and Rohr [424]:

$$\iota_1(\Sigma_g) \propto \frac{det\mathbf{C}_g}{tr\mathbf{C}_g}, \qquad \iota_2(\Sigma_g) \propto det\mathbf{C}_g. \tag{2.85}$$

Considering the matrix $\mathbf{C}_g$ we have

$$\iota_1(\mathbf{C}_g) = tr\mathbf{C}_g, \qquad \iota_2(\mathbf{C}_g) = det\mathbf{C}_g, \tag{2.86}$$

where $\iota_2(\mathbf{C}_g)$ is equivalent to $\iota_2(\Sigma_g)$. Thus, overall we have three different principal invariants of Σ_g and $\mathbf{C}_g$ in the 2D case.

2.5.7   Multi-step Approaches for Subvoxel Localization

The 3D differential operators introduced above are suitable for the detection of 3D anatomical point landmarks. Recently, we have also introduced differential approaches for refined localization of point landmarks (Frantz et al. [176]– [179]). These approaches combine landmark detection with additional steps for refined localization and thus are *multi-step approaches*. With these schemes we yield subvoxel positions of 3D point landmarks. As detection operators we utilize one of the operators $Op3$, $Op3'$, and $Op4$ introduced above, which require only first order image derivatives. Subvoxel positions of the landmarks can be determined by applying a 3D generalization of the 2D differential edge intersection approach of Förstner and Gülch [173], which also requires only first order image derivatives. With the 2D approach in [173] edge curves are locally approximated by tangent lines and these tangent lines are intersected to obtain a refined position. This is formulated as a least-squares problem. For every point within a local window the tangent lines are determined as normals to the image gradient. Since the tangent lines are weighted by the magnitude of the image gradients, it follows that essentially edge points are incorporated. This scheme is most accurate for very sharp tips composed of two straight edge lines (ideal L-corner). For more rounded tips the anatomical structure is approximated and the exact position of the tip is not obtained (see Figure 2.35). However, by reducing the size of the local window we can improve the localization accuracy. On the other hand, we have to take into account the smoothing effect when computing the image gradient by applying derivative filters. Smoothing leads to a displacement of the edge curves. Actually, computing the intersection point for the displaced edge curves (partly) compensates the localization error due to the approximation of the rounded tip (see Figure 2.35 on the right). Note, that the displacement of edge curves due to image smoothing also leads to localization errors in the case of the ideal sharp tip.

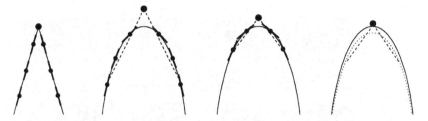

Figure 2.35.   Sketch of localization properties of the differential multi-step approach (from left to right): Sharp tip (L-corner); rounded tip and large window; rounded tip and small window; consideration of edge displacement due to image smoothing.

The 3D case is analogous. Here, the edge surfaces are approximated by tangent planes determined by the 3D image gradient. A refined landmark position is obtained by intersecting these tangent planes. Utilizing the Hessian normal form, the perpendicular distance of a point $\mathbf{x}$ to the tangent plane through $\mathbf{x}_i$ can be written with the image gradient ∇g_i at this point as $d(\mathbf{x}) = (\nabla g_i)^T (\mathbf{x} - \mathbf{x}_i)$. These distances are summed up for all image points inside the window and we want to find the minimum w.r.t. $\mathbf{x}$. Using a least-squares approach this can be stated as

$$S(\mathbf{x}) \; = \; \sum_{i=1}^{m} \left((\nabla g_i)^T (\mathbf{x} - \mathbf{x}_i) \right)^2$$

$$= \; \sum_{i=1}^{m} (\mathbf{x} - \mathbf{x}_i)^T (\nabla g_i (\nabla g_i)^T)(\mathbf{x} - \mathbf{x}_i) \; \to \; min \qquad (2.87)$$

and leads to the following system of linear equations

$$\overline{\nabla g \, (\nabla g)^T} \, \hat{\mathbf{x}} = \overline{\nabla g \, (\nabla g)^T} \, \mathbf{x}, \qquad (2.88)$$

from which the 3D position estimate $\hat{\mathbf{x}}$ can be determined. 'Overline' means average in the local window and $\overline{\nabla g \, (\nabla g)^T}$ is the matrix $\mathbf{C}_g$ as introduced above. An alternative approach for refined localization does not involve the edge intersection scheme and is only based on a 3D detection operator. With this approach, the operator is applied in scale space (e.g., [566],[283],[214]), i.e., derivative filters of different sizes are used to localize points.

In summary, we have investigated the following three multi-step procedures:
i) *Two-step procedure*: Application of a 3D detection operator of large and small scales for robust detection as well as refined localization. Such a procedure has previously been used in the case of 2D images (Dreschler [122], Rohr [424]).
ii) *Two-step procedure*: After landmark detection, the 3D differential edge intersection approach is applied. This procedure yields subvoxel positions and is the 3D extension of the two-step procedure in Förstner and Gülch [173].

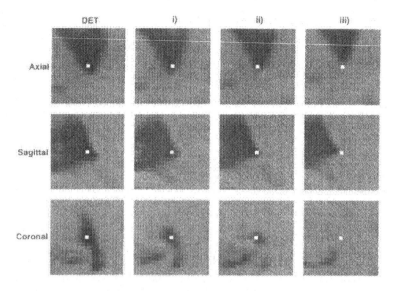

Figure 2.36.   Localized 3D positions for the tip of the left occipital horn of the ventricular system in a 3D MR image using the detection operator alone (DET) and the multi-step procedures i), ii), and iii) in axial, sagittal, and coronal views.

iii) *Three-step procedure*: Combination of the procedures i) and ii).

As an example, in Figure 2.36 we show the result of applying the multi-step procedures for the tip of the left occipital ventricular horn. It can be seen that the localized positions are significantly better than those obtained by applying only a detection operator (abbreviated by DET). A more comprehensive evaluation of the multi-step procedures using 3D synthetic data as well as 3D MR images of the human head is described in Section 3.3.5 below.

As an extension of this approach we have recently developed a statistical scheme which allows to estimate an *optimal size of the region-of-interest (ROI)* for a landmark (Frantz et al. [178]). For related approaches to optimal window and scale selection, see also [387],[309]. Our scheme exploits the covariance matrix of the position estimate of the edge intersection approach. This covariance matrix is related to the Cramér-Rao bound as described above. In our approach, we use the determinant of the covariance matrix as a measure of uncertainty and compute it as a function of the ROI size (starting with a minimal ROI size). If the window is increased then the uncertainty should generally decrease. On the other hand, if some neighboring structure is included in the ROI then the uncertainty significantly increases. Therefore, in our approach we determine such significant changes. This results in reasonable ROI sizes in 2D and 3D while neighboring structures are generally excluded.

2.6 Parametric Approaches

So far we have considered differential operators for the detection and localization of 2D and 3D point landmarks. These operators are very efficient since they evaluate only the *local* neighborhood of a considered image point, e.g., a $5 \times 5 \times 5$ neighborhood. On the other hand, general problems are their sensitivity w.r.t. image noise and the occurrence of systematic localization errors (see also Section 3.2.1 below). Instead, with *semi-global* approaches we can integrate more global image information (see Figure 2.37), which generally increases the robustness against noise and opens the possibility to improve the localization performance. Examples for approaches which act on larger image regions are based on *deformable contour models* or *parametric intensity models* (see also Section 1.5 above). With the latter type of approach we exploit the full information of the image intensities and the estimated parameters have a direct physical meaning. Besides these direct schemes, there are also indirect approaches that first extract edge points, link them together and then operate on the resulting structures. With *global* approaches the result for one image point generally depends on the whole image (e.g., Nitzberg and Shiota [382], Schnörr [471],[470]). These approaches rely on general smoothness assumptions about the image (comparable to deformable contour models), and the primary purpose is robust segmentation of image structures. The resulting image description is well-suited for applying a parametric model in a second step to localize point structures more precisely and to estimate additional attributes (cf. Section 3.3.7).

In this section, we introduce a semi-global approach for landmark extraction based on *parametric intensity models*. These models are based on a radiomet-

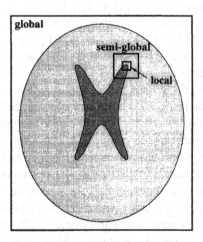

Figure 2.37. Classification of approaches for landmark extraction.

ric model and directly represent the image intensities. The models incorporate more specific knowledge in comparison to differential operators, deformable contour models and global approaches. This allows us to localize point landmarks very precisely without systematic localization errors. Actually it can be shown that with our approach the lower uncertainty bound in estimation theory can be achieved (Cramér-Rao bound; see Section 3.2.2). Also, the approach is relatively robust since it integrates information from larger image regions. The parameters of the models have a physical meaning (e.g., position, orientation, contrast, edge transition width) and are estimated simultaneously by directly fitting the model to the image intensities. As point landmarks we here consider corners of 3D polyhedral objects in 2D images, planar circular landmarks in 2D aerial images, and anatomical landmarks in 2D and 3D tomographic images.

Applications where high-precision localization of landmarks is important are, for example, camera calibration, mensuration tasks, determination of geometric invariants for object recognition (e.g., the cross ratio), scene reconstruction, and image registration. The estimated landmark attributes are relevant for additional applications, e.g., in projection images the estimated width of the intensity transitions can be exploited to estimate the distance to the object (depth-from-focus, e.g., [400]) or other attributes can be used to resolve possibly occurring ambiguities in the interpretation of 3D shape based on, e.g., line drawings. In the case of image registration, estimated attributes can be exploited to further improve the registration accuracy (see also Section 4.7 below).

Previously, fitting procedures using parametric intensity models have been proposed for the extraction of 1D low-level features, particularly image edges (e.g., Hueckel [258], Thurgood and Mikhail [525], Nalwa and Binford [364]). Partly, however, the model is not directly fitted to the image but an orthogonal basis expansion is used, and often the model has not been based on a radiometric model. In Rohr [425]–[427], we have introduced parametric intensity models for the localization of image edges and corners (junctions) in 2D images. These models are based on a radiometric model, incorporate Gaussian image blur, and allow to localize landmarks with subpixel position. Efficient approaches have been described in Rohr [427] as well as in Rohr and Schnörr [440] utilizing partial derivatives of the model for fitting and a B-spline approximation of the Gaussian blurring function. In Drewniok and Rohr [125]–[129] we have extended our scheme for automatic detection and localization of circular point landmarks in 2D aerial images. The extracted landmarks have been used for registration with a geodetic database and for automatic absolute orientation using geometric invariants. For a generalization to other planar point landmarks (e.g., disks and crosses), see particularly [127],[129]. In comparison to our *analytic models, discrete templates,* which have previously been used particularly in the case of aerial images (e.g., Förstner [170]), are not as flexible and also have other disadvantages that result from necessary discretization and filtering. The use of parametric intensity models for feature extraction has recently gained increased attention. Recent approaches are based on, e.g., edge models (e.g., Lai et al. [297], Wang and Binford [550], Chiang and Boult [88], Zhang and Bergholm [578], Wang et al. [549], Hagemann et al. [215]), line models (e.g., Cerneaz and Brady [83], Steger [500], Koller et al. [286], Sato et al. [460], Krissian et al. [289], Noordmans et al. [385]), and corner models (e.g., Deriche and Blaszka [119], Orange and Groen [388], Brand and Mohr [62], Chen et al. [86], Alvarez and Morales [6], Baker et al. [21], Parida et al. [392], Stammberger et al. [499], Rosin [454]). As already mentioned above in Section 1.4, there is a current trend in computer vision to include intensity information to improve the robustness of algorithms (e.g., [360],[365],[45], [103],[264],[275],[366],[477]).

From the above mentioned recent approaches utilizing parametric corner models the closest to our model-fitting approach are the ones in [119],[62], [21],[392]. Therefore, we discuss them in more detail. Deriche and Blaszka [119] have published a slightly modified version of our approach in [425]-[427]. They used the same modelling scheme (L-corner symmetry, superposition of L-corner models), but instead of a Gaussian blurring function they employed an exponential function which, however, has no physical motivation. Also, the model is fitted by using only function values of the model, whereas in our approach function values as well as partial derivatives of the model are used for efficient fitting. Brand and Mohr [62] applied a simplified Gaussian corner model for localizing points on a calibration grid. In comparison to our approach [425]-[427] they only considered L-corners (two intersecting edges) and they assumed a fixed image blur, i.e. this parameter is not optimized. Baker et al. [21] use parametric feature models (e.g., edge, corner, circular disk) and employ a Karhunen-Loève (KL) expansion (similar to Hueckel [258]) to find the closest point w.r.t. a feature manifold defined by the model parameters. Thus, the model is not directly fitted to the image intensities as in our approach. Their focus is on feature detection and as corner model they consider an L-corner model only. It is unclear how the used approximation affects the localization accuracy as well as the accuracy of the other parameters. Parida et al. [392] use a corner model with up to four intersecting edges and apply the minimum description length (MDL) principle to obtain an optimal number of intersecting edges. Their fitting function involves a regularization term based on the gradients of the model and the image. The intensity information in a small neighborhood around the corner point is not taken into account.

In the remainder of this section we first describe the radiometric model and the model of the imaging process utilized in our approach (Section 2.6.1). Then we introduce parametric intensity models comprising edges, corners (junctions), circular landmarks, rectangular landmarks, and 3D landmarks (Sec-

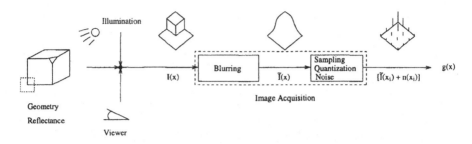

Figure 2.38.   Image formation model.

tion 2.6.2). After that we describe the procedure for directly fitting the models to the image intensities (Section 2.6.3) and present experimental results for real image data (Section 2.6.4).

2.6.1   Radiometric Model and Imaging Process

Our parametric intensity models are based on a radiometric model as described in this section. We first consider corners of 3D polyhedral objects in video images, i.e., projection images. As sketched in Figure 2.38, the observed image intensities $I(\mathbf{x})$ depend on the geometry and the reflectance properties of scene objects, the illumination (position, direction, and type), as well as the position and direction of the viewer. For the scene objects we assume that the borders are ideally sharp and that the surfaces are homogeneous without texture. As *radiometric model* (also denoted as photometric or illumination model) we apply the model of Phong [402] (see also [374],[248],[254]), where the light intensities consist of three parts

$$I(\mathbf{x}) = I_d + I_s + I_a, \qquad (2.89)$$

with

$$
\begin{aligned}
I_d &= \rho_d \left(\mathbf{n}^T \mathbf{1} \right) I_l = \rho_d \cos\theta\, I_l & (2.90) \\
I_s &= \rho_s \left(\mathbf{r}^T \mathbf{v} \right)^m I_l = \rho_s (\cos\psi)^m\, I_l & (2.91) \\
I_a &= \rho_a I_A. & (2.92)
\end{aligned}
$$

I_d represents the diffuse reflection part, which depends on the angle θ between the (normalized) normal vector $\mathbf{n}$ of a surface element and the (normalized) vector $\mathbf{1}$ of the light source as well as the intensity I_l of the light source and the coefficient ρ_d (Figure 2.39). I_d is independent of the viewer (Lambert's law). On the other hand, the specular reflection part I_s depends on the viewer direction $\mathbf{r}$ and the reflection direction $\mathbf{v}$ according to an ideal mirror as well as the coefficient ρ_s and the exponent m ($\mathbf{r}$ and $\mathbf{v}$ are normalized). Finally, I_a represents the ambient light due to extended light sources and multiple

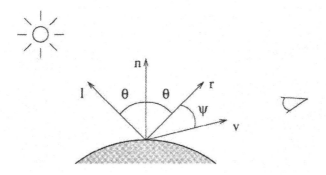

Figure 2.39. Sketch of the illumination model.

reflections from objects in the surroundings, while ρ_a is a coefficient and I_A the basic brightness.

Under certain assumptions we obtain for the image intensities $I(\mathbf{x})$ *planes of constant intensities with ideal step transitions,* which can be explained as follows. First, we assume parallel light rays (point light source at infinity), thus I_d is constant (note, that we consider polyhedral objects). Second, we assume that the distance between the light source and the viewer is large in comparison to the considered section of a depicted object in the scene, then also I_s is constant. Both assumptions can be regarded to be justified in our case, since we are only interested in relatively small image parts compared to the whole image, namely the neighborhood of corners of depicted objects. Finally, I_a only changes the absolute values of the intensities but not the structural variations.

Due to the bandlimiting property of a camera, the ideal step-shaped intensities $I(\mathbf{x})$ are blurred (Figure 2.38). In our case, we describe the blurring by convolution with a Gaussian filter. Note, however, that the point spread function (PSF) corresponding to the *image blur* is generally quite complicated (e.g., Andrews and Hunt [8], Schreiber [475]). Our approximation is particularly justified by the central limit theorem (e.g., Pentland [400]). The image blur results due to a number of single effects (e.g., diffraction, chromatic aberration, lens defocusing) with corresponding point spread functions. The overall point spread function is then obtained by convolving the single functions, while a Gaussian function is obtained in the limit of a large number of independent effects, regardless of the shape of the single functions.

Finally in the image formation model, we have to take into account that the image intensities are sampled, quantized, and disturbed by noise. For the *noise,* we assume additive zero-mean white Gaussian noise that is independent of the signal, which is typically met in real images (e.g., Horn [254]). The Gaussian noise assumption can be justified by the central limit theorem assuming a lot of

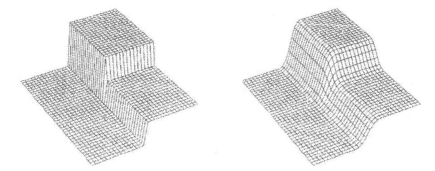

Figure 2.40.   Ideal step-shaped T-corner (left) and Gaussian blurred T-corner (right).

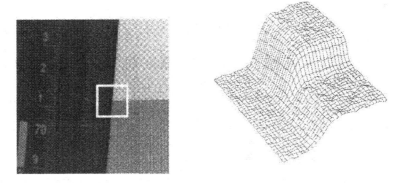

Figure 2.41.   Real image of a T-corner (left) and 3D plot of the marked area (right).

independent noise sources (e.g., Kanatani [271]). Effects due to sampling and quantization will not be considered, besides those that contribute to the image blur and can be integrated into the above mentioned point spread function. Figures 2.40,2.41 demonstrate for a T-corner that our model well describes the intensity variations within a real image.

The above considerations have been made for projected corners of 3D polyhedral objects. This includes object corners, but also corners due to occlusions (an example is a T-corner). Additionally, our consideration is valid for corners created by different reflectance properties on object surfaces and also for corners created by shadows. Moreover, we can describe corners with intersecting edges that have different physical reasons (e.g., intersection of two object edges and one shadow edge). In this case, however, we have to assume that the widths of all edge transitions are equal. Other objects we consider below are planar (2D) scene objects, e.g., landmarks in aerial images. Actually, planar objects are a special case of 3D polyhedra, thus the model from above applies in this case, too.

In the case of 3D tomographic images (e.g., MR, CT), the image formation process is totally different and depends on the imaging modality as well as the imaging parameters. Thus, the image intensities have a different meaning. For example, in CT images the intensities represent the absorption of X-rays and in MR images the intensities represent the magnetic effect of the spin of atomic nuclei (hydrogen atoms). However, also in these cases the same principle as above can be applied to end up with parametric intensity models for landmarks. Here, the key assumption is that the depicted 3D anatomical structures are homogeneous. Then, the image intensities are constant for each structure and we can assume abrupt step-shaped transitions between different structures. Due to the image formation process, which is band-limited, the intensities will be blurred here, too. We can model this blurring by a Gaussian filter again invoking the central limit theorem. Note, however, that for 3D spatial images generally other reasons lead to blurring than in the case of 2D video images as discussed above, e.g., we have partial volume effects and effects due to different resolutions within and between slices (e.g., Barrett and Swindell [27]; see also Back et al. [16]). For the noise we assume as above additive zero-mean white Gaussian noise that is independent of the signal, which is an approximation to the error statistics of medical images (e.g., Barrett and Swindell [27], Abbey et al. [1]). While the assumption of the Gaussian noise model often holds, it has recently been argued in [1] that for large signal-to-noise ratios the dependence of the noise on the signal should be taken into account. However, here we assume that this dependence can be neglected. For landmarks in 2D tomographic images the above considerations also apply, since they are a special case of landmarks in 3D images.

2.6.2 Parametric Intensity Models of Landmarks

Having described the physical process of image formation, we can now derive analytic models for the intensity variations of image features. We consider edges, corners, circular symmetric landmarks as well as other planar landmarks, and 3D landmarks.

2.6.2.1 L-corners and Edges

We first consider an L-corner, i.e. a point landmark with two intersecting straight edges, and parameterize it by an aperture angle β and contrast a (Figure 2.42). This image structure models corners of 3D polyhedral objects, corners of 2D (planar) objects, and also tip-like landmarks in 2D tomographic images of the human brain, for example. Let $E(x,y)$ denote the ideal step-shaped L-corner

$$E(x,y) = \begin{cases} a & \text{if } x \geq 0 \,\wedge\, |y| \leq \tan(\beta/2)\,x \\ 0 & \text{otherwise} \end{cases} \qquad (2.93)$$

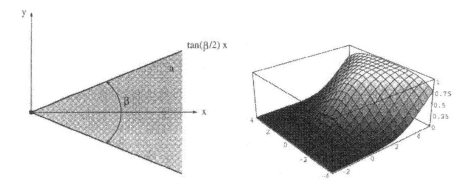

Figure 2.42.   Parameterization of an L-corner and corresponding 3D plot.

and the Gaussian function with $\sigma = 1$

$$G(x,y) = G(x)G(y), \qquad G(x) = \frac{1}{\sqrt{2\pi}} e^{-\frac{x^2}{2}}. \qquad (2.94)$$

Then we obtain the model function for a blurred L-corner by convolution of these two functions:

$$\begin{aligned} g_{ML}(x,y) &= E(x,y) * G(x,y) \\ &= \int\limits_{-\infty}^{\infty} \int\limits_{-\infty}^{\infty} E(\xi,\eta) \, G(x-\xi, y-\eta) \, d\xi d\eta. \qquad (2.95) \end{aligned}$$

The calculations become much easier if we exploit the symmetry of the structure w.r.t. the x-axis. Then, we only have to evaluate the upper part of the L-corner for which we derive the model function $M(x,y)$. The model function for the lower part is then easily obtained by reflecting this function on the x-axis. For the upper part setting $a = 1$ we obtain

$$\begin{aligned} M(x,y) &= \int\limits_{\xi=0}^{\infty} \int\limits_{\eta=0}^{t\xi} G(x-\xi, y-\eta) \, d\xi d\eta \\ &= \phi(x,y) - \int\limits_{-\infty}^{x} G(\xi) \, \phi(t\xi - \zeta_2) d\xi, \qquad (2.96) \end{aligned}$$

with $\phi(x,y) = \phi(x)\phi(y)$, the Gaussian error function $\phi(x) = \int\limits_{-\infty}^{x} G(\xi)d\xi$, and $t = \tan(\beta/2)$, $\zeta_2 = tx - y$. The complete model results from the superposition of the upper and lower model functions, while the contrast a and the parameter σ, characterizing the width of the Gaussian function, introduce as scaling factors (Rohr [425]–[427]):

$$g_{ML}(x, y, \beta, a, \sigma) = a\left(M(\frac{x}{\sigma}, \frac{y}{\sigma}, \beta) + M(\frac{x}{\sigma}, -\frac{y}{\sigma}, \beta)\right). \qquad (2.97)$$

Note, that our model is valid for the whole range of aperture angles, $0^\circ < \beta < 180^\circ$. To compute function values of g_{ML} we apply a rational approximation for $\phi(x)$ (see [2]) and determine the integral in (2.96) by numeric integration using the approach of Romberg [407]. For the special case of the aperture angle $\beta = 180^\circ$ we obtain the model of a step edge

$$g_{MSE}(x, y) = a\,\phi(x). \qquad (2.98)$$

Arbitrary positions (x_0, y_0) and rotations about an angle α of the models are obtained by the substitution

$$x^* = (x - x_0)\cos\alpha + (y - y_0)\sin\alpha \qquad (2.99)$$
$$y^* = -(x - x_0)\sin\alpha + (y - y_0)\cos\alpha. \qquad (2.100)$$

Earlier models of blurred L-corners are only qualitative, i.e. they have been drawn by hand (Dreschler [122], Nagel [362]), or the mathematical formulation is not as elegant as ours since particularly the symmetry of the structure has not been exploited (Berzins [36], Bergholm [32], Guiducci [212], Rangarajan et al. [411]).

2.6.2.2 More Complex Corners

In this section, we derive an analytic corner model with an arbitrary number of intersecting edges. Actually, such much more complex corner structures can easily be modelled by again invoking the superposition principle and using the L-corner model from above as elementary function (Rohr [425]–[427]). Note, that while such structures are often denoted as junctions, we here use the terms *junction* and *corner* synonymously, e.g., L-, T-, Y- and Arrow-junctions are also L-, T-, Y-, and Arrow-corners, respectively (e.g., [427]). In the general case of a number of N intersecting edges we have

$$g_M(x, y) = \left(\sum_{i=1}^{N} E_i(x, y)\right) * G(x, y) = \sum_{i=1}^{N}(E_i(x, y) * G(x, y))$$
$$= a_0 + \sum_{i=1}^{N-1} g_{ML}(x, y, \beta_i, a_i, \sigma), \qquad N \geq 2. \qquad (2.101)$$

Thus, the general model consists of a constant intensity a_0 and a superposition of $N - 1$ L-corner models. For example, corners with three intersecting edges,

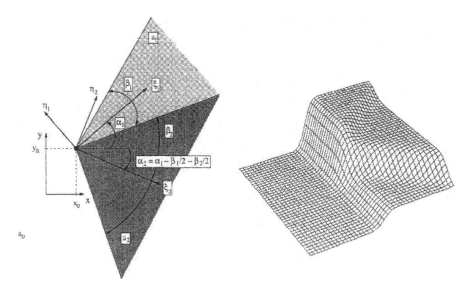

Figure 2.43.   Parameterization of a corner with three intersecting edges (left) and 3D plot of a
K-corner (right).

i.e., T-, Y-, Arrow-corners, are created by superposition of two L-corners.
A parameterization of such a structure is shown in Figure 2.43 on the left.
Actually, we only need two additional parameters (β_2 and a_2) in comparison
to an L-corner to model this structure. Note, that we can exploit the constraint
$\alpha_2 = \alpha_1 - \beta_1/2 - \beta_2/2$ between the orientation and the aperture angles.
Based on the aperture angles β_1 and β_2 we can distinguish the following
different corner types: For a T-corner we have $\beta_1 + \beta_2 = 180^o$, and for Y- and
Arrow-corners $\beta_1 + \beta_2$ is larger or smaller than 180°, respectively, if β_1 and β_2
are the two smaller angles. Corners with four intersecting edges, i.e., $N = 4$,
are obtained analogously. In this case we have PEAK-, K-, X-, MULTI- and
XX-corners using the notation of Waltz [548]. In Figure 2.43 on the right an
example of a K-corner can be seen. $N = 5$ specifies KA- and KX-corners, and
$N \geq 6$ leads to even more complex corners. The number of model parameters
is $n = 3 + 2N$.

Actually, with our general model in (2.101) we can completely describe all
corner types used in the labeling system of Waltz [548]. This model first allowed
to describe mathematically blurred corners with three intersecting edges of
arbitrary aperture angles. Previously, a Y-corner model has been used by De
Micheli et al. [117] as a basis to compare existing edge detection algorithms.
Later, Giraudon and Deriche [194] extended this Y-corner model to corners with
three arbitrary edges, and subsequently Deriche and Blaszka [119] adopted our
model. In Rohr [431] we have extended our model from constant intensity

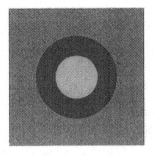

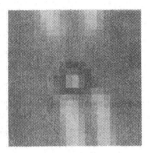

Figure 2.44. Circular symmetric landmark (left) and appearance in aerial images of urban environments (middle and right).

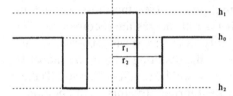
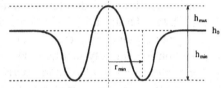

Figure 2.45. Cross-sections of the unblurred (left) and the blurred (right) circular symmetric structure from Fig. 2.44.

plateaus of the unblurred structure to linearly varying intensity variations to cope also with intensity gradients in the scene.

2.6.2.3 Circular Symmetric and Other Planar Landmarks

For the corner models from above the corresponding unblurred structures are characterized by a uniquely defined tip and by the fact that they extend to infinity. Now, we consider landmarks, where the underlying unblurred structures are finite. These image structures primarily correspond to planar landmark objects in the scene. As prominent point of these structures we choose their centerpoint.

We first consider the landmark shown in Figure 2.44 on the left, which is circular symmetric. This type of landmark can be used in many applications, e.g., in remote sensing, neurosurgery, and for car crash tests. In our case, we use a model of this landmark to extract control points from aerial images for image registration applications (Drewniok and Rohr [125]–[129]). A main advantage of this landmark type is that it already exists in urban environments. It corresponds to manhole covers on the road, such that premarking of ground control points is not necessary (Figure 2.44 middle and right). Also, a large number of these landmarks can be found and they are well distributed over the

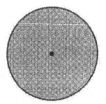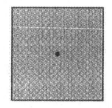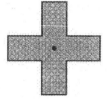

Figure 2.46.   Different types of 2D point landmarks: Disk, square, and cross.

scene. Moreover, geodetic data is usually available from the cadaster of a city's sewerage system. To derive an analytic model we apply the same principle as used above for corners. We start with the ideal step-shaped intensity structure and introduce blurring due to the imaging process (see the cross-sections in Figure 2.45). Doing this, we assume that aerial images are recorded parallel to the ground plane such that the circularity in the image is preserved. This assumption is generally justified. However, the resulting parametric model is rather complicated and landmark extraction would be time-consuming. Therefore, we introduce an approximation of the blurred structure. An additional motivation to use an approximation is that the resolution of the landmarks in our application is rather low, i.e. the landmark is usually represented by a relatively small number of image points. The model we use can be stated as

$$KD(r) = a_0 + (a_1 + a_2 r^2) e^{-\frac{r^2}{2\sigma^2}}, \qquad (2.102)$$

where $r = \sqrt{x^2 + y^2}$, and well describes the exact intensity model. It has a similar shape as the Laplacian-of-Gaussian (e.g., Marr and Hildreth [330]). For the relations between the parameters a_0, a_1, a_2 and those in Figure 2.45 see Section 3.2.2 below as well as [128]. Experimental results using this model function are described in Section 2.6.4 below.

The circular landmark from above can be imagined as the superposition of two concentric disks. As a simpler landmark we could use just one disk as depicted in Figure 2.46 on the left. The blurred disk can be modelled exactly or we can use an approximation by a bivariate Gaussian function which represents a blob:

$$Blob(x, y) = \frac{a}{\sigma_x \sigma_y} G(\frac{x}{\sigma_x}) G(\frac{y}{\sigma_y}), \qquad (2.103)$$

while for $\sigma_x = \sigma_y$ the blob is isotropic. Besides circular landmarks, we can also model rectangular shapes or squares (Figure 2.46 in the middle). The exact model of these structures can be stated as

$$Rect(x,y) = \tag{2.104}$$

$$a\left(\phi(\frac{x+r_x}{\sigma}) - \phi(\frac{x-r_x}{\sigma})\right)\left(\phi(\frac{y+r_y}{\sigma}) - \phi(\frac{y-r_y}{\sigma})\right),$$

while for a square we have the half widths $r_x = r_y = r$. Another often used type of landmark is a cross (Figure 2.46 on the right). Actually, this type of landmark can be modelled by superposition of rectangular shapes based on (2.104). Analogously, by using the superposition principle, we can model a large variety of other point landmarks (see also Drewniok and Rohr [127], [129]). Besides point landmarks we can also model 1D features such as lines, for example (see also Section 3.2 where we use such models for performance characterization of landmark operators).

2.6.2.4 3D Landmarks

While above we have focussed on point landmarks in 2D images, we now describe landmarks in 3D spatial images. Primarily we are interested in modelling anatomical point landmarks in 3D tomographic images of the human brain (e.g., MR, CT), however, our models are also applicable to 3D spatial images of other domains, e.g., geology or industrial inspection. As already discussed in Section 2.6.1 we use the same principle as before to derive parametric intensity models for 3D landmarks. We generally start out from ideal step-shaped structures and smooth them by a Gaussian filter. The assumption is that the depicted 3D anatomical structures are homogeneous and that blurring can be modelled by convolution with a trivariate Gaussian filter. For some of the structures we use approximations.

In this manner we can derive analytic models for 3D edges, 3D ridges, or 3D lines which can be stated as follows (see also Section 3.2.3 below):

$$Edge3D(x,y,z) = a\phi(\frac{x}{\sigma}) \tag{2.105}$$

$$Ridge3D(x,y,z) = a\phi(\frac{x}{\sigma})\phi(\frac{y}{\sigma}) \tag{2.106}$$

$$Line3D(x,y,z) = \frac{a}{\sigma_x\sigma_z}G(\frac{x}{\sigma_x})G(\frac{z}{\sigma_z}). \tag{2.107}$$

Note, that for edges and ridges we have exact models while for lines we have used an approximation. By combining the structures in (2.105)-(2.107) unique points can be defined. For example, point landmarks can be defined as line-line intersections. By additionally introducing a coordinate transformation also curving structures can be modelled. An example for a line-line (curve-curve) intersection is the optic chiasm within the human brain. Also, we can define point landmarks as line-plane intersections or intersections of planes utilizing the 3D line model and a plane model based on the 3D edge model. An example for a line-plane intersection is the intersection between the midsaggital plane and the commissura anterior within the human brain.

Direct models of 3D point landmarks can be derived by extending the 2D structures from above to 3D. For example, an L-corner in a 3D image can be modelled by

$$L3D(x, y, z) = a\phi(\frac{x}{\sigma})\phi(\frac{y}{\sigma})\phi(\frac{z}{\sigma}), \tag{2.108}$$

while a T-corner in 3D can be stated as

$$T3D(x, y, z) = a_0 + \phi(\frac{x}{\sigma})\left((a_2 - a_0) + (a_1 - a_2)\phi(\frac{y}{\sigma})\right)\phi(\frac{z}{\sigma}). \tag{2.109}$$

For both of these structures we assumed that all occurring angles have an aperture of 90°. An extension of a rectangular structure is a 3D box, which can be modelled by

$$\begin{aligned}
Box3D(x, y, z) = \; & a\left(\phi(\frac{x + r_x}{\sigma}) - \phi(\frac{x - r_x}{\sigma})\right)\left(\phi(\frac{y + r_y}{\sigma}) - \phi(\frac{y - r_y}{\sigma})\right) \\
& \times \left(\phi(\frac{z + r_z}{\sigma}) - \phi(\frac{z - r_z}{\sigma})\right).
\end{aligned} \tag{2.110}$$

Note, that these 3D corner and box models seem primarily suited to describe fiducial markers or also bony landmarks, but not the generally rather curved point landmarks within the human brain. More closer to the shapes of curving structures within the human brain is a 3D blob which can be modelled by a trivariate Gaussian function

$$Blob3D(x, y, z) = \frac{a}{\sigma_x \sigma_y \sigma_z}G(\frac{x}{\sigma_x})G(\frac{y}{\sigma_y})G(\frac{z}{\sigma_z}). \tag{2.111}$$

For sketches of these 3D landmarks see Figures 3.23–3.25 in Section 3.2.3 below.

2.6.3 Model Fitting

The parametric intensity models introduced above are applied for landmark extraction as described in this section. The central idea is that we directly fit the models to the image intensities. We do not use a basis expansion (e.g., Hueckel [258]) but directly work with the original intensities. By this we exploit the full information of the image intensities. Another application of the models is to use them for performance characterization of computer vision algorithms (see Section 3.2 below).

We apply a fitting procedure, where all free parameters $\mathbf{p} = (p_1, ..., p_n) \in \mathbb{R}^n$ of the model $g_M(\mathbf{x}, \mathbf{p})$ are estimated simultaneously, yielding precise geometric and radiometric information about the considered image structure. As similarity measure we employ the sum of the squared differences between the model and the image intensities $g(\mathbf{x})$, i.e. the (squared) l_2-norm

$$S(\mathbf{p}) = \sum_{i=1}^{m} (g(\mathbf{x}_i) - g_M(\mathbf{x}_i, \mathbf{p}))^2 \rightarrow min. \qquad (2.112)$$

We assume that we have no statistical a priori knowledge about the parameters and that we have additive zero-mean white Gaussian noise, which is independent of the parameters. In this case, the *least-squares approach* in (2.112) is equivalent to *maximum-likelihood estimation* and shares the same asymptotic properties: For $m \rightarrow \infty$ the estimate is unbiased, efficient, and Gaussian distributed. Since in our approach the model is fitted within semi-global image regions, a relatively large number of measurements is used, e.g., $m = 25 \times 25$ pixels $= 625$ pixels in the 2D case. Thus, the validity of the asymptotic properties can well be assumed. Since our models are nonlinear, we have to apply an iterative scheme for solving (2.112). A standard optimization procedure is the one by Powell [406],[407]. This method is based on conjugate directions and only requires function values for multidimensional minimization. If we have both function values and partial derivatives of the model, then we can apply the method of Levenberg-Marquardt [326],[407], which is the standard procedure for least-squares minimization in this case. This procedure varies smoothly between the steepest descent method and the Gauss-Newton method, and is much more efficient in comparison to using function values alone. Note, that the numeric solution depends on the starting values as is the case with all *nonlinear optimization* procedures. In our case, we determine an initial parameter vector $\mathbf{p}_0$ by applying local operators, which yielded quite good experimental results (see [426]).

An important advantage of our model-fitting approach is that we can use the computed sum-of-squared differences between the model and the intensities as direct measure for *model deviations*. This is important in practical applications, where we want to check the validity of the model. Another possibility to determine model deviations is to apply the fitting approach in scale space. This means that we fit the model not only to the original image but also to Gaussian blurred versions of it. If the model is correct, then the estimated parameters should be independent of prior blurring. This property also holds for the parameter characterizing the width of the intensity transitions, if we reconstruct the width in the original image using the relation

$$\sigma_0 = \sqrt{\sigma^2 - \sigma_F^2}, \qquad (2.113)$$

where σ is the estimated parameter and σ_F characterizes prior Gaussian image blur.

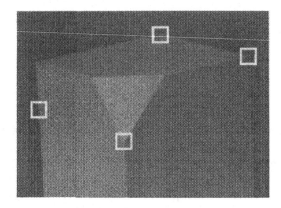

Figure 2.47.   Original image of a cut cube with marked image features.

2.6.4   Experimental Results

We now describe experimental results of applying our approach to real image data. We consider edges and corners in images of 3D polyhedra as well as circular landmarks in 2D aerial images. Experiments for landmarks in 3D images are currently underway.

An example of a depicted 3D polyhedra is shown in Figure 2.47. We first consider the step edge marked on the left in this figure and use a 20×20 portion of the image to fit the model function given in (2.98). The result is shown in Figure 2.48. On the left is a 3D plot of the original intensities and on the right is the fitted model. It can be seen that the agreement is fairly well. The involved parameters are the position x_0, the orientation α, the heights of the intensity plateaus a_0 and a_1 as well as the transition width σ. The estimated parameter values have been listed in Table 2.4 as a function of a prior Gaussian blur of σ_F. Also, we have computed the reconstructed transition width σ_0 in the original image. If we have no prior blur ($\sigma_F = 0$), then the mean error (positive root of the mean squared error) between the model and the intensities computes to $\bar{e} = 2.48$ and agrees well with the standard deviation of the image noise. It can also be seen that the estimated parameters are nearly independent of σ_F (except for σ which is what we expect). The mean error $\bar{e}$ decreases with increasing σ_F since the image noise is accordingly reduced. For an example where the step edge model is not valid, see Rohr [427]. Experimental comparisons with other approaches for estimating edge attributes (contrast and transition width) have been performed by Bergholm and Rohr [33] as well as Hagemann et al. [215]. There, on the basis of synthetic and real images, our approach has been compared with the differential approaches of Back et al. [16] as well as Zhang and Bergholm [577],[578]. These investigations showed that the accuracy in estimating attributes using our approach is very good.

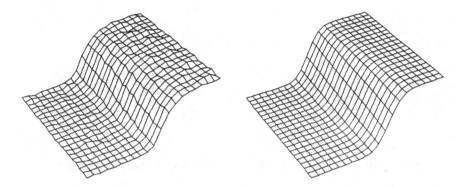

Figure 2.48.   Step edge marked in Fig. 2.47 (left) and estimated model (right).

σ_F	x_0	α	a_0	a_1	σ	$\bar{e}$	σ_0
0.0	11.87	3.87	16.15	115.09	1.52	2.48	1.52
0.5	11.87	3.97	16.13	114.92	1.59	1.98	1.51
1.0	11.86	4.27	16.25	114.03	1.82	1.02	1.52
1.5	11.89	4.24	16.08	114.66	2.13	0.60	1.52

Table 2.4.   Estimation result for the step edge marked in Fig. 2.47.

Next we show experimental results for the Y-corner in Figure 2.47 in the middle. With this more complex structure we have used a 25×25 image portion for fitting. The starting values for the minimization procedure have been determined by applying the differential corner detector $det\mathbf{C}_g$ (Rohr [424]; see Section 2.5.1), an edge detector (Canny [79], Korn [287]) as well as other local operations (see [426]). For numeric minimization we have investigated both the methods of Powell [406] and Levenberg-Marquardt [326]. Note, that the latter one is much faster, but it requires the partial derivatives of the corner model w.r.t. all parameters. However, since our general corner model is created by superposition of L-corner models, this calculation is enormously reduced. Also it turns out, that, in comparison to the model function, all partial derivatives of it can be stated analytically without a remaining integral (see also [427]). In our investigation, both optimization methods [406] and [326] yielded the same results for the estimated parameters. This remained true even in the case if we applied an approximation for the model function using B-splines to further improve the efficiency (see [427],[440]). The original intensities of the Y-corner and the fitted model according to (2.97),(2.101) are shown in Figure 2.49. The values for the estimated parameters have been listed in Table 2.5 and correspond to the position (x_0, y_0), the orientation α, the aperture angles β_1,β_2, the heights of the intensity plateaus a_0,a_1,a_2, as well as the transition widths σ and σ_0. Also in this example the model agrees well

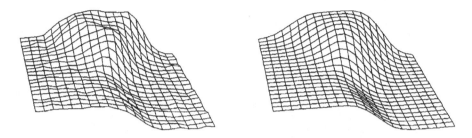

Figure 2.49.   Y-corner marked in Fig. 2.47 (left) and estimated model (right).

σ_F	x_0	y_0	α	β_1	β_2	a_0	a_1	a_2	σ	$\bar{e}$	σ_0
0.0	29.60	26.30	91.42	59.31	146.00	124.41	177.50	59.66	1.46	2.87	1.46
0.5	29.65	26.25	91.19	58.88	145.40	124.32	177.97	59.82	1.55	2.41	1.46
1.0	29.69	26.20	91.17	58.70	144.56	124.09	179.05	59.66	1.87	1.69	1.58
1.5	29.68	26.23	91.30	58.50	145.17	124.15	179.72	59.38	2.18	1.15	1.58

Table 2.5.   Estimation result for the Y-corner marked in Fig. 2.47.

and the parameters are (nearly) independent of image blur and prior Gaussian smoothing. Actually, what we determine are the parameters of the unblurred ideal wedge shaped structure. This is particularly important for estimating the (subpixel) position of the structure, since the tip of the unblurred structure represents the exact geometric position of the corner. In comparison to that, existing differential corner detectors lead to systematic localization errors due to blurring effects (see Section 3.2.1 below). Based on the estimated parameters we can reconstruct the image edges as shown in Figure 2.50 on the right. In comparison to the result of a standard edge detector (Figure 2.50 on the left), in our case we have no gaps, the position is uniquely defined, and the edges are better aligned with the intensity structure. Note, that the highest plateau of the original structure is perturbed by a more or less elliptic region (see Figure 2.49 on the left). However, since we integrate a relatively large image region, such perturbations have a minor influence on the result.

In our last example, we describe experimental results for the circular symmetric landmark shown in Figure 2.44 on the left. The model function is given in (2.102). We already mentioned above, that we can use this landmark type to extract ground control points in aerial images of urban environments (Drewniok and Rohr [125]–[129]; see also Drewniok [124] for further details). A major difficulty in this application is that the image resolution of the landmarks is rather low as can be seen in Figure 2.44 (middle and right). Therefore, indirect approaches for landmark detection based on image edges generally fail. In-

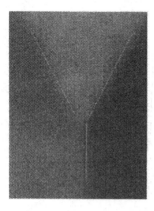 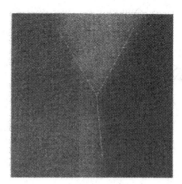

Figure 2.50. Y-corner from Fig. 2.47: Result of a standard edge detector (left) and reconstructed edges based on model fitting (right).

stead, with our approach it is possible to detect the landmarks robustly and to localize them very precisely. For landmark detection we use a prototype model which is generated from a few representative examples during a training phase. This prototype model is given analytically, but the parameters are fixed and represent the mean values over the training examples. The prototype model is used for automatic landmark detection, for providing starting values for model fitting, and for determining thresholds in a final verification step. In Figure 2.51 we show the result of model fitting for the landmark shown in Figure 2.44 in the middle. This example demonstrates the agreement between the model and the observed image intensities. The overall approach has been applied to an aerial image of 3072×3072 pixels, for example, from which a 170×170 subimage is shown in Figure 2.52 on the left. In this subimage five manhole covers are visible which correspond to our circular symmetric landmark type. Out of the five landmarks, four landmarks have automatically been detected and localized by applying our model-fitting approach. The fifth landmark has not been detected since its appearance differs significantly from the standard appearance (the surrounding dark ring is much larger compared to the mean shape). For further experimental results, see particularly [128]. Based on this model-fitting scheme we have developed an approach for automatic exterior orientation of aerial images, i.e. for determining a transformation between the image and the world coordinate system. This requires to match the detected landmark constellations with the entries of a cadastral database. For this task we employ geometric invariants and apply a hypothesize-and-test mechanism for verification ([126],[127]).

In Drewniok and Rohr [127],[128] we have also analyzed the localization precision of fitting landmark models in more detail. Using circular symmetric and cross-type models we experimentally obtained a rather high precision of

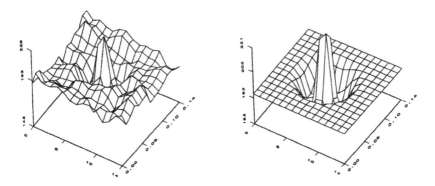

Figure 2.51.   3D plot of the circular landmark in Fig. 2.44 middle (left) and estimated model (right).

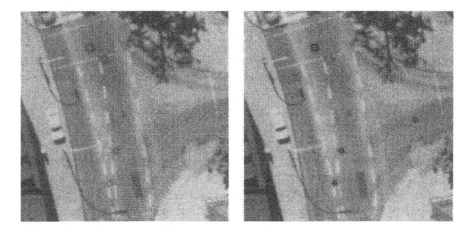

Figure 2.52.   170 × 170 subimage of an aerial image (left) and automatically detected and localized manhole covers (right).

$\sigma_{\hat{x}} < 0.1 pix$, where $\sigma_{\hat{x}}$ denotes the standard deviation and pix the spatial unity. We also verified that the location estimate is unbiased. Additionally, we compared the experimentally obtained values for the precision with theoretically derived values and found a remarkable agreement (cf. Section 3.2.2).

2.7   Summary and Conclusion

In this chapter, we have introduced computational schemes for the detection and localization of 2D and 3D point landmarks. Our focus has been on the extraction of 3D anatomical point landmarks of the human head. To arrive at operators of predictable performance we have worked along a methodic framework with clearly distinguishable modelling steps. First, we have analyzed in detail the anatomical structure of point landmarks and have characterized their geometry. Then, we discussed suitable mathematical descriptions of these structures. Based on this investigation we have developed 3D differential operators for extracting anatomical point landmarks. These operators require only low-order image derivatives in comparison to previous schemes for landmark extraction. Therefore, our operators are computationally efficient and they do not suffer from instabilities of computing high order derivatives.

One principal approach to develop landmark operators is based on isocontour curvature properties. The assumption is that isocontours well approximate the landmark's surface. We have described 3D differential operators which are based on the mean and Gaussian curvature of isocontours. These operators consist of first and second order partial derivatives of an image. In a principally different approach we have generalized existing differential corner operators from 2D to 3D. These operators extract general prominent points and require image derivatives of first and second order, while some of them require only first order derivatives. Actually, the operators based on first and second order derivatives can be related to the 3D operators based on isocontour curvature properties. The class of operators based on only first order image derivatives belong to the most efficient differential operators that exist and we have studied them in more detail. We have shown that for these operators a statistical interpretation in terms of the Cramér-Rao bound exists. The considered operators of this class represent measures for the size of the error ellipsoid characterizing the minimal localization uncertainty, i.e., these operators extract points with highest localization precision. Additionally, we have shown that these operators can also be derived on the basis of invariance principles. The operators are invariant under similarity transformations and form a complete set of principal invariants. The considered corner operators have also been extended to nD, i.e., for arbitrary image dimension. While the above differential operators have been designed for the detection of point landmarks, we have also described multi-step differential procedures for refined localization. These approaches require only first order image derivatives and yield subvoxel positions. Experimental results of the different approaches have been reported for 3D MR as well as CT images. In Chapter 3 below we study the performance of the 3D differential landmark operators in more detail. In Chapter 4 we will use the localized landmarks for point-based registration of 3D medical images.

Besides differential operators we have also described parametric approaches to landmark extraction. Parametric approaches are more time-consuming, but on the other hand integrate more global image information and more specific knowledge, which allows to improve the detection and localization performance.

The work described in this chapter is a step towards the formalization of 3D anatomical landmarks and the design of applicable algorithms for landmark detection and localization. As already indicated above, there are many fundamental problems. In our opinion, the solution to these problems requires an interdisciplinary cooperation between experts from anatomy, neurosurgery, radiology, and computer vision.

Chapter 3

Performance Characterization of Landmark Operators

Within the field of computer vision the development of algorithms with predictable performance is of major concern. Before using a certain algorithm we like to know how well it performs and whether it is suitable at all for a given task. To answer these questions, we need quantitative characterizations of the performance of algorithms. This includes a statement of obtained results for certain performance measures (e.g., the localization accuracy) as well as the specification for which image classes and under which assumptions this performance can be guaranteed. On the one hand, such a characterization is a major step towards a sound description of algorithms as well as the foundation of the field of computer vision. On the other hand, it serves a clear practical need. To solve a certain task it is generally required that we have to select certain existing algorithms which solve a subtask (e.g., edge detection). However, in computer vision there are often a large number of approaches and algorithms which have been designed to solve the same subtask. Since often only scarce information is given on the performance of a certain algorithm and also comprehensive comparisons with other schemes can hardly be found, the selection of a suitable algorithm is very difficult and can actually be compared with 'playing dice'. In practical applications it is therefore often necessary to implement several algorithms and to find out on his own which algorithm is best suited. Due to the above-stated reasons *performance characterization in computer vision* has recently gained increased attention (e.g., Jain and Binford [262], Haralick [224], Christensen and Förstner [95], Bowyer and Phillips [58], Klette et al. [281]).

In this chapter, we describe our work on the performance characterization of algorithms designed for the detection and localization of *point landmarks*. In Chapter 2 above we have developed 3D operators for landmark extraction and here we want to find out, which of these operators perform best, and we

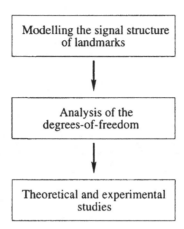

Figure 3.1.   General approach to performance characterization of landmark operators.

also want to quantify the performance. This study is thus concerned with the last step of our general framework for the development of landmark operators as sketched in Figure 2.4 above (Section 2.1.2). The 3D operators have been designed for the extraction of anatomical point landmarks from 3D spatial images. Additionally, we study in this chapter the performance of 2D corner operators. These operators are relevant for extracting corners of 3D polyhedral objects in 2D projection images, but are also relevant for extracting anatomical landmarks in 2D spatial images. Below, we first discuss the general problem as well as our approach to the validation and evaluation of landmark operators (Section 3.1). Then we describe analytic studies (Section 3.2) and experimental evaluations (Section 3.3). We are primarily concerned with the localization accuracy, the localization precision, as well as the detection performance of 2D as well as 3D landmark operators. We utilize both geometric and intensity models of landmarks.

3.1   General Approach

Our general approach to the validation and evaluation of landmark operators is depicted in Figure 3.1 and consists of three principal steps (Rohr et al. [449]). Central to this scheme is the *formalization of the signal structure* which in our opinion is a key to the design of algorithms with predictable performance. Examples for point landmarks are corners in 2D projection images or point landmarks in 3D tomographic images of the human brain. In the latter case a prerequisite is a careful analysis of brain anatomy. In either case, we have to find a mathematical description of the landmarks, e.g., in terms of differential geometry.

A second main step is a detailed *analysis of the degrees-of-freedom*. Here, a fundamental problem is that the number of the degrees-of-freedom is often very large. Particularly, this is true in the case of 3D landmark operators, where we can classify the degrees-of-freedom w.r.t. (i) anatomy (landmark type, scale, anatomical variability, etc.), (ii) imaging (contrast, noise, resolution, modality, etc.), as well as (iii) the algorithm (operator type, filter widths, thresholds, etc.). Therefore, in experimental studies it is often only possible to analyze the performance w.r.t. a subset of the degrees-of-freedom. Priorities may be set, for example, on the basis of application scenaria and requirement analyses.

Third, *theoretical as well as experimental studies* should be performed. A theoretical analysis of operator performance should be carried out as far as possible since this reduces the number of experiments. However, experimental studies are indispensable for performance prediction w.r.t. real applications. To this end, we advocate an incremental approach building upon a hierarchy of test data (e.g., Neumann and Stiehl [371]). By this, we mean an experimental strategy that starts out from synthetic ideal signal structures of landmark prototypes and incrementally increases the complexity of the test data by incorporating, e.g., image blur, noise, and further degradations. The usage of synthetic images at first, in comparison to real images, has the advantage that *ground truth* is available.

A central issue in these studies is the selection of suitable criteria for performance characterization. Examples for criteria are: Localization accuracy, precision, robustness, fault tolerance, detection performance, controllability, parameter dependence, predictability as a function of algorithmic parameters, reproducibility, efficiency, or applicability in interactive application scenaria. For these criteria we have to find suitable quantitative measures. A problem is that generally there are different measures for one criterion, e.g., for the detection performance as we will discuss below.

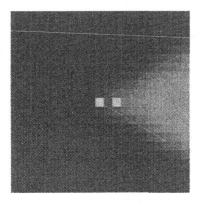 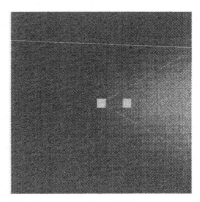

Figure 3.2.   Result of a corner operator applied to an L-corner while using different sizes of Gaussian derivative filters: $\sigma = 1$ (left) and $\sigma = 2$ (right).

3.2   Analytic Studies

The studies on the performance characterization of landmark operators in this section are based on *analytic models* of the intensity variations at landmarks. These *intensity models* are used to derive closed-form expressions for the performance of landmark operators. We start with an investigation of the localization accuracy of 2D corner operators and analyze the systematic errors, i.e., the bias (Section 3.2.1). Then, we investigate the minimal localization uncertainty of the position estimate under image noise for 2D as well as 3D images (Sections 3.2.2 and 3.2.3).

3.2.1   Localization Accuracy

We theoretically analyze the localization accuracy of existing 2D operators for extracting corners. We primarily consider corners in 2D images of 3D polyhedral objects, however, this study is also relevant for images of planar objects as well as for 2D slices of 3D tomographic images. The general problem is illustrated by Figure 3.2. We here have applied a corner detector to an image of an L-corner. The L-corner is represented by the left-most marked point and the corresponding two lines. The point to the right is obtained by the corner operator and we see that the position is displaced towards the inner part of the sector of the L-corner. Thus, we have a localization error. The same is observed in 3D tomographic image data (e.g., see Figure 2.36 on the left). If we use different sizes for the applied Gaussian derivative filters ($\sigma = 1$ and $\sigma = 2$ on the left and right of Figure 3.2, respectively), then we see that the localization error increases with increasing filter widths. In summary, this gives an indication that there is a systematic localization error (bias) which depends on the filter width.

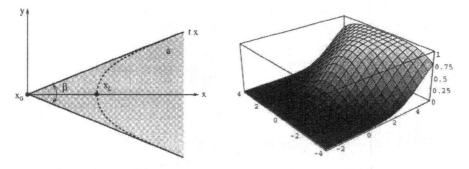

Figure 3.3.   Model of an L-corner.

To quantify this bias we perform a theoretical study which is based on an analytic model of the intensities of an L-corner in Rohr [425],[427]. This model is a prototype for a tip-like structure. We consider ten well-known differential corner detectors and analyze the dependence of the localization accuracy on all model parameters given the full range of the parameter values (Rohr [428],[430]). Another analytic study of corner operators by Deriche and Giraudon [118] only considered special aperture angles of an L-corner (45° and 90°) to compare three different operators. In alternative studies, the performance of 2D corner operators has been investigated experimentally, either by visual judgement of the results (e.g., Kitchen and Rosenfeld [280]), by applying statistical measures (e.g., Zuniga and Haralick [581]), by using projective invariants (e.g., Coelho et al. [98], Heyden and Rohr [242]), or by computing the number of corresponding points under elastic transformations (e.g., Hartkens et al. [232]) and projective transformations of planar scenes (e.g., Schmid et al. [468]), see also Section 3.3 below.

We model an L-corner by Gaussian convolution of a wedge-shaped structure (see Section 2.6.2 above and Figure 3.3). Taking advantage of the symmetry of this structure, we can derive an analytic model which can be written as the superposition of two functions:

$$g_{ML}(x, y, \beta, a, \sigma) = a \left(M(\frac{x}{\sigma}, \frac{y}{\sigma}, \beta) + M(\frac{x}{\sigma}, -\frac{y}{\sigma}, \beta) \right), \qquad (3.1)$$

where β is the aperture angle, a the contrast, and σ represents the degree of image blur. The point we want to localize is the tip of the unblurred wedge, i.e., the point x_0 in Figure 3.3 where $x = y = 0$. As alternative reference position, we also compute the (exact) curvature extremum x_L along the edge curve given by $\Gamma = g_x^2 g_{xx} + 2g_x g_y g_{xy} + g_y^2 g_{yy} = 0$. This edge criterion defines points of maximal gradient magnitude in the direction of the gradient (Canny [79]) and is often used as basis for designing corner operators. In Section 2.3.1 above we saw that the corresponding differential operator consists of several

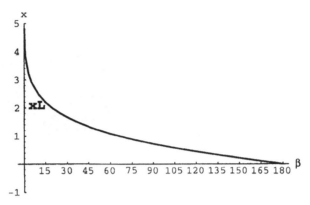

Figure 3.4.   Positions of the curvature extremum along the edge curve as a function of the aperture angle β and for $\sigma = 1$.

hundred terms comprising partial derivatives up to the fifth order. However, for this operator we can indeed derive a relatively simple equation from which the localized positions for our analytic corner model can be determined (Rohr [427],[430]). Due to the symmetry of the L-corner the position is localized on the symmetry line $y = 0$ and thus we only have to compute the x-coordinate (see Figure 3.3 on the left). With $x' = x/q$, $q = \sqrt{1 + t^2}$ and $t = \tan(\beta/2)$, this equation can be stated as

$$G(x') - t^2 x' \phi(x') = 0. \tag{3.2}$$

We here have an implicit equation which determines the position x_L as a function of the aperture angle β. Figure 3.4 depicts the computed positions for $0^o < \beta < 180^o$ setting $\sigma = 1$. It can be seen that the smaller the angle the larger is the difference to the tip position x_0. The positions are independent of the contrast a of the corner. For different image blurs σ we obtain the positions by using the linear relation $x_L(\sigma) = x_L \cdot \sigma$ (which is just a scaling of the coordinates), where x_L is the position for a certain aperture angle β. This can easily be seen from (3.2).

We now consider the localization properties of existing differential corner operators. These operators require partial image derivatives up to order one, two, or three. We have analyzed the approaches of Beaudet [28], Dreschler and Nagel [123], Kitchen and Rosenfeld [280], Zuniga and Haralick [581] , Nagel [362], Förstner [168], Harris (see Noble [383]), Rohr [424], Blom et al. [47], and Brunnström et al. [74]. It can be shown that the cornerness measure in Zuniga and Haralick [581] does not localize corners without incorporating edge points (Rohr [430]). Since we are interested in direct schemes which do not rely on prior segmentation of the image, we do not consider this operator further. On the other hand, most other direct operators could also be modified

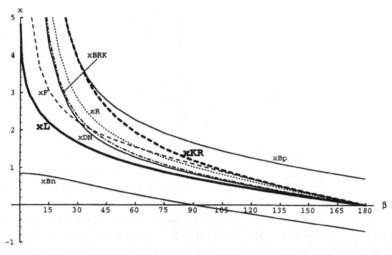

Figure 3.5. Localization accuracy of differential corner operators as a function of the aperture angle β and for $\sigma = 1$.

and applied in conjunction with prior segmented edges. In addition, we have shown that the corner conditions in Nagel [362] are overdetermined and actually do not yield a corner point. Furthermore, the operators of Förstner [168] and Harris (Noble [383]) as well as those of Blom et al. [47] and Brunnström et al. [74] can be shown to be equivalent. Thus, in total we have six different corner operators left which actually localize corners (see Section 2.5.1 above and Rohr [430] for the formulas of the operators). For all these operators we have derived implicit equations which determine the localized positions. The dependence on all model parameters (aperture angle, contrast, image blur) can be stated as follows:

- $x(\beta)$ is nonlinear (see Figure 3.5),

- $x(a) = const.$,

- $x(\sigma) = x \cdot \sigma$.

From Figure 3.5 we see that the operator of Beaudet [28] yields two positions for the corner model (denoted by x_{Bp} and x_{Bn} and represented by the solid curves). The other operators yield only one position and are abbreviated and depicted as follows: Dreschler and Nagel [123] by x_{DN} and the solid curve, Kitchen and Rosenfeld [280] by x_{KR} and the boldfaced dashed curve, Förstner [168] by x_F and the dashed curve, Rohr [424] by x_R and the dotted curve, and Blom et al. [47] by x_{BRK} and the dashed dotted curve. For all operators we have systematic localization errors w.r.t. the tip of the structure as well as w.r.t. the curvature extremum along the edge line (denoted by x_L and represented

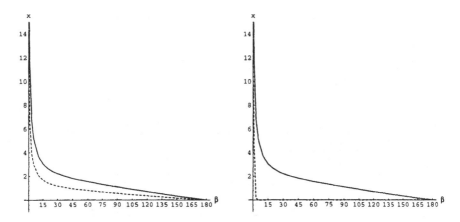

Figure 3.6. Localization of an L-corner by the two-step approach of Förstner and Gülch [173] (dashed curve) in comparison to applying the detection operator alone (solid curve; positions x_F in Fig. 3.5) for different sizes of the local window: 3×3 pixels (left) and 15×15 pixels (right).

by the bold-faced curve) and these errors depend on the model parameters β and σ. The errors in Figure 3.5 are given in pixel units. Particularly for small angles large errors occur. The best result w.r.t. x_L is achieved by the operators of Förstner [168] and Blom et al. [47] (hereby we have disregarded the approach in [123] since there additional postprocessing steps are necessary in comparison to solely computing extrema of cornerness measures as is the case with the remaining approaches). Note, however, that particularly w.r.t. the tip x_0, the localization errors are significant. Also note, that a model-based approach to the localization of corners (Rohr [425],[427]) is able to determine the correct position x_0 independently of all three parameters β, a, and σ (see also Section 2.6 above).

Based on the above results we can calculate the displacement of the positions when smoothing with Gaussian filters of different widths. Consider, for example, the positions x_{Bp} of the operator in Beaudet [28] and assume the blur of the original image to be $\sigma_0 = 1$. Then, for an aperture angle of $\beta = 10^o$ we have $x_{Bp} \approx 11.5$ pixels and processing the image with a Gaussian filter of $\sigma_F = 1\,(2)$ leads to a displacement of the positions of $\Delta x = (\sqrt{\sigma_0^2 + \sigma_F^2} - \sigma_0)\,x_{Bp} \approx 4.8\,(14.2)$ pixels. Thus, due to these significant displacements, corner operators that rely on tracking such points in scale space (e.g., Deriche and Giraudon [118]) generally have problems.

Recently, we have shown that the localization errors of differential corner operators can significantly be reduced by applying multi-step approaches (Frantz et al. [177]; see also Section 2.5.7 above). Using the same analytic model as above we have analyzed the two-step approach of Förstner and Gülch

[173]. This approach combines a corner detector as considered above with a differential edge intersection approach applied in a local window. It turns out that the larger this window the more accurate is the localized position. Even for small window sizes, e.g., 3 × 3 pixels, we obtain a significant improvement, while for a window size of 15 × 15 pixels, the localization error is nearly zero (Figure 3.6). Moreover, also for curved structures such as the tip of an ellipse, the localization errors can significantly be reduced (see [177]).

3.2.2 Localization Precision in 2D Images

Above in Section 3.2.1, we have analyzed the systematic localization errors of local operators for detecting corners. These errors are inherently due to the differential structure of the operators and, in general, are enlarged by discretization and noise effects. Here, we take the statistical point of view to analyze the localization errors caused by noisy data. We consider a continuous image model that represents the blur as well as noise introduced by an imaging system. In general, the systematic intensity variations are nonlinear functions of the location parameters. For this model we derive analytic results stating lower bounds for the localization uncertainty of image features such as corners and edges. The lower bounds are evaluated for explicitly given feature models. We show that the precision of localization in general depends on the noise level, on the size of the observation window, on the width of the intensity transitions, as well as on other parameters describing the systematic intensity variations.

Our study on the positional random errors is based on nonlinear estimation theory and the Cramér-Rao bound (CRB). As explicitly given models of image features we first investigate 2D corners as well as other 2D image features, e.g., edges. The edge models under consideration are general step edges and ramp edges. This generalizes the work of Kakarala and Hero [266] which deals with the special case of a step edge with constant intensity plateaus. A further generalization is the consideration of corners which in contrast to edges are 2D features, i.e. they have intensity variations in two dimensions. Therefore, two parameters are necessary to describe their position in comparison to one parameter for edges. Here, we study the precision of localizing corners for analytic L- and T-corner models. We also point out that the uncertainty lower bounds in localizing these image features can in principle be attained by fitting parametric models directly to the image intensities as done in Rohr [425], [427]. To give an impression of the achievable accuracy numeric examples are presented and also experimental investigations are reported. The work in this section is based on Rohr [433] where we have derived uncertainty lower bounds for 2D edge and corner models. Below, we also state bounds for lines, rectangles, blobs, and circular point landmarks. In Section 3.2.3 we further extend this work and derive analytic results for 3D image features. Recently, Cramér-Rao bounds have also been considered in the case of circular arc and curve fitting to extracted edge points (Chan and Thomas [84], Kanatani [272]) and in the context of information-preserving object recognition (Betke and Makris [40]).

3.2.2.1   Nonlinear Estimation of Single Parameters

We here derive analytic results for the highest possible precision (minimal uncertainty) in localizing 1D features in 2D images, namely edges and lines. We assume that these image features have intensity variations only in one dimension, thus a single parameter determines their location. The features are modelled as systematic intensity variations which are disturbed by an additive noise process. Signal measurements are available within finite regions of an image. As far as it will be needed, we shortly review nonlinear estimation theory for single parameters (van Trees [533]) and then analyze a general step edge model, a model of a ramp edge, as well as two different models of a line.

Our observations $g(x)$ are continuous functions extended over certain intervals. We deal with space-dependent random variables, i.e. random processes. The model $g_M(x, p)$ describing the systematic signal variations depends on a single parameter p and, in general, is nonlinear. The interference $n(x)$ will be assumed to be a sample function from an additive zero-mean white Gaussian noise process with spectral power density $L_n(u) = \sigma_n^2$.

$$g(x) = g_M(x, p) + n(x), \quad x_1 \leq x \leq x_2. \tag{3.3}$$

Note that by choosing a particular space point $x = x_i$ a random variable $n(x_i)$ with variance σ_n^2 is defined. In the following we suppose to have no statistical a priori knowledge about p and therefore treat p as a non-random variable. In this case, the maximum-likelihood method gives a useful estimate $\hat{p}_{ml}$. This estimate is the one, that most likely caused the given data:

$$\Lambda_1(p) \rightarrow max, \tag{3.4}$$

with $\Lambda_1(p)$ being the likelihood function which is defined in van Trees [533] using a K-coefficient approximation to $g(x)$:

$$g_K(x) = \sum_{i=1}^{K} g_i \varphi_i(x), \quad x_1 \leq x \leq x_2, \tag{3.5}$$

where

$$g_i = \int_{x_1}^{x_2} g(x)\varphi_i(x)dx,$$

and the $\varphi_i(x)$ belong to an arbitrary complete orthonormal set of functions. The necessary condition for the estimate in (3.4) is obtained by letting $K \rightarrow \infty$

and equating the partial derivative of $\Lambda_1(p)$ or, equivalently the logarithm of it, to zero.

$$\frac{\partial \ln \Lambda_1(p)}{\partial p} = \frac{1}{\sigma_n^2} \int_{x_1}^{x_2} (g(x) - g_M(x,p)) \frac{\partial g_M(x,p)}{\partial p} dx = 0. \qquad (3.6)$$

For any unbiased estimate $\hat{p}$, for which we have $E\{\hat{p}\} = p$ (where $E\{\cdot\}$ denotes the expectation operation), the following inequality provides a lower bound on the variance of the estimated parameter.

$$\sigma_{\hat{p}}^2 = Var\{\hat{p}\} = E\{(\hat{p}-p)^2\} \geq \left(-E\left\{ \frac{\partial^2 \ln \Lambda_1(p)}{\partial p^2} \right\} \right)^{-1}.$$

This inequality is usually referred to as *Cramér-Rao bound (CRB)*. In our case we have

$$E\left\{ \frac{\partial^2 \ln \Lambda_1(p)}{\partial p^2} \right\} = \frac{1}{\sigma_n^2} \left(E\left\{ \int_{x_1}^{x_2} (g(x) - g_M(x,p)) \frac{\partial^2 g_M(x,p)}{\partial p^2} dx \right\} \right.$$
$$\left. - E\left\{ \int_{x_1}^{x_2} \left(\frac{\partial g_M(x,p)}{\partial p} \right)^2 dx \right\} \right).$$

Since $E\{g(x) - g_M(x,p)\} = E\{n(x)\} = 0$, we finally obtain

$$\sigma_{\hat{p}}^2 \geq CRB_{\hat{p}} = \frac{\sigma_n^2}{\displaystyle\int_{x_1}^{x_2} \left(\frac{\partial g_M(x,p)}{\partial p} \right)^2 dx} \qquad (3.7)$$

This lower bound can be compared with the actual variance of a certain estimation scheme. For an efficient estimate, (3.7) is satisfied with equality. However, this is only the case if $g_M(x,p)$ depends linearly on p. Then, the maximum-likelihood estimate is the estimate with minimum variance. It is possible that, under certain conditions, the variance in the nonlinear case approaches this bound (see below).

Analogously to (3.7) which holds for 1D signals, a lower bound for 2D signals $g_M(\mathbf{x}, p)$ with $\mathbf{x} = (x, y)$ can be derived as

$$\sigma_{\hat{p}}^2 \geq CRB_{\hat{p}} = \frac{\sigma_n^2}{\displaystyle\int_{x_1}^{x_2} \int_{y_1}^{y_2} \left(\frac{\partial g_M(\mathbf{x},p)}{\partial p} \right)^2 d\mathbf{x}} \qquad (3.8)$$

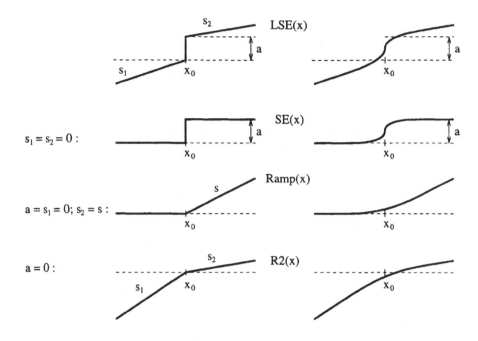

Figure 3.7.   Linear step edge model and some specializations (cross-sections).

3.2.2.2 Edges

The formulas above are now applied to derive lower bounds for the localization uncertainty of explicitly given edge transitions. We analyze a general model of Gaussian smoothed step edges which, for other purposes, has also been used in, e.g., Asada and Brady [14], Nalwa and Binford [364], and Ulupinar and Medioni [535]. This model represents several typical edge transitions (see the unblurred and corresponding blurred profiles in Figure 3.7 and the 3D plot in Figure 3.8). $SE(\mathbf{x})$ is the classical step edge model (see also Figure 3.9) and $Ramp(\mathbf{x})$ and $R2(\mathbf{x})$ commonly appear in range images. We also analyze a ramp edge model $RE(\mathbf{x})$ depicted in Figure 3.10, which is a valid model for intensity transitions in CT and MR images (e.g., Neumann et al. [373]).

We arbitrarily assume the edges to have grey-value variations only along the x-axis and denote their location by x_0. This means that we consider model functions of the type $g_M(\mathbf{x}, p) = g_M(x - x_0, y)$. The minimal uncertainty for estimating x_0 is obtained by using (3.8). To simplify the calculations we

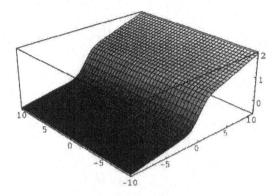

Figure 3.8. 3D plot of the linear step edge model ($a = 1$; $s_1 = 0.05$; $s_2 = 0.1$; $\sigma = 1$).

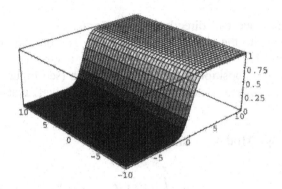

Figure 3.9. 3D plot of the classical step edge model ($a = 1$; $\sigma = 1$).

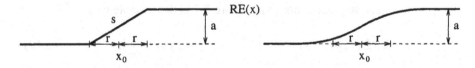

Figure 3.10. Ramp edge model (cross-section).

choose the coordinate system in such a way that $x_0 = 0$. Then we have

$$
\left(\frac{\partial g_M(x - x_0, y)}{\partial x_0} \right)^2 \Bigg|_{x_0=0} = \left(\frac{\partial g_M(x - x_0, y)}{\partial x} \cdot (-1) \right)^2 \Bigg|_{x_0=0}
$$

$$
= \left(\frac{\partial g_M(\mathbf{x})}{\partial x} \right)^2 \tag{3.9}
$$

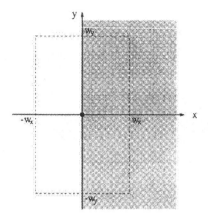

Figure 3.11.   Coordinate system and observation window.

which means that we can directly use the partial derivatives of the model functions to evaluate the lower bound in (3.8). The observation window is described by the half-widths w_x and w_y and is assumed to be symmetric around x_0 and some position $y_0 = 0$ in y-direction (see Figure 3.11). In the discrete case, w_x and w_y determine the number of pixels that are taken into account.

Linear Step Edge Model.   Using

$$G(x) = \frac{1}{\sqrt{2\pi}} e^{-\frac{x^2}{2}}, \quad \phi(x) = \int\limits_{-\infty}^{x} G(\xi)d\xi, \quad R(x) = G(x) + x\phi(x)$$

the general linear step edge model in Figure 3.7 is describable by

$$LSE(x, y) = s_1 x + a\phi(\frac{x}{\sigma}) + (s_2 - s_1)\sigma R(\frac{x}{\sigma}), \tag{3.10}$$

where s_1, s_2 denote the slopes of the linear transitions and σ the width of a Gaussian filter characterizing the blur of an imaging system.

Although this model depends on several parameters we are only interested in deriving an uncertainty lower bound for the location. Therefore, in the following, we may assume that all model parameters except the ones for the location are known. On the other hand, if all parameters are unknown and thus have to be estimated then the Fisher information matrix can be used (cf. Section 3.2.2.4). However, as shown by Scharf [464], pp. 231-233, in this case the resulting bound can only increase. Therefore, the bounds derived here are indeed lower bounds.

The partial derivative of $LSE(\mathbf{x})$ w.r.t. x is

$$LSE_x(x,y) = s_1 + \frac{a}{\sigma}G(\frac{x}{\sigma}) + (s_2 - s_1)\phi(\frac{x}{\sigma}),$$

and after some calculations we get the lower bound for the uncertainty of the location estimate:

$$\sigma^2_{\hat{x}_0,LSE} \geq \frac{\sigma^2_n}{\int\limits_{-w_x}^{w_x}\int\limits_{-w_y}^{w_y} LSE_x^2(\mathbf{x})d\mathbf{x}} = \tag{3.11}$$

$$\frac{1}{2(2s_1 s_2 w_x + \frac{a^2}{2\sqrt{\pi}\sigma}\mathrm{erf}(\frac{w_x}{\sigma}) + a(s_1 + s_2)\mathrm{erf}(\frac{w_x}{\sqrt{2}\sigma}) + (s_2 - s_1)^2\sigma U(\frac{w_x}{\sigma}))} \cdot \frac{\sigma^2_n}{w_y}$$

with the auxiliary functions

$$U_1(x) = (G(x) + R(x))\phi(x) - \frac{1}{2\sqrt{\pi}}\mathrm{erf}(x) \tag{3.12}$$

$$U(x) = x + 2(U_1(x) - R(x)) \tag{3.13}$$

and where

$$\mathrm{erf}(x) = \frac{2}{\sqrt{\pi}}\int\limits_0^x e^{-\xi^2}d\xi = 2\phi(\sqrt{2}x) - 1. \tag{3.14}$$

Considering the special case of the classical step edge (setting $s_1 = s_2 = 0$)

$$SE(x,y) = a\phi(\frac{x}{\sigma}) \tag{3.15}$$

we have

$$\sigma^2_{\hat{x}_0,SE} \geq \frac{\sqrt{\pi}\sigma}{a^2\mathrm{erf}(\frac{w_x}{\sigma})} \cdot \frac{\sigma^2_n}{w_y} \tag{3.16}$$

which agrees with (5) in Kakarala and Hero [266] when we simplify their result by exploiting $\phi(-x) = 1 - \phi(x)$ and using $\mathrm{erf}(x)$ as given in (3.14) (Note that we assumed $x_0 = 0$).

The lower bound for the ramp transition in Figure 3.7 ($a = s_1 = 0; s_2 = s$)

$$Ramp(x,y) = s\sigma R(\frac{x}{\sigma}) \tag{3.17}$$

is

$$\sigma^2_{\hat{x}_0,Ramp} \geq \frac{1}{2s^2\sigma U(\frac{w_x}{\sigma})} \cdot \frac{\sigma^2_n}{w_y}, \tag{3.18}$$

and for the double ramp ($a = 0$)

$$R2(x, y) = s_1 x + (s_2 - s_1)\sigma R(\frac{x}{\sigma})$$ (3.19)

we obtain

$$\sigma^2_{\hat{x}_0, R2} \geq \frac{1}{2(2s_1 s_2 w_x + (s_2 - s_1)^2 \sigma \, U(\frac{w_x}{\sigma}))} \cdot \frac{\sigma^2_n}{w_y}.$$ (3.20)

To interpret the derived formulas we evaluate approximations of them by assuming the width w_x of the observation window in x-direction to be much larger than the width of the Gaussian filter σ (this means that the significant grey-value variations due to the blur essentially lie within the window). Then we have

$$\frac{w_x}{\sigma} \gg 1: \quad G(\frac{w_x}{\sigma}) \approx 0, \quad \phi(\frac{w_x}{\sigma}) \approx \phi(\sqrt{2}\frac{w_x}{\sigma}) \approx 1,$$

$$\mathrm{erf}(\frac{w_x}{\sigma}) \approx \mathrm{erf}(\sqrt{2}\frac{w_x}{\sigma}) \approx 1,$$ (3.21)

$$R(\frac{w_x}{\sigma}) \approx \frac{w_x}{\sigma}, \quad U(\frac{w_x}{\sigma}) \approx \frac{w_x}{\sigma}$$

and the uncertainty bound for the linear step edge model simplifies to

$$CRB_{\hat{x}_0, LSE} \approx \frac{1}{2(\frac{a^2}{2\sqrt{\pi}\sigma} + a(s_1 + s_2) + (s_1^2 + s_2^2)w_x)} \cdot \frac{\sigma^2_n}{w_y}$$ (3.22)

For the special cases of the classical step edge, the ramp transition, and the double ramp we obtain

$$CRB_{\hat{x}_0, SE} \approx \frac{\sqrt{\pi}\sigma}{a^2} \cdot \frac{\sigma^2_n}{w_y}$$ (3.23)

$$CRB_{\hat{x}_0, Ramp} \approx \frac{1}{2s^2 w_x} \cdot \frac{\sigma^2_n}{w_y}$$ (3.24)

$$CRB_{\hat{x}_0, R2} \approx \frac{1}{2(s_1^2 + s_2^2)w_x} \cdot \frac{\sigma^2_n}{w_y}.$$ (3.25)

We see that all bounds are proportional to the ratio σ^2_n/w_y of the noise level and the width of the observation window in y-direction. In the discrete case w_y corresponds to the number of measurements in this direction. It is worth noting that this result agrees with the uncertainty for the mean of a random variable $\bar{z} = \frac{1}{m}\sum_{i=1}^{m} z_i$ for independent and identically distributed observations. In this case the variance is given by $\sigma_{\bar{z}}^2 = \sigma_z^2/m$, that is the ratio between the noise level and the overall number of measurements.

For $SE(\mathbf{x})$ the height a has a large influence on the precision since it appears (inverse) quadratically. The approximate bound depends linearly on the width of the grey-value transition σ. We also see that if the grey-value variations are essentially captured in x-direction then the precision cannot be improved by increasing w_x. In the expressions for $Ramp(\mathbf{x})$ and $R2(\mathbf{x})$ the slopes enter inverse quadratically and correspond to the height a for $SE(\mathbf{x})$. As opposed to the approximation for $SE(\mathbf{x})$, here σ has no influence. Since these two edge models have infinitely extended slopes, the precision can be improved by increasing w_x.

Ramp Edge Model.   Whereas the unblurred edge models in Figure 3.7 have one significant position x_0, for the ramp edge $RE(\mathbf{x})$ in Figure 3.10 there are two such positions. Therefore, we treat this model separately. Choosing $x_0 = 0$ to be the center of these two points we have the advantage that the observation window around x_0 is symmetric w.r.t. the slope transition $s = a/(2r)$. With

$$RE(\mathbf{x}) = s\sigma(R(\frac{x+r}{\sigma}) - R(\frac{x-r}{\sigma})) \qquad (3.26)$$

$$RE_x(\mathbf{x}) = s(\phi(\frac{x+r}{\sigma}) - \phi(\frac{x-r}{\sigma}))$$

$$RE_{xx}(\mathbf{x}) = \frac{s}{\sigma}(G(\frac{x+r}{\sigma}) - G(\frac{x-r}{\sigma}))$$

it can easily be verified that the first partial derivative of the model has an extremum in x_0 ($RE_{xx}(\mathbf{x}) = 0$ for $x = x_0 = 0$). This agrees with the usual definition of edges. Note, that for the linear step edge model $LSE(\mathbf{x})$ the position x_0, in general, is not an extremum of the gradient. However, in all cases (and in particular for corners) an unbiased estimate of the position can be obtained by fitting parametric models as done in [425],[427].

For $RE(\mathbf{x})$, using the abbreviations $w_1 = w_x - r$ and $w_2 = w_x + r$, the lower bound for the localization uncertainty of $\hat{x}_0$ computes to

$$\sigma_{\hat{x}_0,RE}^2 \geq \frac{\sigma_n^2}{\int\limits_{-w_x}^{w_x} \int\limits_{-w_y}^{w_y} RE_x^2(\mathbf{x})dx} =$$

$$\frac{1}{2s^2\sigma\left(U(\frac{w_1}{\sigma}) + U(\frac{w_2}{\sigma}) - 2\int\limits_{\frac{-w_1}{\sigma}}^{\frac{w_2}{\sigma}} \phi(x)\phi(x - \frac{2r}{\sigma})dx\right)} \cdot \frac{\sigma_n^2}{w_y} \qquad (3.27)$$

Differing from the edge models above, for $RE(\mathbf{x})$ there is one integral left which we cannot calculate analytically. To derive an approximation of (3.27) we assume that $r \gg \sigma$. In this case the characteristic form of the unblurred ramp edge dominates. Then we have

$$\int\limits_{-w_x}^{w_x} RE_x^2(x)dx \approx s^2 \left(\int\limits_{-w_x}^{0} \phi^2(\frac{x+r}{\sigma})dx + \int\limits_{0}^{w_x} \left(1 - \phi(\frac{x-r}{\sigma})\right)^2 dx \right)$$

which leads to

$$CRB_{\hat{x}_0,RE} \approx \frac{1}{2s^2\sigma(\frac{w_2}{\sigma} - 2R(\frac{w_1}{\sigma}) + U(\frac{w_1}{\sigma}))} \cdot \frac{\sigma_n^2}{w_y}. \tag{3.28}$$

Assuming, in addition, $w_1 \gg \sigma$ (i.e., $w_x \gg r$) and using the approximations in (3.21) as before we finally obtain

$$CRB_{\hat{x}_0,RE} \approx \frac{r}{a^2} \cdot \frac{\sigma_n^2}{w_y}. \tag{3.29}$$

We see that the lower bound for the ramp edge is also proportional to σ_n^2/w_y. The precision increases for larger values of a and smaller values of r. In comparison to the classical step edge $SE(\mathbf{x})$ in (3.23) we obtain the same precision if we have $r = \sqrt{\pi}\sigma_{SE}$, where σ_{SE} denotes the blur of $SE(\mathbf{x})$.

3.2.2.3 Lines

Next, we consider two different analytic models of lines. The cross-section of the first one is modelled by a Gaussian function and represents a ridge structure. The second model is a Gaussian blurred bar structure (e.g., [32],[373]).

The first line model (Figure 3.12 on the left) can be written as

$$Line(x,y) = \frac{a}{\sigma}G(\frac{x}{\sigma}). \tag{3.30}$$

The minimal localization uncertainty computes to

$$\sigma_{\hat{x}_0,Line}^2 \geq \frac{2\sqrt{\pi}\sigma^3}{a^2(-2\sqrt{2}\frac{w_x}{\sigma}G(\frac{\sqrt{2}w_x}{\sigma}) + \mathrm{erf}(\frac{w_x}{\sigma}))} \cdot \frac{\sigma_n^2}{w_y} \tag{3.31}$$

and assuming $w_x \gg \sigma$ we obtain

$$CRB_{\hat{x}_0,Line} \approx \frac{2\sqrt{\pi}\sigma^3}{a^2} \cdot \frac{\sigma_n^2}{w_y}, \tag{3.32}$$

while the length of the line is given by $l = 2w_y$. The derived formula is similar to the one for the classical step edge in (3.23). Besides a factor of two the main

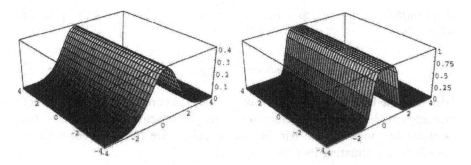

Figure 3.12. 3D plots of a Gaussian line (left) and a bar line (right).

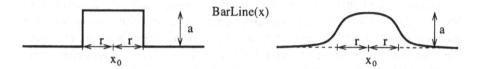

Figure 3.13. Bar line model (cross-section).

difference is that here the parameter σ has a larger influence since it enters with the third power while for the step edge it enters only linearly. For a value of $\sigma = 1$ the uncertainty for the line is two times larger than for the step edge, but note that this parameter has a different meaning. For the step edge, σ represents the blur of an imaging system while for the line this parameter comprises the ideal systematic intensity variations and the image blur.

As a second model of a line we consider a Gaussian blurred bar structure (Figure 3.12 on the right and Figure 3.13). This structure can be written as

$$BarLine(x,y) = a\left(\phi(\frac{x+r}{\sigma}) - \phi(\frac{x-r}{\sigma})\right).\tag{3.33}$$

The computation of the localization uncertainty for this model is more complicated than for the Gaussian line model. Analogous to the derivation for the ramp edge $RE(\mathbf{x})$ above we introduce the approximation $r \gg \sigma$ to obtain an analytic result. Then, we have

$$\int_{-w_x}^{w_x} BarLine_x^2(x)dx \approx \frac{a^2}{\sigma^2}\left(\int_{-w_x}^{0} G^2(\frac{x+r}{\sigma})dx + \int_{0}^{w_x} G^2(\frac{x-r}{\sigma})dx\right)$$

and the uncertainty bound evaluates to

$$CRB_{\hat{x}_0,BarLine} \approx \frac{\sqrt{\pi}\sigma}{2a^2\phi(\frac{\sqrt{2}(w_x-r)}{\sigma})}\cdot\frac{\sigma_n^2}{w_y}.\tag{3.34}$$

If we further assume $w_x \gg r$ and use the approximations in (3.21) as before we obtain

$$CRB_{\hat{x}_0, BarLine} \approx \frac{\sqrt{\pi}\sigma}{2a^2} \cdot \frac{\sigma_n^2}{w_y}. \tag{3.35}$$

Also here the length of the bar line is $l = 2w_y$. In comparison to the classical step edge in (3.23) the localization uncertainty is a factor of two smaller. This is plausible, since for the bar line we actually have two step edges which contribute to estimating its position.

3.2.2.4   Nonlinear Estimation of Multiple Parameters

The results above are valid for the case of estimating a single parameter. Below, we consider 2D features where it is necessary to estimate two parameters to fix their position. Therefore, we now have to deal with the case of multiple parameter estimation. After introducing the general formalism we investigate the precision of localizing L- and T-corners, rectangles, squares, blobs, and circular point landmarks.

In the case of multiple parameter estimation, the uncertainties of a parameter vector $\hat{\mathbf{p}} = (\hat{p}_1, ..., \hat{p}_n)$ are represented by the covariance matrix (van Trees [533])

$$\Sigma = cov\{\hat{\mathbf{p}}\} = E\{(\hat{\mathbf{p}} - \mathbf{p})(\hat{\mathbf{p}} - \mathbf{p})^T\} = \begin{pmatrix} \sigma_{\hat{p}_1}^2 & \cdots & \sigma_{\hat{p}_1\hat{p}_n} \\ \vdots & \ddots & \vdots \\ \sigma_{\hat{p}_n\hat{p}_1} & \cdots & \sigma_{\hat{p}_n}^2 \end{pmatrix}$$

The diagonal elements of this matrix represent the mean-squared errors and the off-diagonal elements are the covariances between different parameters. Lower bounds for the elements of this matrix are determined by using the *Fisher information matrix*

$$\mathbf{F} = \frac{1}{\sigma_n^2} \int_{x_1}^{x_2} \int_{y_1}^{y_2} \frac{\partial g_M(\mathbf{x}, \mathbf{p})}{\partial \mathbf{p}} \cdot \left(\frac{\partial g_M(\mathbf{x}, \mathbf{p})}{\partial \mathbf{p}}\right)^T dx.$$

If $\hat{\mathbf{p}}$ is an unbiased estimate of $\mathbf{p}$ then the errors are bounded by the inverse of $\mathbf{F}$:

$$\Sigma \geq \mathbf{F}^{-1} \tag{3.36}$$

which means that the symmetric matrix $\Sigma - \mathbf{F}^{-1}$ is positive semidefinite. Since the diagonal elements of positive semidefinite matrices are larger or equal to zero, the uncertainty of an element of $\hat{\mathbf{p}}$ is bounded by

$$\sigma_{\hat{p}_i}^2 \geq (\mathbf{F}^{-1})_{ii}, \tag{3.37}$$

where $(\mathbf{F}^{-1})_{ii}$ is the ii-th element of $\mathbf{F}^{-1}$. In our application we want to determine the uncertainties in estimating the position of point landmarks in 2D images. Since the location of such 2D features is described by two parameters $\mathbf{p} = (p_1, p_2)$, the Fisher information matrix is the 2×2-matrix

$$\mathbf{F} = \begin{pmatrix} F_{11} & F_{12} \\ F_{21} & F_{22} \end{pmatrix},$$

where

$$F_{11} = \frac{1}{\sigma_n^2} \int_{x_1}^{x_2} \int_{y_1}^{y_2} \left(\frac{\partial g_M(\mathbf{x}, \mathbf{p})}{\partial p_1} \right)^2 d\mathbf{x} \tag{3.38}$$

$$F_{12} = F_{21} = \frac{1}{\sigma_n^2} \int_{x_1}^{x_2} \int_{y_1}^{y_2} \frac{\partial g_M(\mathbf{x}, \mathbf{p})}{\partial p_1} \cdot \frac{\partial g_M(\mathbf{x}, \mathbf{p})}{\partial p_2} d\mathbf{x} \tag{3.39}$$

$$F_{22} = \frac{1}{\sigma_n^2} \int_{x_1}^{x_2} \int_{y_1}^{y_2} \left(\frac{\partial g_M(\mathbf{x}, \mathbf{p})}{\partial p_2} \right)^2 d\mathbf{x}. \tag{3.40}$$

With the determinant of $\mathbf{F}$

$$det\mathbf{F} = F_{11} F_{22} - F_{12}^2,$$

the inverse of $\mathbf{F}$ is

$$\mathbf{F}^{-1} = \frac{1}{det\mathbf{F}} \begin{pmatrix} F_{22} & -F_{12} \\ -F_{12} & F_{11} \end{pmatrix}$$

Bounds for the uncertainties of $\hat{p}_1$ and $\hat{p}_2$ are then given by

$$\sigma_{\hat{p}_1}^2 \geq CRB_{\hat{p}_1} = \frac{F_{22}}{det\mathbf{F}} \tag{3.41}$$

$$\sigma_{\hat{p}_2}^2 \geq CRB_{\hat{p}_2} = \frac{F_{11}}{det\mathbf{F}}. \tag{3.42}$$

3.2.2.5 Corners

L-corner Model. The simplest corner is created if two straight edges meet in a point. For such an L-corner the systematic intensity variations can be modelled as a wedge-shaped structure smoothed by a Gaussian filter. Assuming constant grey-value plateaus and a Gaussian image blur of $\sigma = 1$ the corresponding model function can be described by (see Rohr [427], Figure 3.14, and Section 2.6.2 above)

$$g_{ML}(\mathbf{x}) = a \left(\phi(x) - m(\mathbf{x}) - m(\mathbf{x}^{\#}) \right), \tag{3.43}$$

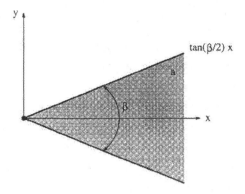

Figure 3.14.   L-corner characterization.

where

$$m(\mathbf{x}) = \int\limits_{-\infty}^{x} D(\xi, t\xi - \zeta_2)d\xi,$$

$D(\mathbf{x}) = G(x)\phi(y), \mathbf{x}^{\#} = (x, -y), t = \tan(\beta/2)$, and $\zeta_2 = tx - y$. Using, in addition, $\zeta_1 = x + ty$, $\zeta_1^{\#} = x - ty$, $\zeta_2^{\#} = tx + y$, $\zeta = (\zeta_2/q, \zeta_1/q)$, $\zeta^{\#} = (\zeta_2^{\#}/q, \zeta_1^{\#}/q)$, and $q = \sqrt{1 + t^2}$, the first partial derivatives of $g_{ML}(\mathbf{x})$ compute to

$$g_{MLx}(\mathbf{x}) = \frac{a\,t}{q}\left(D(\zeta) + D(\zeta^{\#})\right)$$
$$g_{MLy}(\mathbf{x}) = \frac{a}{q}\left(D(\zeta^{\#}) - D(\zeta)\right).$$

Since we deal with constant plateaus of the unsmoothed grey-value structure, the L-corner model for different amounts of blur σ can easily be obtained by scaling the model function. Note, that this is not possible in the general case, e.g., for the linear step edge model $LSE(\mathbf{x})$ analyzed above. To determine lower bounds for the uncertainties of estimating $\mathbf{x}_0$, we arbitrarily assume the origin of the corner to be located at $\mathbf{x}_0 = (x_0, y_0) = (0, 0)$ and use a symmetric observation window around this point. Then we have to evaluate

$$
F_{11} = \frac{1}{\sigma^2 \sigma_n^2} \int\limits_{-w_x}^{w_x} \int\limits_{-w_y}^{w_y} g_{MLx}^2 (\frac{\mathbf{x}}{\sigma}) d\mathbf{x}
$$

$$
= \frac{a^2 t^2}{q^2 \sigma^2 \sigma_n^2} \int\limits_{-w_x}^{w_x} \int\limits_{-w_y}^{w_y} \left(D^2(\frac{\zeta}{\sigma}) + 2D(\frac{\zeta}{\sigma}) D(\frac{\zeta^{\#}}{\sigma}) + D^2(\frac{\zeta^{\#}}{\sigma}) \right) d\mathbf{x}
$$

$$
F_{12} = \frac{1}{\sigma^2 \sigma_n^2} \int\limits_{-w_x}^{w_x} \int\limits_{-w_y}^{w_y} g_{MLx}(\frac{\mathbf{x}}{\sigma}) g_{MLy}(\frac{\mathbf{x}}{\sigma}) d\mathbf{x}
$$

$$
= \frac{a^2 t}{q^2 \sigma^2 \sigma_n^2} \int\limits_{-w_x}^{w_x} \int\limits_{-w_y}^{w_y} \left(D^2(\frac{\zeta^{\#}}{\sigma}) - D^2(\frac{\zeta}{\sigma}) \right) d\mathbf{x}
$$

$$
F_{22} = \frac{1}{\sigma^2 \sigma_n^2} \int\limits_{-w_x}^{w_x} \int\limits_{-w_y}^{w_y} g_{MLy}^2 (\frac{\mathbf{x}}{\sigma}) d\mathbf{x}
$$

$$
= \frac{a^2}{q^2 \sigma^2 \sigma_n^2} \int\limits_{-w_x}^{w_x} \int\limits_{-w_y}^{w_y} \left(D^2(\frac{\zeta^{\#}}{\sigma}) - 2D(\frac{\zeta}{\sigma}) D(\frac{\zeta^{\#}}{\sigma}) + D^2(\frac{\zeta}{\sigma}) \right) d\mathbf{x}.
$$

The lower bounds are then obtained using (3.41) and (3.42). We cannot calculate the above integrals analytically, but we can do this numerically. However, we are interested in analytic solutions. Setting the aperture angle to $\beta = 90^\circ (t = 1)$ we obtain the simplification $D(\zeta/\sigma) = G((x-y)/(\sqrt{2}\sigma))\phi((x+y)/(\sqrt{2}\sigma))$ and $D(\zeta^{\#}/\sigma) = G((x+y)/(\sqrt{2}\sigma))\phi((x-y)/(\sqrt{2}\sigma))$ but still the resulting integrals cannot be evaluated analytically.

The corner description above has the nice property that it is symmetric w.r.t. the x-axis. Therefore, the symmetry line is just $y = 0$ and the calculation of the partial derivatives becomes easier. However, assuming $\beta = 90^\circ$ and rotating the corner about $\alpha = 45^\circ$ (see Figure 3.15) we found that then the resulting integrals can be solved analytically. The reason for this is that in this case the space coordinates are decoupled. This model is given by

$$
g_{ML}(x, y) = a\phi(x)\phi(y) \tag{3.44}
$$

and with

$$
\begin{aligned}
g_{MLx}(x, y) &= aG(x)\phi(y) \\
g_{MLy}(x, y) &= a\phi(x)G(y)
\end{aligned}
$$

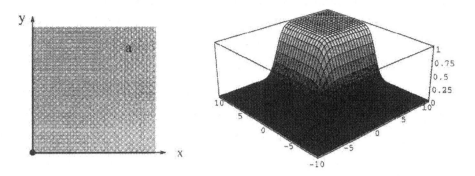

Figure 3.15.   L-corner with aperture angle $\beta = 90°$ and rotated about $\alpha = 45°$ (left), and corresponding 3D plot for $a = 1, \sigma = 1$ (right).

we obtain

$$F_{11} = \frac{a^2}{\sigma^2\sigma_n^2} \int_{-w_x}^{w_x} G^2(\frac{x}{\sigma})dx \int_{-w_y}^{w_y} \phi^2(\frac{y}{\sigma})dy = \frac{a^2}{2\sqrt{\pi}\sigma_n^2}\text{erf}(\frac{w_x}{\sigma})U(\frac{w_y}{\sigma})$$

$$F_{12} = \frac{a^2}{\sigma^2\sigma_n^2} \int_{-w_x}^{w_x} G(\frac{x}{\sigma})\phi(\frac{x}{\sigma})dx \int_{-w_y}^{w_y} G(\frac{y}{\sigma})\phi(\frac{y}{\sigma})dy = \frac{a^2}{4\sigma_n^2}\text{erf}(\frac{w_x}{\sqrt{2}\sigma})\text{erf}(\frac{w_y}{\sqrt{2}\sigma})$$

$$F_{22} = \frac{a^2}{\sigma^2\sigma_n^2} \int_{-w_x}^{w_x} \phi^2(\frac{x}{\sigma})dx \int_{-w_y}^{w_y} G^2(\frac{y}{\sigma})dy = \frac{a^2}{2\sqrt{\pi}\sigma_n^2}U(\frac{w_x}{\sigma})\text{erf}(\frac{w_y}{\sigma})$$

using $U(x)$ and the error function $\text{erf}(x)$ as introduced in (3.13) and (3.14). With (3.41) and (3.42) the uncertainty bounds for estimating x_0 and y_0 are

$$\sigma_{\hat{x}_0,L}^2 \geq \frac{F_{22}}{F_{11}F_{22} - F_{12}^2} = \frac{1}{F_{11} - \frac{F_{12}^2}{F_{22}}} =$$

$$\frac{2\sqrt{\pi}\sigma_n^2}{a^2\left(\text{erf}(\frac{w_x}{\sigma})U(\frac{w_y}{\sigma}) - \frac{\pi}{4}\frac{\text{erf}^2(\frac{w_x}{\sqrt{2}\sigma})\text{erf}^2(\frac{w_y}{\sqrt{2}\sigma})}{U(\frac{w_x}{\sigma})\text{erf}(\frac{w_y}{\sigma})}\right)} \tag{3.45}$$

$$\sigma_{\hat{y}_0,L}^2 \geq \frac{F_{11}}{F_{11}F_{22} - F_{12}^2} = \frac{1}{F_{22} - \frac{F_{12}^2}{F_{11}}} =$$

$$\frac{2\sqrt{\pi}\sigma_n^2}{a^2\left(U(\frac{w_x}{\sigma})\text{erf}(\frac{w_y}{\sigma}) - \frac{\pi}{4}\frac{\text{erf}^2(\frac{w_x}{\sqrt{2}\sigma})\text{erf}^2(\frac{w_y}{\sqrt{2}\sigma})}{\text{erf}(\frac{w_x}{\sigma})U(\frac{w_y}{\sigma})}\right)} \tag{3.46}$$

To interpret the results we derive an approximation of the above expressions by assuming $w_x \gg \sigma$ and use the simplifications in (3.21) as done above in the case of edges. Since here we deal with 2D features we also assume $w_y \gg \sigma$. Then, for the lower bounds we obtain

$$CRB_{\hat{x}_0,L} \approx \frac{2\sqrt{\pi}\sigma}{a^2} \cdot \frac{\sigma_n^2}{w_y} \tag{3.47}$$

$$CRB_{\hat{y}_0,L} \approx \frac{2\sqrt{\pi}\sigma}{a^2} \cdot \frac{\sigma_n^2}{w_x}. \tag{3.48}$$

Interestingly, the uncertainty bound in (3.47) is the same as that for the classical step edge in (3.23) but is twice as large:

$$CRB_{\hat{x}_0,L} \approx 2 \cdot CRB_{\hat{x}_0,SE}. \tag{3.49}$$

However, this is plausible since in x-direction the grey-value transitions of the L-corner represent about one half of the transitions of the classical step edge. The precision increases by increasing a^2 or w_y and by decreasing σ or σ_n^2. Increasing w_x does not improve the precision. The result in (3.48) is analogous to that in (3.47).

T-corner Model. More complex corners, e.g. T-, Y-, or Arrow-corners, can be modelled as suggested in Rohr [427] by the superposition of L-corner models:

$$g_M(\mathbf{x}, \mathbf{p}) = \sum_{i=0}^{N-1} g_{ML}(\mathbf{x}, \mathbf{p}_i), \qquad N \geq 2,$$

where N denotes the number of intersecting edges (number of adjacent regions). $N = 2$, for example, characterizes an L-corner while $N = 3$ describes T-, Y-, and Arrow-corners. The vectors $\mathbf{p}_i$ represent a subset of the overall parameters $\mathbf{p}$. The partial derivatives of the general model are

$$g_{Mx}(\mathbf{x}, \mathbf{p}) = \sum_{i=0}^{N-1} g_{MLx}(\mathbf{x}, \mathbf{p}_i)$$

$$g_{My}(\mathbf{x}, \mathbf{p}) = \sum_{i=0}^{N-1} g_{MLy}(\mathbf{x}, \mathbf{p}_i)$$

and consist of linear combinations of partial derivatives of the L-corner. Therefore, the calculation of uncertainty bounds for more complex corners is a straightforward extension to that of the L-corner. The bounds are obtained analogously as described above.

However, since already for L-corners in the general case it was not possible to evaluate the resulting expressions analytically, in the following, we will

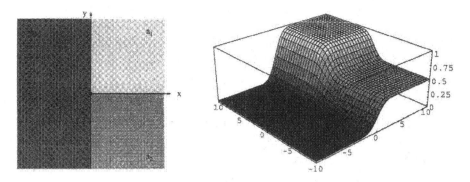

Figure 3.16.   T-corner (left) and corresponding 3D plot for $a_0 = 0, a_1 = 1, a_2 = 0.5, \sigma = 1$ (right).

concentrate on a simplified T-corner model shown in Figure 3.16. Introducing $a_{20} = a_2 - a_0$ and $a_{12} = a_1 - a_2$ the model function is

$$g_{MT}(x, y) = a_0 + \phi(x)(a_{20} + a_{12}\phi(y)) \tag{3.50}$$

and the first partial derivatives compute to

$$
\begin{aligned}
g_{MTx}(x, y) &= G(x)(a_{20} + a_{12}\phi(y)) \\
g_{MTy}(x, y) &= a_{12}\phi(x)G(y).
\end{aligned}
$$

With $a_{10} = a_1 - a_0$, a Gaussian image blur of σ, and

$$
\begin{aligned}
F_{11} &= \frac{1}{2\sqrt{\pi}\sigma_n^2}\mathrm{erf}(\frac{w_x}{\sigma})\left(2a_{10}a_{20}\frac{w_y}{\sigma} + a_{12}^2 U(\frac{w_y}{\sigma})\right) \\
F_{12} &= \frac{a_{12}}{4\sigma_n^2}(a_{10} + a_{20})\mathrm{erf}(\frac{w_x}{\sqrt{2}\sigma})\mathrm{erf}(\frac{w_y}{\sqrt{2}\sigma}) \\
F_{22} &= \frac{a_{12}^2}{2\sqrt{\pi}\sigma_n^2}U(\frac{w_x}{\sigma})\mathrm{erf}(\frac{w_y}{\sigma})
\end{aligned}
$$

for the lower bounds we get

$$
\sigma_{\hat{x}_0,T}^2 \geq \frac{2\sqrt{\pi}\sigma_n^2}{\mathrm{erf}(\frac{w_x}{\sigma})\left(2a_{10}a_{20}\frac{w_y}{\sigma} + a_{12}^2 U(\frac{w_y}{\sigma})\right) - \frac{\pi}{4}\frac{(a_{10}+a_{20})^2\mathrm{erf}^2(\frac{w_x}{\sqrt{2}\sigma})\mathrm{erf}^2(\frac{w_y}{\sqrt{2}\sigma})}{U(\frac{w_x}{\sigma})\mathrm{erf}(\frac{w_y}{\sigma})}} \tag{3.51}
$$

$$
\sigma_{\hat{y}_0,T}^2 \geq \frac{2\sqrt{\pi}\sigma_n^2}{a_{12}^2\left(U(\frac{w_x}{\sigma})\mathrm{erf}(\frac{w_y}{\sigma}) - \frac{\pi}{4}\frac{(a_{10}+a_{20})^2\mathrm{erf}^2(\frac{w_x}{\sqrt{2}\sigma})\mathrm{erf}^2(\frac{w_y}{\sqrt{2}\sigma})}{\mathrm{erf}(\frac{w_x}{\sigma})\left(2a_{10}a_{20}\frac{w_y}{\sigma} + a_{12}^2 U(\frac{w_y}{\sigma})\right)}\right)} \tag{3.52}
$$

For $w_x \gg \sigma$ and $w_y \gg \sigma$ we have the approximations

$$CRB_{\hat{x}_0,T} \approx \frac{2\sqrt{\pi}\sigma}{(a_{10}^2 + a_{20}^2)} \cdot \frac{\sigma_n^2}{w_y} \tag{3.53}$$

$$CRB_{\hat{y}_0,T} \approx \frac{2\sqrt{\pi}\sigma}{a_{12}^2} \cdot \frac{\sigma_n^2}{w_x} \tag{3.54}$$

which show the dependence on the noise level, the size of the window, the intensity contrasts, and the width of the transitions. Increasing w_y (w_x) leads to a higher precision for $\hat{x}_0$ ($\hat{y}_0$). Choosing, in addition, equal intensity contrasts $a_{12} = a_{20} = a/2$ ($a_{10} = a$) as indicated by the 3D plot in Figure 3.16 we finally obtain

$$CRB_{\hat{x}_0,T} \approx \frac{8\sqrt{\pi}\sigma}{5a^2} \cdot \frac{\sigma_n^2}{w_y} \tag{3.55}$$

$$CRB_{\hat{y}_0,T} \approx \frac{8\sqrt{\pi}\sigma}{a^2} \cdot \frac{\sigma_n^2}{w_x}. \tag{3.56}$$

Note, that we set the overall contrast between the highest and the lowest intensity plateau to a, so that our results are directly comparable to the lower bounds for the classical step edge in (3.23) and for the L-corner in (3.47) and (3.48). In comparison to these structures we have

$$CRB_{\hat{x}_0,T} \approx \frac{8}{5} \cdot CRB_{\hat{x}_0,SE} \approx \frac{4}{5} \cdot CRB_{\hat{x}_0,L} \tag{3.57}$$

$$CRB_{\hat{y}_0,T} \approx 4 \cdot CRB_{\hat{y}_0,L}. \tag{3.58}$$

Thus, for the T-corner the precision in estimating x_0 is somewhat better than for the L-corner, but the precision in estimating y_0 is four times worse. This is plausible as the following consideration shows. The T-corner in x-direction is mainly a combination of two L-corners with intensity contrasts a and $a/2$. Since the contrast enters quadratically in the formulas for the lower bound of the L-corner this leads to $CRB_{\hat{x}_0,T} \approx \left(\frac{1}{1+\frac{1}{4}}\right) \cdot CRB_{\hat{x}_0,L}$ which agrees with (3.57). In y-direction only the intensity contrast $a/2$ contributes to the uncertainty bound. Therefore, we have a factor of 4 as in (3.58).

To visualize the derived localization uncertainties for the classical step edge, the L-corner, and the T-corner, in Figure 3.17 we have depicted the corresponding uncertainty ellipses which have been normalized by the uncertainty for the classical step edge.

3.2.2.6 Rectangles

Next, we analyze the minimal uncertainties in localizing rectangles (Figures 3.18 and 3.19). In comparison to corners, these 2D image structures

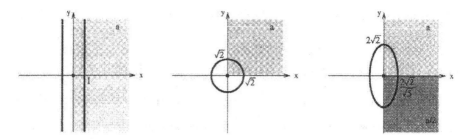

Figure 3.17.   Comparison of uncertainty ellipses for a step edge, an L-corner, and a T-corner normalized to the uncertainty for the step edge.

are finite in the unblurred case. We take the center of the rectangles as the point we want to localize. The Gaussian blurred rectangle reads

$$Rect(x, y) = a \left(\phi(\frac{x + r_x}{\sigma}) - \phi(\frac{x - r_x}{\sigma}) \right) \left(\phi(\frac{y + r_y}{\sigma}) - \phi(\frac{y - r_y}{\sigma}) \right) \quad (3.59)$$

Introducing analogous assumptions as in the case of the ramp edge $RE(\mathbf{x})$ and the bar line above, i.e., $r_x, r_y \gg \sigma$ and $w_x \gg r_x, w_y \gg r_y$ we obtain

$$CRB_{\hat{x}_0, Rect} \approx \frac{\sqrt{\pi} \sigma \sigma_n^2}{2 a^2 r_y} \quad (3.60)$$

$$CRB_{\hat{y}_0, Rect} \approx \frac{\sqrt{\pi} \sigma \sigma_n^2}{2 a^2 r_x} \quad (3.61)$$

The result can directly be related to that of an L-corner. The difference is only a factor of four which can be explained as follows. In x-direction we have two step edges for the rectangle, thus the precision is a factor of two better than the L-corner. Additionally, the term $2 r_y$ in (3.60) represents the length of the step edges and thus corresponds to w_y in the case of the L-corner. Taking this together makes a factor of four. The same holds true for the y-direction. In the special case of a square ($r_x = r_y = r$) we have

$$CRB_{\hat{x}_0, Rect} = CRB_{\hat{y}_0, Rect} \approx \frac{\sqrt{\pi} \sigma \sigma_n^2}{2 a^2 r} \quad (3.62)$$

3.2.2.7   Blobs and circular point landmarks

We now consider blobs as 2D image features (Figures 3.20 and 3.21) and model them by an anisotropic bivariate Gaussian function

$$Blob(x, y) = \frac{a}{\sigma_x \sigma_y} G(\frac{x}{\sigma_x}) G(\frac{y}{\sigma_y}). \quad (3.63)$$

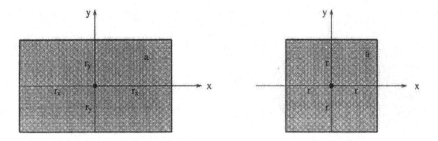

Figure 3.18. Rectangle and square.

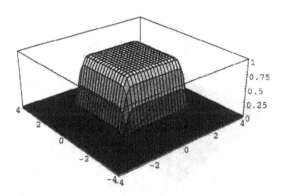

Figure 3.19. 3D plot of a rectangle (square).

The minimal localization uncertainty of localizing the centerpoint of the blob computes to

$$\sigma^2_{\hat{x}_0,Blob} \geq \frac{8\pi\sigma_x^3\sigma_y\,\sigma_n^2}{a^2\left(-2\sqrt{2}\frac{w_x}{\sigma_x}G(\frac{\sqrt{2}w_x}{\sigma_x}) + \mathrm{erf}(\frac{w_x}{\sigma_x})\right)\mathrm{erf}(\frac{w_y}{\sigma_y})} \qquad (3.64)$$

$$\sigma^2_{\hat{y}_0,Blob} \geq \frac{8\pi\sigma_x\sigma_y^3\,\sigma_n^2}{a^2\,\mathrm{erf}(\frac{w_x}{\sigma_x})\left(-2\sqrt{2}\frac{w_y}{\sigma_y}G(\frac{\sqrt{2}w_y}{\sigma_y}) + \mathrm{erf}(\frac{w_y}{\sigma_y})\right)}. \qquad (3.65)$$

Assuming $w_x \gg \sigma_x, w_y \gg \sigma_y$ we obtain the much simpler relations

$$CRB_{\hat{x}_0,Blob} \approx \frac{8\pi\sigma_x^3\sigma_y\,\sigma_n^2}{a^2} \qquad (3.66)$$

$$CRB_{\hat{y}_0,Blob} \approx \frac{8\pi\sigma_x\sigma_y^3\,\sigma_n^2}{a^2}. \qquad (3.67)$$

The result is partly comparable to that for the Gaussian line derived in (3.32) above. The uncertainty in x-direction, for example, is proportional to σ_n^2 and $1/a^2$ and also depends on the third power of σ_x. Additionally, we have a linear

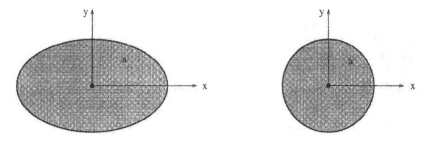

Figure 3.20.   Elliptic and circular symmetric blob.

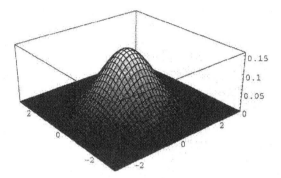

Figure 3.21.   3D plot of a circular symmetric blob.

dependence on σ_y. In the case of a circular symmetric blob ($\sigma_x = \sigma_y = \sigma$) we obtain

$$CRB_{\hat{x}_0,Blob} = CRB_{\hat{y}_0,Blob} \approx \frac{8\pi\sigma^4 \sigma_n^2}{a^2}. \qquad (3.68)$$

As a related circular point landmark we consider the one depicted in Figure 3.22 (see also Section 2.6 above). This type of landmark has successfully been used for automatic landmark extraction in aerial images (Drewniok and Rohr [125]–[129]). Note, however, that this landmark type is also relevant in medical applications. We model this landmark by

$$KD(r) = a_0 + (a_1 + a_2 r^2) e^{-\frac{r^2}{2\sigma^2}}, \qquad (3.69)$$

which has a similar shape as the Laplacian-of-Gaussian (LoG). The minimal localization uncertainty of this landmark computes to

$$\sigma_{\hat{x}_0,KD}^2 = \sigma_{\hat{y}_0,KD}^2 \geq \frac{2\sigma_n^2}{\pi(2\sigma^4 a_2^2 + a_1^2)}, \qquad (3.70)$$

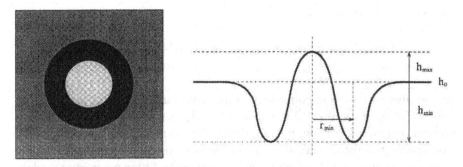

Figure 3.22. Circular point landmark (left) and corresponding cross-section intensities (right).

which shows that the uncertainty is proportional to σ_n^2 and inverse proportional to σ^4, a_2^2, and a_1^2 (see [128]). The relations between these parameters and the landmark characteristics in Figure 3.22 are as follows: $h_{max} = a_1$, $h_{min} = 2\sigma^2 a_2 e^{-(2\sigma^2 a_2 - a_1)/(2\sigma^2 a_2)}$, and $r_{min} = \sqrt{2\sigma^2 - a_1/a_2}$. In simulations with synthetic data we have shown that the theoretically derived minimal localization uncertainties can actually be obtained by fitting this model directly to the image intensities (see [128] as well as the next section).

3.2.2.8 Localization Uncertainties when Fitting Parametric Models

In Section 2.6 above, we have introduced an approach for extracting image features by fitting parametric intensity models directly to the image. While originally this approach has been applied for edges and corners (Rohr [425], [427]), application to other image structures such as lines, rectangles, blobs, and circular point landmarks is straightforward (see Drewniok and Rohr [128]). With this approach, the model parameters $\mathbf{p} = (p_1, ..., p_n)$ characterize the location of the image structures as well as other attributes like the orientation, the heights of the grey-value plateaus, and the width of the grey-value transitions. All parameters are estimated simultaneously by a least-squares fit of the model $g_M(\mathbf{x}, \mathbf{p})$ to the image intensities $g(\mathbf{x})$:

$$S(\mathbf{p}) = \int_{x_1}^{x_2} \int_{y_1}^{y_2} (g(\mathbf{x}) - g_M(\mathbf{x}, \mathbf{p}))^2 \, d\mathbf{x} \;\rightarrow\; min. \qquad (3.71)$$

In the following we assume that the model is valid and that all model parameters except the ones for the location are known. For edges (as well as other 1D image features such as lines) we have one location parameter $\mathbf{p} = p = x_0$. Considering, in addition, a 1D signal, then for the least-squares approach in (3.71) we obtain

$$\frac{\partial S(p)}{\partial p} = -2 \int_{x_1}^{x_2} (g(x) - g_M(x,p)) \frac{\partial g_M(x,p)}{\partial p} dx = 0. \tag{3.72}$$

Indeed, this condition is equivalent to the maximum-likelihood condition in (3.6) which has been derived in van Trees [533] using a K-coefficient approximation. On the other hand, the maximum-likelihood scheme in the nonlinear case approaches the Cramér-Rao bound for large signal-to-noise ratios [533]. Therefore, the Cramér-Rao bound can be achieved by fitting parametric models as done in [425],[427] (at least in principle). In other words, in order to calculate the precision of the model fitting approach for special 1D signals we can use the general formula in (3.7). Analogously, we can use (3.8) to calculate the precision of this approach when considering 2D signals (images). Note, that the requirement of large signal-to-noise ratios in the continuous case corresponds to the asymptotically efficient estimates in the case of discrete measurements where a large number of measurements is required [533].

For 2D image features (e.g., corners, rectangles, squares, blobs, and circular point landmarks), the model fitting approach yields two location parameters $\mathbf{p} = (p_1, p_2) = (x_0, y_0)$. In this case, from (3.71) we obtain the following system of equations

$$\frac{\partial S(\mathbf{p})}{\partial \mathbf{p}} = -2 \int_{x_1}^{x_2} \int_{y_1}^{y_2} (g(\mathbf{x}) - g_M(\mathbf{x}, \mathbf{p})) \frac{\partial g_M(\mathbf{x}, \mathbf{p})}{\partial \mathbf{p}} d\mathbf{x} = \mathbf{0}, \tag{3.73}$$

which is equivalent to the maximum-likelihood condition in the multiple parameter case in [533]. Therefore, also for 2D image features the lower bounds for the localization uncertainty can be approached by fitting parametric models. The precision of this approach can thus be calculated using the general formulas in (3.41) and (3.42).

Note, that the above relation agrees with the result of Kakarala and Hero [266] who showed for the special case of the classical step edge $SE(\mathbf{x})$ that the Cramér-Rao bound can be achieved by the maximum-likelihood estimate. Note also, that the result above agrees with the work of Förstner [166],[167] (see also Ryan et al. [458] and Okutomi and Kanade [387]). In [166], Förstner derives the precision of estimating the location by digital template matching resulting from a least-squares solution. This is done for the 1D case assuming the same model as we have used in (3.3). In [167] the precision for the 2D case is calculated. Actually, the obtained expressions in [166] and [167] are discrete approximations of the Cramér-Rao bounds given in (3.7), (3.41), and (3.42). Since for our result we assumed that only the location parameters are estimated, this is indeed equivalent to template matching as investigated by

Förstner. However, by using the discrete expressions in [166],[167] it would not have been possible or at least it would have been much more tedious to derive analytic results which state the localization precision as a function of all model parameters.

Numeric Examples. In the following, we give some numeric examples of the achievable precision for the feature models studied above. We focus on edge and corner models and use typical parameter values from the experiments in [427]. As mentioned above, we assume that the signal-to-noise ratio is large. To give an idea of the numeric values, we present the precision in terms of the image grid by identifying the units of the space coordinates with pixel positions. The pixel spacing in x- and y-direction will be denoted by pix, but note that we still deal with the continuous case. The grey values will be characterized by the dimension gr. For the noise process we assumed in (3.3) a constant spectral power density of $L_n(u) = \sigma_n^2$. Using the abbreviations just introduced the dimension of $L_n(u)$ for a 1D signal is $[gr^2 \cdot pix]$ and in the 2D case is $[gr^2 \cdot pix^2]$. On the other hand, the dimension of σ_n^2 as the variance of a random variable $n(x_i)$ is $[gr^2]$. Therefore, when using dimensions the spectral power density should be more precisely stated as $L_n(u) = \sigma_n^2 \cdot pix$ or $L_n(u) = \sigma_n^2 \cdot pix^2$ for the 1D and 2D case, respectively. This has to be kept in mind when applying the continuous formulas for the uncertainty lower bounds to evaluate numeric values associated with dimensions. Note also, that for range images the pixel spacing as well as the grey values can both be measured in the unit $meter$.

First we consider the classical step edge $SE(\mathbf{x})$. For edges, the window in [427] has been chosen to 21×21 pixels, which means that $w_x = w_y = 10pix$. For the height of $SE(\mathbf{x})$ we take $a \approx 100gr$ and for the width of the transition we choose $\sigma \approx 1pix$. The noise level is assumed to be $\sigma_n^2 \approx (3gr)^2$. Then, using the approximation in (3.23), which is valid since $w_x = 10pix \gg \sigma = 1pix$, the precision for localizing $SE(\mathbf{x})$ computes to

$$\sigma_{\hat{x}_0, SE} \approx 0.013pix.$$

Note, that in the numeric examples we present the uncertainties in terms of the standard deviation (square root of the variance) in order to be better comparable with the space coordinates. It should also be noted that the subpixel precision above can only be achieved if a and σ (and the orientation of the edge) are determined correctly and surely only if the model is valid. However, the obtained precision which is better than $2/100pix$ is amazing. If we consider the 1D case (assuming the window is extended only in x-direction), we nevertheless get

$$\sigma_{\hat{x}_0, SE} \approx 0.056pix. \tag{3.74}$$

With the same parameter values as above but for a 5×5 pixel window ($w_x = w_y = 2pix$) which is often used for local operators, we calculate a precision of

$$\sigma_{\hat{x}_0,SE} \approx 0.028pix. \tag{3.75}$$

Since in (3.74) and (3.75) about the same number of measurements is used (21 and $5 \cdot 5 = 25$, respectively) we see that with a 2D window the achievable precision is twice as good in this example.

For the double ramp $R2(\mathbf{x})$ we use typical parameter values from a measurement task in an industrial application where range images are analyzed. We assume a 1D observation window with $w_x = 2mm$. For the slopes we take $s_1 = 1$ and $s_2 = 0.7$ which correspond to slope angles of $\varphi_1 = 45^o$ and $\varphi_2 = 55^o$, respectively, measured against the vertical axis. The noise level has been determined to be $\sigma_n^2 \approx (0.02mm)^2$. Then, supposing $w_x \gg \sigma$ (e.g., $\sigma = 0.1mm$), we obtain a precision of

$$\sigma_{\hat{x}_0,R2} \approx 0.012mm,$$

which satisfies the required precision for this task.

For the ramp edge $RE(\mathbf{x})$ we have the same precision as for $SE(\mathbf{x})$ if $r \gg \sigma_{RE}$ and if we let $r = \sqrt{\pi}\sigma_{SE}$, where σ_{RE} and σ_{SE} denote the corresponding blur of the structures. In this case we therefore can take the numeric examples for $SE(\mathbf{x})$ as given above.

Next we consider the localization uncertainties for the corner models studied above. We use the same parameter setting as above for the step edge (21×21 window, $a \approx 100gr$, $\sigma \approx 1pix$, $\sigma_n^2 \approx (3gr)^2$). For the L-corner sketched in Figure 3.15 and by using (3.47) and (3.48) we then obtain

$$\sigma_{\hat{x}_0,L} \approx \sigma_{\hat{y}_0,L} \approx \sqrt{2} \cdot \sigma_{\hat{x}_0,SE} \approx 0.018pix.$$

For the T-corner sketched in Figure 3.16 with intensity contrasts a and $a/2$ and by using (3.55) and (3.56) we have

$$\sigma_{\hat{x}_0,T} \approx \frac{2\sqrt{2}}{\sqrt{5}} \cdot \sigma_{\hat{x}_0,SE} \approx 0.016pix$$

$$\sigma_{\hat{y}_0,T} \approx 2\sqrt{2} \cdot \sigma_{\hat{x}_0,SE} \approx 0.036pix.$$

We see that in both cases the achievable precision is very high. Assuming $a \approx 50gr$ which is also typical in the experiments in [427] then the uncertainties above are enlarged by a factor of two but they are still much better than $1/10pix$.

Experimental investigations.   Actually, experimental investigations in [127], [128] and [62] have shown that the above derived theoretical values for the localization precision can indeed be achieved by model fitting. Below, we

SNR^2	10	5	2	1
Theoretical	0.017	0.024	0.038	0.054
Experimental	0.018	0.024	0.038	0.053

Table 3.1. Localizing a circular symmetric landmark by model fitting: Standard deviation of the precision (in *pix*) as a function of the signal-to-noise ratio (SNR).

briefly summarize the results from the study in Drewniok and Rohr [127],[128]. In this study, we analyzed the approximate model for the circular symmetric landmark depicted in Figure 3.22 above. The study is based on synthetic images of this landmark with added Gaussian noise of different signal-to-noise ratios (SNR) as well as randomly generated positions of the landmark. From this experiment it turned out that the position estimate is unbiased, i.e., the systematic error is zero. The results for the precision of the position estimate applying the model-fitting approach has been listed in Table 3.1. The table gives the standard deviation of the precision in *pix* (pixel units) as a function of SNR^2. In comparison, we have also listed the analytically derived values based on the Cramér-Rao bound in (3.70). It can be seen that the agreement between the theoretical and the experimental values is very good. The agreement is even more remarkable since the analytic derivation does not consider discretization effects due to sampling and quantization, while in the experiments naturally discrete images have to used.

The here considered circular symmetric landmark has been applied in [127], [128] to extract ground control points from aerial images. Assume for the airplane a height of $h = 1500m$ and that one pixel corresponds to ca. $15 \times 15 cm^2$ on the ground, which are typical values. Then it follows that the standard deviation of the precision for localizing ground control points is actually only about $1cm$.

3.2.3 Localization Precision in 3D Images

Having studied the minimal uncertainties for localizing features in 2D images, we now generalize this work and derive analytic results for 3D image features. We consider 3D point landmarks (3D corners, 3D boxes, and 3D blobs) as well as other image features (3D edges, 3D ridges, and 3D lines). The investigated feature models are examples for 0D, 1D, and 2D features. This means that we have to estimate the following number of positional parameters: Three for 3D point landmarks, two for 3D ridges and 3D lines, and one for 3D edges. To derive analytic results for 3D image features the same principle can be used as in the 2D case above, however, the calculations are more extensive.

Given the model function $g_M(\mathbf{x}, \mathbf{p})$ with $\mathbf{x} = (x, y, z)$ and where $\mathbf{p} = (p_1, ..., p_n)$ is the vector of the positional parameters to be estimated, our analysis is based on the Fisher information matrix in the 3D case:

$$\mathbf{F} = \frac{1}{\sigma_n^2} \int_{x_1}^{x_2} \int_{y_1}^{y_2} \int_{z_1}^{z_2} \frac{\partial g_M(\mathbf{x}, \mathbf{p})}{\partial \mathbf{p}} \cdot \left(\frac{\partial g_M(\mathbf{x}, \mathbf{p})}{\partial \mathbf{p}}\right)^T dx. \tag{3.76}$$

For general 3D image features we have a symmetric 3×3 matrix

$$\mathbf{F} = \begin{pmatrix} F_{11} & F_{12} & F_{13} \\ F_{21} & F_{22} & F_{23} \\ F_{31} & F_{32} & F_{33} \end{pmatrix}, \tag{3.77}$$

where $F_{21} = F_{12}$, $F_{31} = F_{13}$, and $F_{23} = F_{32}$. Lower bounds for the estimated parameters are given by the diagonal elements of $\mathbf{F}$, i.e.,

$$\sigma_{\hat{p}_i}^2 \geq (\mathbf{F}^{-1})_{ii}. \tag{3.78}$$

With

$$\begin{aligned} det\mathbf{F} &= F_{11}(F_{22}F_{33} - F_{23}^2) - F_{12}(F_{12}F_{33} - F_{23}F_{13}) \\ &\quad + F_{13}(F_{12}F_{23} - F_{22}F_{13}) \end{aligned}$$

we thus have for the positional parameters $\hat{x}_0, \hat{y}_0, \hat{z}_0$ the following bounds

$$\sigma_{\hat{x}_0}^2 \geq CRB_{\hat{x}_0} = \frac{F_{22}F_{33} - F_{23}^2}{det\mathbf{F}} \tag{3.79}$$

$$\sigma_{\hat{y}_0}^2 \geq CRB_{\hat{y}_0} = \frac{F_{11}F_{33} - F_{13}^2}{det\mathbf{F}} \tag{3.80}$$

$$\sigma_{\hat{z}_0}^2 \geq CRB_{\hat{z}_0} = \frac{F_{11}F_{22} - F_{12}^2}{det\mathbf{F}}. \tag{3.81}$$

Analogous to the 2D case we specify the observation window by the half-widths w_x, w_y, and w_z (cf. Figure 3.11).

3.2.3.1   3D Edges

First, we consider a plane edge in 3D (Figure 3.23 on the left). The model function of this image feature is identical to the 2D case in (3.15) and is given by

$$Edge3D(x, y, z) = a\phi\left(\frac{x}{\sigma}\right). \tag{3.82}$$

For this model there is one uniquely defined location parameter, thus we only have to determine one element of the Fisher information matrix. The lower bound for the location parameter calculates to

$$\sigma_{\hat{x}_0, Edge3D}^2 \geq \frac{\sqrt{\pi}\sigma}{2a^2 \mathrm{erf}\left(\frac{w_x}{\sigma}\right)} \cdot \frac{\sigma_n^2}{w_y w_z} \tag{3.83}$$

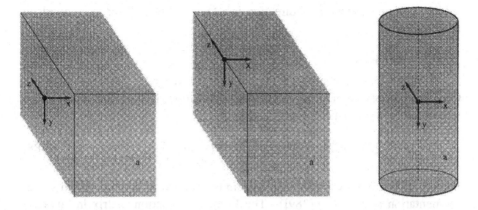

Figure 3.23.   Models of a 3D edge point (left), a 3D ridge point (middle), and a 3D line point (right).

and assuming $w_x \gg \sigma$ we obtain

$$CRB_{\hat{x}_0, Edge3D} \approx \frac{\sqrt{\pi}\sigma}{2a^2} \cdot \frac{\sigma_n^2}{w_y w_z}. \tag{3.84}$$

In comparison to the 2D case in (3.16) and (3.23), we now can improve the localization precision by extending the window in z-direction, i.e. by enlarging w_z.

3.2.3.2   3D Ridges

Next we consider a model of a 3D ridge structure. This structure is a 1D feature and its extremal points define a line in 3D images. Actually such a structure can be modelled by extending the 2D L-corner model to 3D. We use an L-corner with an aperture angle of 90° and assume that we have no variation in z-direction (Figure 3.23 in the middle). Thus, we can directly apply the same model as in the 2D case in (3.44):

$$Ridge3D(x, y, z) = a\phi(\frac{x}{\sigma})\phi(\frac{y}{\sigma}). \tag{3.85}$$

Assuming that $w_x, w_y \gg \sigma$, the analytic lower bounds for the two positional parameters compute to

$$CRB_{\hat{x}_0, Ridge3D} \approx \frac{\sqrt{\pi}\sigma}{a^2} \cdot \frac{\sigma_n^2}{w_y w_z} \tag{3.86}$$

$$CRB_{\hat{y}_0, Ridge3D} \approx \frac{\sqrt{\pi}\sigma}{a^2} \cdot \frac{\sigma_n^2}{w_x w_z}. \tag{3.87}$$

Also here the result is analogous to the 2D L-corner in (3.47),(3.48), but additionally we can reduce the positional uncertainty by enlarging w_z. The localization uncertainty in x-direction is a factor of two larger in comparison to the 3D edge.

3.2.3.3   3D Lines

3D (straight) lines are also 1D features in 3D images. We here analyze a Gaussian model of a 3D line extended in y-direction (Figure 3.23 on the right) which can be written as

$$Line3D(x, y, z) = \frac{a}{\sigma_x \sigma_z} G(\frac{x}{\sigma_x}) G(\frac{z}{\sigma_z}).$$ (3.88)

Such models are relevant, for example, in the context of cerebral blood vessel segmentation (e.g., [460],[289]). The Fisher information matrix in this case consists of two elements and for the lower bounds we obtain

$$\sigma^2_{\hat{x}_0, Line3D} \geq \frac{4\pi\sigma_x^3\sigma_z}{a^2\left(-2\sqrt{2}\frac{w_x}{\sigma_x}G(\frac{\sqrt{2}w_x}{\sigma_x}) + \text{erf}(\frac{w_x}{\sigma_x})\right)\text{erf}(\frac{w_z}{\sigma_z})} \cdot \frac{\sigma_n^2}{w_y}$$ (3.89)

$$\sigma^2_{\hat{z}_0, Line3D} \geq \frac{4\pi\sigma_x\sigma_z^3}{a^2\text{erf}(\frac{w_x}{\sigma_x})\left(-2\sqrt{2}\frac{w_z}{\sigma_z}G(\frac{\sqrt{2}w_z}{\sigma_z}) + \text{erf}(\frac{w_z}{\sigma_z})\right)} \cdot \frac{\sigma_n^2}{w_y}.$$ (3.90)

Assuming $w_x \gg \sigma_x, w_z \gg \sigma_z$ we derive

$$CRB_{\hat{x}_0, Line3D} \approx \frac{4\pi\sigma_x^3\sigma_z}{a^2} \cdot \frac{\sigma_n^2}{w_y}$$ (3.91)

$$CRB_{\hat{z}_0, Line3D} \approx \frac{4\pi\sigma_x\sigma_z^3}{a^2} \cdot \frac{\sigma_n^2}{w_y},$$ (3.92)

where the length of the line is given by $l = 2w_y$. In comparison to the result for the 2D Gaussian line model in (3.32), we here have for $\hat{x}_0$ ($\hat{y}_0$) a dependence on the parameter σ_z (σ_x) which enters linearly.

3.2.3.4   3D Corners

Now we analyze 3D point landmarks, i.e. uniquely defined points in 3D images. Our first model is a 3D corner, which can be defined as a generalization of a 2D corner

$$L3D(x, y, z) = a\phi(\frac{x}{\sigma})\phi(\frac{y}{\sigma})\phi(\frac{z}{\sigma}).$$ (3.93)

This model is also an extension of the 3D ridge model from above. All involved angles have 90° (Figure 3.24 on the left). For this model we have to compute all elements of the 3×3 Fisher information matrix in (3.77). Assuming

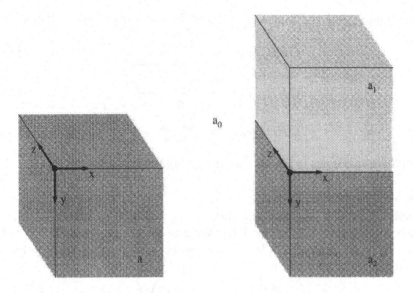

Figure 3.24. Models of a 3D L-corner (left) and a 3D T-corner (right).

$w_x, w_y, w_z \gg \sigma$ we finally obtain

$$CRB_{\hat{x}_0,L3D} \approx \frac{2\sqrt{\pi}\sigma}{a^2} \cdot \frac{\sigma_n^2}{w_y w_z} \qquad (3.94)$$

$$CRB_{\hat{y}_0,L3D} \approx \frac{2\sqrt{\pi}\sigma}{a^2} \cdot \frac{\sigma_n^2}{w_x w_z} \qquad (3.95)$$

$$CRB_{\hat{z}_0,L3D} \approx \frac{2\sqrt{\pi}\sigma}{a^2} \cdot \frac{\sigma_n^2}{w_x w_y}. \qquad (3.96)$$

In comparison to the 2D case in (3.47),(3.48) we can improve the precision by enlarging the window in the two directions orthogonal to the respective coordinate directions x, y, or z. In comparison to the 3D ridge model, the localization uncertainty in x-direction, for example, is a factor of two larger.

A more complicated model of a 3D point landmark is a 3D generalization of a T-corner (Figure 3.24 on the right). Using the same parameter values for the contrasts as in the 2D case, i.e. $a_{12} = a_{20} = a/2$, $a_{10} = a$, we can model such a structure by

$$T3D(x,y,z) = \frac{a}{2}\phi(\frac{x}{\sigma})(1 + \phi(\frac{y}{\sigma}))\phi(\frac{z}{\sigma}). \qquad (3.97)$$

Assuming $w_x, w_y, w_z \gg \sigma$ we can derive the following analytic relations

$$CRB_{\hat{x}_0,T3D} \approx \frac{8\sqrt{\pi}\sigma}{5a^2} \cdot \frac{\sigma_n^2}{w_y w_z} \qquad (3.98)$$

$$CRB_{\hat{y}_0,T3D} \approx \frac{8\sqrt{\pi}\sigma}{a^2} \cdot \frac{\sigma_n^2}{w_x w_z} \qquad (3.99)$$

$$CRB_{\hat{z}_0,T3D} \approx \frac{8\sqrt{\pi}\sigma}{5a^2} \cdot \frac{\sigma_n^2}{w_x w_y} \qquad (3.100)$$

which are analogous to the 2D case in (3.55),(3.56).

3.2.3.5   3D Boxes

Another type of a 3D point landmark can be modelled as a Gaussian blurred 3D box (cf. Figure 3.25 on the left). We take the center of the 3D box as the point we want to localize. The model can be written analogously to the 2D rectangle model in (3.59) as

$$Box3D(x,y,z) = a \left(\phi(\frac{x+r_x}{\sigma}) - \phi(\frac{x-r_x}{\sigma}) \right) \left(\phi(\frac{y+r_y}{\sigma}) - \phi(\frac{y-r_y}{\sigma}) \right)$$
$$\times \left(\phi(\frac{z+r_z}{\sigma}) - \phi(\frac{z-r_z}{\sigma}) \right). \qquad (3.101)$$

Introducing analogous assumptions, $r_x, r_y, r_z \gg \sigma$ and $w_x \gg r_x, w_y \gg r_y, w_z \gg r_z$, we finally obtain the following lower bounds

$$CRB_{\hat{x}_0,Box3D} \approx \frac{\sqrt{\pi}\sigma\sigma_n^2}{4a^2 r_y r_z} \qquad (3.102)$$

$$CRB_{\hat{y}_0,Box3D} \approx \frac{\sqrt{\pi}\sigma\sigma_n^2}{4a^2 r_x r_z} \qquad (3.103)$$

$$CRB_{\hat{z}_0,Box3D} \approx \frac{\sqrt{\pi}\sigma\sigma_n^2}{4a^2 r_x r_y}. \qquad (3.104)$$

Here, enlargement of the structure in the two directions orthogonal to the respective coordinate directions x, y, or z improves the localization precision. For the special case of a cube ($r_x = r_y = r_z = r$) we have

$$CRB_{\hat{x}_0,Box3D} = CRB_{\hat{y}_0,Box3D} = CRB_{\hat{z}_0,Box3D} \approx \frac{\sqrt{\pi}\sigma\sigma_n^2}{4a^2 r^2}. \qquad (3.105)$$

If we relate this result to that for the square in the 2D case in (3.62), which is a special case of the 2D rectangle, then we can write

$$CRB_{\hat{x}_0,Box3D} = \frac{1}{2r} \cdot CRB_{\hat{x}_0,Rect}. \qquad (3.106)$$

Since generally $r \gg 1$ we see that the localization precision for the 3D box is significantly higher than that for the 2D square.

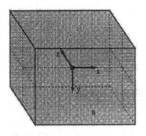 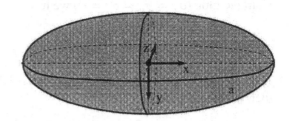

Figure 3.25. Models of a 3D box (left) and a 3D blob (right).

3.2.3.6 3D Blobs

Finally, we consider 3D anisotropic blobs as point landmarks in 3D images (Figure 3.25 on the right). We take the centerpoint as the point we want to localize and model such structures by a trivariate Gaussian function

$$Blob3D(x,y,z) = \frac{a}{\sigma_x \sigma_y \sigma_z} G(\frac{x}{\sigma_x}) G(\frac{y}{\sigma_y}) G(\frac{z}{\sigma_z}). \tag{3.107}$$

For this model we only have to compute the three diagonal elements of the Fisher information matrix since $F_{12} = F_{13} = F_{23} = 0$. The localization uncertainty for this structure computes to

$$\sigma_{\hat{x}_0,Blob3D}^2 \geq \frac{16\pi^{\frac{3}{2}}\sigma_x^3\sigma_y\sigma_z\,\sigma_n^2}{a^2\left(-2\sqrt{2}\frac{w_x}{\sigma_x}G(\frac{\sqrt{2}w_x}{\sigma_x}) + \mathrm{erf}(\frac{w_x}{\sigma_x})\right)\mathrm{erf}(\frac{w_y}{\sigma_y})\mathrm{erf}(\frac{w_z}{\sigma_z})} \tag{3.108}$$

$$\sigma_{\hat{y}_0,Blob3D}^2 \geq \frac{16\pi^{\frac{3}{2}}\sigma_x\sigma_y^3\sigma_z\,\sigma_n^2}{a^2\,\mathrm{erf}(\frac{w_x}{\sigma_x})\left(-2\sqrt{2}\frac{w_y}{\sigma_y}G(\frac{\sqrt{2}w_y}{\sigma_y}) + \mathrm{erf}(\frac{w_y}{\sigma_y})\right)\mathrm{erf}(\frac{w_z}{\sigma_z})} \tag{3.109}$$

$$\sigma_{\hat{z}_0,Blob3D}^2 \geq \frac{16\pi^{\frac{3}{2}}\sigma_x\sigma_y\sigma_z^3\,\sigma_n^2}{a^2\,\mathrm{erf}(\frac{w_x}{\sigma_x})\,\mathrm{erf}(\frac{w_y}{\sigma_y})\left(-2\sqrt{2}\frac{w_z}{\sigma_z}G(\frac{\sqrt{2}w_z}{\sigma_z}) + \mathrm{erf}(\frac{w_z}{\sigma_z})\right)} \tag{3.110}$$

Assuming $w_x \gg \sigma_x, w_y \gg \sigma_y, w_z \gg \sigma_z$, we obtain the relatively simple formulas

$$CRB_{\hat{x}_0,Blob3D} \geq \frac{16\pi^{\frac{3}{2}}\sigma_x^3\sigma_y\sigma_z\,\sigma_n^2}{a^2} \tag{3.111}$$

$$CRB_{\hat{y}_0,Blob3D} \geq \frac{16\pi^{\frac{3}{2}}\sigma_x\sigma_y^3\sigma_z\,\sigma_n^2}{a^2} \tag{3.112}$$

$$CRB_{\hat{z}_0,Blob3D} \geq \frac{16\pi^{\frac{3}{2}}\sigma_x\sigma_y\sigma_z^3\,\sigma_n^2}{a^2} \tag{3.113}$$

For $\hat{x}_0$, for example, the precision depends on the third power of σ_x while σ_y and σ_z enter linearly. The result for $\hat{y}_0$ and $\hat{z}_0$ is analogous. In the case of an isotropic blob ($\sigma_x = \sigma_y = \sigma_z = \sigma$) we have

$$\sigma^2_{\hat{x}_0,Blob3D} = \sigma^2_{\hat{y}_0,Blob3D} = \sigma^2_{\hat{z}_0,Blob3D} \approx \frac{16\pi^{\frac{3}{2}}\sigma^5\sigma^2_n}{a^2}. \qquad (3.114)$$

If we compare this result with the precision for the isotropic 2D blob in (3.68), then we have the relation

$$\sigma^2_{\hat{x}_0,Blob3D} = 2\sqrt{\pi}\sigma \cdot \sigma^2_{\hat{x}_0,Blob}. \qquad (3.115)$$

Thus, for $\sigma = 1$, for example, the localization uncertainty for a 3D blob is $2\sqrt{\pi} \approx 3.54$ times higher in comparison to a 2D blob, while for $\sigma = 0.1$ the localization uncertainty is a factor of 0.35 lower.

3.3 Experimental Studies

In this section, we describe our experimental investigations on the performance of point landmark operators. We are primarily concerned with 3D differential operators, but partially also deal with 2D operators. The studies are based on 3D synthetic data (e.g., tetrahedra and ellipsoids), for which ground truth is available, as well as on 3D tomographic images of the human brain (MR and CT images). We start with a brief analysis of operator responses of nine 3D differential operators, which we have introduced in Sections 2.4 and 2.5 above. Then, we consider the detection performance of these operators in more detail. We introduce statistical measures to quantify the detection performance. In addition, we suggest a certain type of detection performance visualization and also introduce a scalar performance measure, which combines the number of false detections with the significance of the detections. After that, we report about our investigations concerning the localization accuracy. Then, we briefly describe other performance studies of 3D operators. We have analyzed the image registration accuracy under affine transformations as well as the number of corresponding points under elastic deformations and noise. For other studies, which have investigated 3D ridge curve based operators (Section 2.3.2 above), see Thirion [521]. There, the rigid registration accuracy and the number of matched points under rigid registration have been determined. Finally in this section, we use projective invariants to assess the performance of 2D corner operators.

3.3.1 Operator Responses

We here analyze the operator responses of nine different 3D differential operators for detecting anatomical point landmarks in 3D images. The 3D operators have been introduced above in Chapter 2 and for some of the operators we have already visually judged the detection result. There, the detections have been visualized by marked points in the original images. Here, we analyze the operator responses in more detail. First, we briefly recapitulate the considered operators. Since most of these operators are 3D extensions of 2D corner operators we denote them also by the names of the corresponding authors, who introduced the 2D operators, and use the suffix '3D'. H and H^* denote the mean curvature and the gradient-weighted mean curvature of isocontours, respectively (Section 2.4). H^* can be written as $H^* = H \cdot 2|\nabla g|^3$, with $|\nabla g|$ being the 3D image gradient, and is actually identical to the 3D corner operator $Op2$ (or $Blom3D$) in Section 2.5. In addition, we consider the corner operator $Op1$ (or $KitchenRosenfeld3D$) which is also based on the mean curvature and can be written as $Op1 = H \cdot 2|\nabla g|$ (Section 2.5). K and K^* are the Gaussian curvature and the gradient-weighted Gaussian curvature (Section 2.4), where $K^* = K \cdot |\nabla g|^4$. Related to these two operators is a 3D extension of the corner operator of Beaudet [28] defined by *Beaudet3D* $= det\mathbf{H}_g$, where $\mathbf{H}_g$ is the Hessian matrix of the image function in 3D. In Section 2.5 we saw that the 2D operator generally yields two detections for one landmarks. This behavior can also be observed in the 3D case below. Finally, we consider the 3D corner operators from Section 2.5 which are based on only first order partial derivatives, namely $Op3 = det\mathbf{C}_g/tr\,\mathbf{C}_g$, $Op3' = 1/tr\mathbf{C}_g^{-1}$, and $Op4 = det\mathbf{C}_g$. Since $Op3'$ and $Op4$ are the direct extensions of the 2D corner operators of Förstner [168] and Rohr [424], we also denote them by *Förstner3D* and *Rohr3D*, respectively.

The operator responses of the above-mentioned nine 3D operators applied to the landmark 'frontal ventricular horn' in a 3D MR image are shown in Figure 3.26 (Hartkens et al. [235]). We have used a ROI of size $40 \times 40 \times 40$ voxels and represent the result by three orthogonal sections (sagittal, axial, coronal) at the landmark. We immediately see that for the operators H and K there are no significant operator responses and thus they are unsuited for landmark extraction. The reason seems to be that these operators represent curvature properties of single isocontours, while in Figure 3.26 their responses have been computed for all image points, i.e., we have not selected a certain isocontour. This behavior is analogous to the 2D case when directly using the curvature κ of isocontour curves (without multiplication of some power of the gradient magnitude). Also in the 2D case there is no prominent point (see Rohr [430]). Multiplying H and K by the gradient magnitude (operators $Op1$, $Op2$ (H^*), and K^*) significantly improves the result. For the operators $Op1$ and $Op2$, which are based on the mean curvature, we have significant operator responses at the tip of the landmark. However, we also have large operator values along the contour surface of the landmark. With the operator K^* the response is better concentrated at the tip of the landmark. The same is true for the operator *Beaudet3D*, but in this case we have positive as well as negative values and thus we do not have a unique detection (see also [430] for the 2D case). For the operators $Op3$, $Op4$, and $Op3'$ the responses are well concentrated at the tip of the landmark, while the results of $Op3$ and $Op4$ appear to be superior. For these three operators the discrimination between the landmark and the background seems to be better than for the other approaches (grey vs. black for the background). Additional examples of the operator responses for other synthetic as well as real images can be found in Hartkens et al. [235],[231].

3.3.2   Statistical Measures for the Detection Performance

Above in Section 2.5 we saw that the 3D operators yield a large number of 3D anatomical landmarks, but there are also a number of false detections. The detection performance is very important in practical applications (e.g., when using a semi-automatic procedure as in our case), and the reliability and ac-

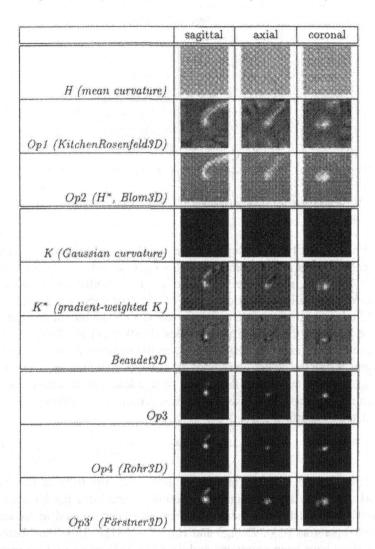

Figure 3.26. Operator responses of nine different 3D operators at the landmark 'frontal ventricular horn' in a 3D MR image.

curacy of subsequent procedures (e.g., image registration) strongly depend on this criterion. Therefore, we here analyze the detection performance of the operators in more detail. While so far we have only visually judged the performance of the different 3D operators, in this section, we introduce quantitative measures for the detection performance. We apply statistical measures for performance characterization while using 3D synthetic data as well as 3D MR and CT images.

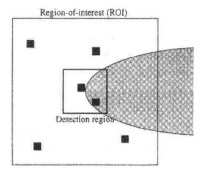

Figure 3.27.   Landmark with corresponding ROI and detection region as well as detected landmark candidates.

To compute statistical measures for the detection performance, we consider around each landmark a ROI ($25 \times 25 \times 25$ voxels) as well as a detection region ($7 \times 7 \times 7$ voxels), see Figure 3.27. The usage of a detection region has the advantage that small localization errors of the operators (see Sections 3.2.1 and 3.3.5) do not falsify the detection performance. The measures used in our study are based on the following quantities (Hartkens et al. [233]–[235]): n_d as the overall number of detections, $n_{d,in}$ as the number of correct detections (detections inside the detection region), n_l as the overall number of landmarks, and $n_{l,detect}$ as the number of landmarks with at least one detection inside the detection region. Based on these quantities we compute the following measures for the detection performance:

$$P_{in} = \frac{n_{d,in}}{n_d}, \qquad P_{detect} = \frac{n_{l,detect}}{n_l}, \qquad P_{multiple} = \frac{n_{d,in}}{n_l}, \qquad (3.116)$$

which represent the fraction of correct detections, the fraction of detected landmarks, and the average number of multiple detections per landmark, respectively. Previously, statistical measures have been applied in the case of 2D corner operators (e.g., Zuniga and Haralick [581]). However, there only two measures have been employed and detection regions around corners have not been considered. Thus, the resulting detection performance in that work depends more strongly on the localization accuracy.

In the case of 3D synthetic images (tetrahedra, ellipsoids, hyperbolic paraboloids), we have analyzed the measures in (3.116) as a function of the parameters of the modelled landmarks as well as the noise level. Tetrahedra and ellipsoids model different types of tips while hyperbolic paraboloids model saddle points. An example is given in Figure 3.28. We show the result of applying the operator $Op3$ to the tip of an ellipsoid. Note, that the figure represents mean values over different parameters of the ellipsoid (different lengths of the semi-axes). Depicted are the overall number of detections (for all landmarks and

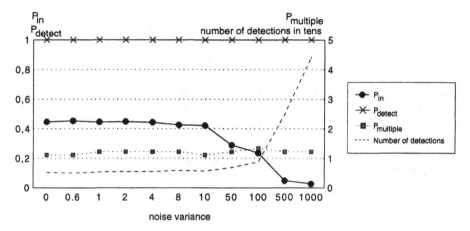

Figure 3.28.   Statistical detection performance measures as a function of the image noise for the 3D operator *Op*3 applied to the tip of an ellipsoid (mean values over differently parameterized ellipsoids).

images) as well as the obtained mean values for the statistical measures as a function of the image noise variance σ_n^2 (note the different units on the left and right side of the diagram). We see that the overall number of detections is nearly constant for low noise levels, but significantly increases for large noise levels. The fraction of detections inside the window P_{in} is also nearly constant for low noise levels but gets strongly worse for large noise levels. P_{detect} is always equal to one which means that the landmark has been detected in all cases. The average number of multiple detections $P_{multiple}$ is approximately 1, which supports that we here have a good detection performance. Results for the other operators as well as for additional synthetic data are provided in Hartkens et al. [235],[231].

In the case of 3D MR and CT images, we have computed mean values of the measures for all considered landmarks. As landmarks we have used the external occipital protuberance, the tips of the frontal, occipital, and temporal ventricular horns, as well as the junction at the top of pons (see Figures 2.11,2.12 above). Since the ventricular horns can be found in both hemispheres of the human brain, we have in total eight landmarks. The corresponding ROIs and detection regions have been placed around manually specified positions. Figure 3.29 shows the result for the case of MR images. We have used MR images of four different persons and the result represents mean values over all landmarks as well as all MR images. It turns out, that the operators based on only first order partial derivatives of an image (*Op*3, *Rohr3D*, *Förstner3D*) yield the best results. Although the fraction of detected landmarks P_{detect} in Figure 3.29 is comparable for all operators, the fraction of correct detections P_{in} is significantly higher for the mentioned three operators. Additionally,

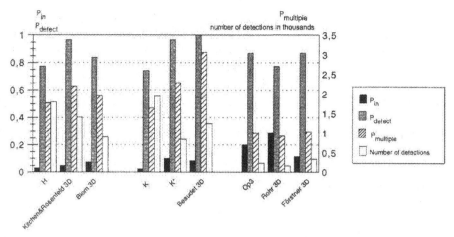

Figure 3.29.   Detection performance of the nine investigated 3D operators for MR images (mean values over different landmarks as well as different images).

the average number of multiple detections is $P_{multiple} \approx 1$ for these operators which is much better in comparison to the other operators (note the different units on the left and right side of the diagram). The results for the operators on the basis of the CT images are comparable (see Hartkens et al. [233]-[235]).

In total, we have analyzed 242 synthetic and 43 real images, where image here means subimage volumes (ROIs) around the considered landmarks. In summary, the operators *Op3, Rohr3D, Förstner3D* yield the best results while *Op3* and *Rohr3D* show superior performance.

3.3.3   Detection Performance Visualization and Measure ψ

The semi-automatic procedure for 3D landmark localization as described in Section 2.1.3 above can be applied most efficiently and reliably if the number of false detections is small (in the ideal case there should be only one correct detection), but moreover if the operator response of the correct detection is much larger than the operator responses corresponding to the false detections. Then, we can sort the landmark candidates on the basis of the operator response beginning with the largest response and generally the first candidate is correct. Sorting thus simplifies the selection of candidates. In comparison to the study of the detection performance in Section 3.3.2 above, we here take into account the strengths of the operator responses at the detections. Note, that landmark candidates with very low operator responses can be excluded by applying a relatively low threshold. However, since still there would be false detections left, such a procedure would not principally solve the problem of landmark selection. Also note, that since we deal with 3D images, which are displayed on a slice-by-slice basis in practice, it is generally difficult to distinguish false detections from correct detections. In the 2D case, the selection is generally no problem since, for example, we can mark all detections in the original image and display the whole result on the screen. To improve the selection procedure in the case of 3D images, below we describe a certain type of performance visualization and also introduce a quantitative performance measure (Rohr [437]).

3.3.3.1 Performance Visualization

To aid a user in distinguishing correct from false detections in the case of 3D images, we suggest to use a certain performance visualization which gives an indication of the detection performance. With this visualization we first compute the Euclidean distances $\|\mathbf{x}_i - \mathbf{x}_{ROI}\|_2$ between the positions $\mathbf{x}_i$ of the detected candidates and the manually specified center of the ROI, abbreviated by $\mathbf{x}_{ROI}$. Then, the computed distances are represented together with the operator responses (cf. Figures 3.30-3.32). Thus, this representation combines the information of the number of false detections with the significance of the detections. Also, we obtain an indication of how the locations of the detections are distributed w.r.t. $\mathbf{x}_{ROI}$. However, a disadvantage is that we loose the full information of the distribution in 3D space.

3.3.3.2 Performance Measure ψ

Whereas the performance visualization described above gives a visual impression, we are also interested in quantitative measures for the detection performance. One measure is the number of false detections, however, with this measure the strength of the operator responses is not taken into account. Instead, we suggest using another measure (Rohr [437]). Suppose we have a number of n detections within a ROI and let the operator responses be denoted by $R_i = Op(\mathbf{x}_i), i = 1...n$, where the maximal operator response is $R_{max} = Op(\mathbf{x}_{max})$. For the candidates a threshold may be applied

$$\Omega = \{\mathbf{x}_i | R_i \geq \epsilon \cdot R_{max}\}, \tag{3.117}$$

where ϵ is user-defined, e.g., $\epsilon = 0.01$. For this set of candidates we can compute the following measure

$$\psi = \begin{cases} 0 & n = 0 \\ \sum_{i=1}^{n} \dfrac{R_i}{R_{max}} & n \geq 1. \end{cases} \tag{3.118}$$

If there are no detections at all, then we have $\psi = 0$. Alternatively, if there is only one detection we obtain $\psi = 1$, and additional false detections with low operator responses yield a value of $\psi \approx 1$. In this case, the correct detection can clearly be distinguished from the false detections. On the other hand, if there are operator responses with similar values as the maximal operator response, then ψ is much larger than 1. Thus, in summary we here have a scalar quantity which gives an indication of the detection performance. Additionally, we can employ the mean value $\overline{\psi} = \psi/n$. In the case of several exclusively similar operator values, where we have $\psi \gg 1$, we obtain $\overline{\psi} \approx 1$. In the case of one strong response and a large number of low responses which also sum up to $\psi \gg 1$, we instead obtain $\overline{\psi} \ll 1$. Note, that for the operators $Op3$, $Op3'$, and $Op4$ the responses R_i are always larger or equal to zero and thus (3.118) can directly be applied. When computing ψ for operators which yield positive as well as negative responses, then absolute values of R_i should be used.

3.3.3.3   Experimental Results

We now apply the performance visualization and the measure ψ to assess the performance of 3D landmark operators. We focus on the class of operators which are based on only first order image derivatives, namely $Op3$, $Op3'$ (*Förstner3D*), and $Op4$ (*Rohr3D*), and which showed superior performance in the previous study in Section 3.3.2. The plots on the left side of Figure 3.30 show the detection performance visualization described above for three different anatomical landmarks within a 3D MR image of the human brain (on the right side are the results for another 3D MR dataset). The landmarks are located at the ventricular system and the skull base. We have used the operator $Op3$ and Gaussian derivative filters of $\sigma = 1.5$ to compute the partial derivatives of an image. The size of the ROI has been chosen to $21 \times 21 \times 21$ voxels and the center of the ROI is the position due to manual localization. Thus, we take the manually selected position as ground truth, although we know that this position may be prone to error. In our case, we have alleviated this problem by using landmark positions which have been specified in agreement with the judgement of three to four persons (no medical experts, however). To further reduce the subjectivity in our experiments we have used no thresholds at all. For the landmark on the top left of Figure 3.30 (external occipital protuberance), we see that we have a detected landmark candidate close to the manually specified position. However, we also have a number of false detections with relatively large responses. Thus, the detection performance for this landmark is relatively bad and it will be difficult and time-consuming for a user to select the correct candidate. Instead, for the landmark in the middle left of Figure 3.30 (tip of left frontal ventricular horn), we have a perfect detection result with only one strong candidate within the whole 3D ROI. For the landmark on the bottom left of Figure 3.30 (tip of left occipital ventricular horn), we essentially have two strong operator responses of similar values, where one of them is closer to the manually specified position. Inspection of the original image reveals that the double detection is due to the individual anatomy of the imaged person. Here, the occipital ventricular horn of this

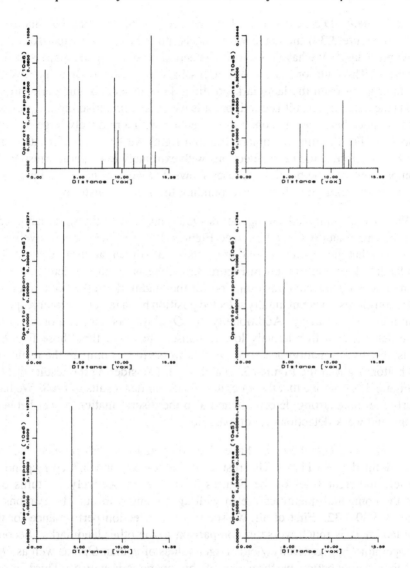

Figure 3.30.   Operator responses of *Op*3 for landmarks external occipital protuberance (top), left frontal ventricular horn (middle), and left occipital ventricular horn (bottom) in two different 3D MR datasets (left and right).

person actually is a 'double horn' consisting of two tips. We already discussed this deviation from normal anatomy in Section 2.2.1 above (see also Figure 2.6 above). In this case, both landmarks are suited for use in registration and the user has to decide which of the landmarks should be used. In Figure 3.30 on the right are displayed the results for the same landmarks as before but for a different 3D MR dataset. Here, we see that for the first landmark (top right of Figure 3.30) the detection result is much better in comparison to the previous dataset. We have one strong detection close to the manually specified position. The additional false detections have lower operator responses and are farer away from the landmark position. For the second landmark (middle right) the detection result is good, but it is worse in comparison to the previous dataset, since here we have one false detection with a relatively large operator response. For the third landmark (bottom right) we have a perfect detection result apart from some false detections with extremely low operator responses. Comparison with the previous dataset shows that we here have a unique tip of the occipital ventricular horn corresponding to 'normal' anatomy.

We have also applied the operators $Op3'$ and $Op4$ to the same landmarks and the same datasets as above (see Figures 3.31 and 3.32, respectively). It turns out, that the results of $Op3'$ are somewhat worse than those of $Op3$. For the landmark on the top left in Figure 3.31 there is no strong detection close to the manually selected position, and for the landmark on the bottom left the detection closest to the manually selected position has a lower operator response than the one farer away. Additionally, for $Op3'$ the operator responses of the false detections with relatively low responses are larger than those for $Op3$. Thus, the discrimination power of $Op3'$ is worse (e.g., compare the results on the bottom right of the Figures 3.30 and 3.31). Considering the results of $Op4$ in Figure 3.32, we see that this operator yields similar results as $Op3$. We have nearly the same strong detections and also the discrimination power between strong and weak detections is comparable.

For all examples above we have also computed the performance measure ψ as defined in (3.118). The results in Tables 3.2 and 3.3 correspond to the left and right sides of the Figures 3.30-3.32, respectively. It turns out, that the computed quantities are in well agreement with our observations in Figures 3.30-3.32. First of all, we see that the detection performance for the first landmark is much worse in comparison to the other landmarks. Second, the operator $Op3'$ generally yields larger values of ψ than $Op3$ as well as $Op4$ and thus the detection performance of this operator is worse. Third, it can also be seen that $Op3$ and $Op4$ yield very similar results. We also note, that the measure ψ is a much better performance characterization than the number of false detections alone. For example, for $Op3$ in Table 3.3 we have for the first and third landmark exactly the same number of false detections (7 false detections). However, the detection performance for the third landmark is much better than that for the first one, since for the third landmark the false detections have much lower operator responses than the correct detection. This fact is clearly quantified by the corresponding values of ψ which are in accordance with the performance visualizations on the top and bottom right of Figure 3.30.

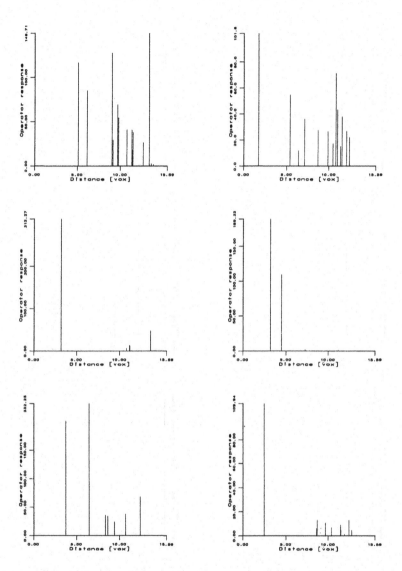

Figure 3.31. Same as Fig. 3.30 but for the operator *Op3'*.

In summary, we have seen that the detection performance strongly differs for different landmarks and thus some landmarks seem to be better suited for semi-automatic extraction than others. Also it turned out, that the operators *Op3* and *Op4* (*Rohr3D*) yield similar results and that they are superior to the operator *Op3'* (*Förstner3D*). These conclusions are confirmed by a more comprehensive study in Hartkens et al. [235],[231], where the measure ψ has been used to assess the performance of all nine 3D differential operators from

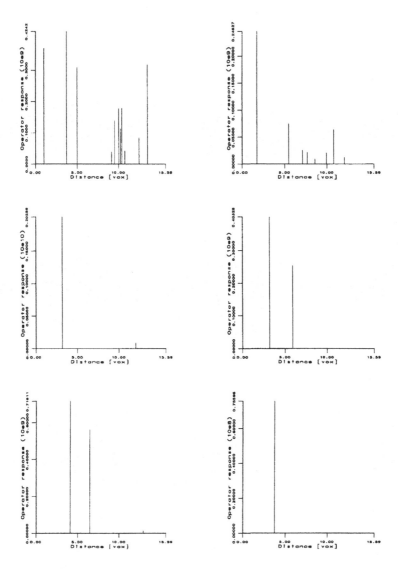

Figure 3.32.   Same as Fig. 3.30 but for the operator *Op*4.

Section 3.3.1 above. In Figure 3.33 we show the result for eight landmarks each
visible in four different 3D MR datasets (external occipital protuberance, tips
of the frontal, occipital, and temporal ventricular horns, as well as the junction
at the top of pons; note that the tips of the ventricular horns are visible in both
brain hemispheres and thus count double). The figure shows the mean values
over all landmarks as well as all MR images. ROIs of size $20 \times 20 \times 20$ voxels
around the landmarks have been used. It can clearly be seen that the results

Landmark	Op3	Op3'	Op4
external occipital protuberance	4.82	6.38	5.17
frontal ventricular horn	1.01	1.31	1.04
occipital ventricular horn	2.14	2.93	1.81

Table 3.2. Performance measure ψ for landmarks in a 3D MR dataset.

Landmark	Op3	Op3'	Op4
external occipital protuberance	2.58	4.84	1.93
frontal ventricular horn	1.56	1.60	1.63
occipital ventricular horn	1.06	1.62	1.01

Table 3.3. Same as Tab. 3.2 but for a different 3D MR dataset.

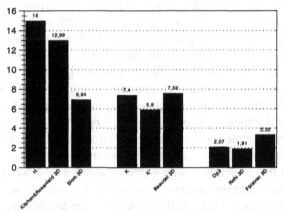

Figure 3.33. Detection performance measure ψ for nine 3D operators in the case of MR images (mean values over different landmarks as well as different images).

of the operators *Op3*, *Op4* (*Rohr3D*), and *Op3'* (*Förstner3D*) are much better than the results of the other operators (note that $\psi = 1$ is the ideal case). It also turns out that *Op3* and *Op4* are superior to *Op3'*.

3.3.3.4 Improvement of the Detection Performance

The performance visualization as described above is also useful to study the effectiveness of modifications and extensions of the landmark operators. Below, we consider two possibilities to improve the detection performance. First, we study the resulting detections in scale space to see whether the performance can be improved by adjusting an optimal scale. Second, we employ additional knowledge about the geometry and the intensities at a landmark to improve the performance.

So far, we have applied the 3D landmark operators while using a constant width of the derivative filters. However, for tiny landmarks generally a smaller filter is more adequate, while for extended landmarks a larger filter is optimal. Below, we thus study the detection performance as a function of the width of the derivative filters, i.e., we perform a *scale space* analysis. In our case, we use 3D Gaussian filters of $\sigma = 0.5, 1, 1.5, 2, 2.5$, and 3, where σ denotes the standard deviation. The considered region-of-interest (ROI) has been set to $21 \times 21 \times 21$ voxels around a manually specified landmark position. As an example, we show in Figure 3.34 the results of the operator $Op3$ for the landmark 'frontal ventricular horn' in a 3D MR image. We see that for filter widths of $\sigma = 0.5$ and 1 (top-left and top-right, respectively) there are false detections with significant operator responses besides the correct detection. Using a filter width of $\sigma = 1.5$, however, we have a perfect detection result with only one strong detection. Further increasing the filter width also yields a good detection result, but the position of the detection is displaced away from the correct position. Thus, in this case a filter width of $\sigma = 1.5$ would be optimal. Another example is given in Figure 3.35 which shows the result of $Op3$ for the landmark 'occipital ventricular horn'. Also here, a filter width of $\sigma = 0.5$ is too small since we obtain several significant detections. For $\sigma = 1$ and 1.5 we have essentially two strong detections. These two detections correspond to the 'double horn' which actually has two tips and which we have already discussed above. For $\sigma = 2$ and 2.5 one of these strong detections becomes dominant while for $\sigma = 3$ only one strong detection remains. On the other hand, for values of $\sigma \geq 1.5$ the localization error increases significantly. In summary, in this example a filter width of about $\sigma = 1$ would be optimal. Generally, we saw that the detection performance improves when increasing the size of the Gaussian filter. At the same time, the localization performance gets worse. Thus, to select an optimal σ one has to make a compromise between these two effects. These effects have clearly been observed with the introduced performance visualization.

Another approach to reduce the number of false detections is to use *additional knowledge* about the geometry as well as the intensity variations of landmarks (Frantz et al. [180],[182]). For landmark detection we first apply the operator $Op3$. This operator detects general points of high intensity variations or, more precisely, points of minimal localization uncertainty (Section 2.5.5). However, with our semi-automatic procedure we know in advance which landmark we want to localize, i.e., whether we have a tip or a saddle. Actually, these two types can be distinguished on the basis of the principal curvatures of isocontours. For a tip both principal curvatures have the same sign (the Gaussian curvature is positive), while for a saddle they have opposite signs (the Gaussian curvature is negative), see Section 2.4. Additionally, if we know the image modality (e.g., MR or CT) as well as certain imaging parameters (e.g., T_1- or T_2-

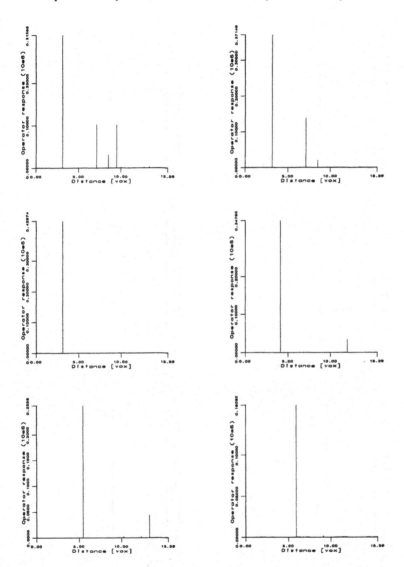

Figure 3.34. Operator responses of *Op*3 in scale space ($\sigma = 0.5, 1, 1.5, 2, 2.5, 3$) for the landmark 'frontal ventricular horn' in a 3D MR image.

weighting for MR images) which is generally the case, then we can exploit this additional knowledge, too. For a tip we then can decide whether we have a dark tip or a bright tip (on a bright or dark background, respectively). This distinction on the 'polarity' of landmarks can also be made using the principal curvatures. In the first case the principal curvatures are both positive, and in the second case they are both negative. For saddle points such a

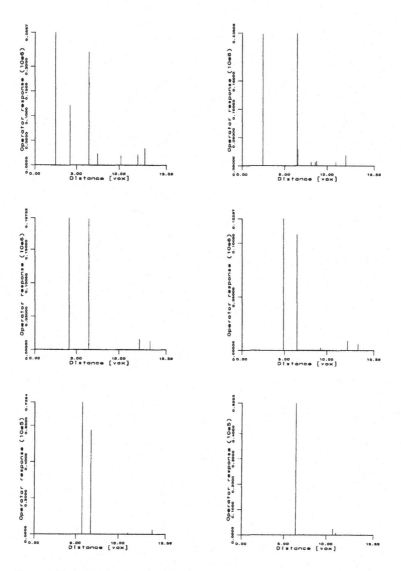

Figure 3.35.   Same as Fig. 3.34 but for the landmark 'occipital ventricular horn'.

distinction is not possible. In summary, this approach is a combination of the 3D corner operator approach (Section 2.5) with the approach based on isocontour curvature information (Section 2.4). We now show examples of applying the combined approach to the detection of the landmarks 'tip of 4th ventricle roof' and 'saddle point at zygomatic bone'. Figure 3.36 shows the detection result of applying the operator $Op3$ alone, and in Figure 3.37 are the remaining detections when utilizing additional knowledge about the geometry

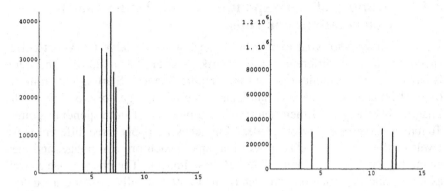

Figure 3.36.   Detection performance for landmark 'tip of 4th ventricle roof' (left) and 'saddle point at zygomatic bone' (right).

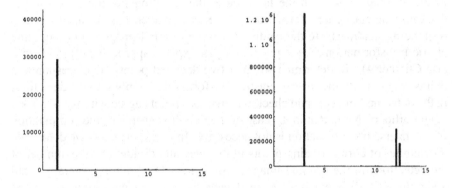

Figure 3.37.   Same as Fig. 3.36 but with incorporation of additional knowledge about the geometry and polarity.

as well as the polarity of the landmarks. We see that the number of false detections has been reduced significantly by employing additional knowledge, while the detection close to the landmark is preserved. The improvement is also reflected by the performance measure ψ. For the first landmark this measure changed from $\psi = 5.65$ to $\psi = 1.00$, and for the second landmark we have a change from $\psi = 2.11$ to $\psi = 1.39$ (note, that $\psi = 1$ is the ideal case). For further investigations using this approach to the reduction of false detections, see Frantz et al. [180]-[182].

3.3.4   Number of Corresponding Points Under Elastic Deformations and Noise

We now analyze to what extent the 3D operators are able to extract corresponding points in different images (Hartkens et al. [233]–[235]). The study is based on 3D synthetic and 3D tomographic images. Starting out from the original images with specified landmarks, we add image noise or deform the images elastically, and then determine the number of corresponding points. To reduce the probability of accidental matches we apply three different noise levels or three different elastic deformations to each original image, and then count the corresponding points in all of these images. The image noise as well as the elastic deformations are determined automatically utilizing a random generator. In the experiments w.r.t. the image noise the random generator is applied to the image intensities, while in the experiments w.r.t. the elastic deformations the random generator is applied to the positions of the landmarks in the original image. In the latter case, the resulting positions are used to determine an elastic transformation, where we consider these positions as corresponding landmarks to the landmarks in the original image. For computing elastic transformations we apply a thin-plate spline approach [49],[443] (see also Chapter 4). To determine whether two detected points are corresponding points we compute the inverse elastic transformation, apply it to the detections in the deformed images, and check whether two points agree within a $3 \times 3 \times 3$ neighborhood. Note, that in the case of the noise experiments, the computation of the inverse transformation is not necessary. In all experiments we determine the number of corresponding points in this way and divide it by the number of the detections in the original images. Since the 3D operators generally yield a significantly different number of detections, this normalization makes the results better comparable.

We have applied this evaluation scheme to 3D synthetic images of tetrahedra, ellipsoids, and hyperbolic paraboloids. From this study it turns out that the operators *Op3*, *Op4 (Rohr3D)*, and *Op3' (Förstner3D)* yield the best result among the investigated nine 3D operators (see also Section 3.3.1). The operator K^* (gradient-weighted Gaussian curvature) performs also well. Significantly worse in comparison to the other operators are the operators H (mean curvature) and K (Gaussian curvature). The results in the case of 3D MR images are shown in Figure 3.38. As above we have investigated eight landmarks in four different 3D MR datasets. The part of experiments dealing with image noise reveals that the operators *Op3*, *Op4*, and *Op3'* are best, while *Blom3D* and K^* also perform well (Figure 3.38 on the top). Under elastic deformations the operators *Op3* and *Op4* yield the best results. The operators *Blom3D*, K^*, *Blom3D*, and *Op3'* are somewhat worse (Figure 3.38 on the bottom). Interestingly, the results of the operators H and K are not so bad as in the case of synthetic images. An explanation is that these operators detect a very large number of points,

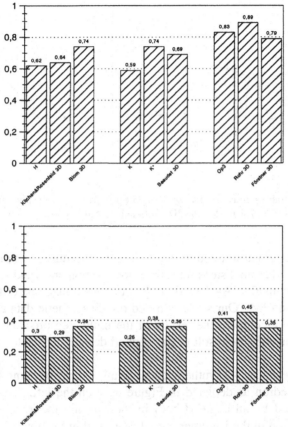

Figure 3.38.   Mean values of the fraction of corresponding points in 3D MR images under image noise (top) and elastic deformations (bottom).

particularly when there is noise in the image (which we always have in real images). Therefore, a large number of points correspond randomly. For 3D CT images we obtained comparable results.

In summary, it turns out that the operators based on only first order image derivatives ($Op3$, $Op4$, and $Op3'$) yield the best result while $Op3$ and $Op4$ are superior. This finding agrees with a previous study of the performance of the corresponding 2D operators on the basis of 2D synthetic as well as 2D tomographic images (Hartkens et al. [232]).

3.3.5 Localization Accuracy

Having studied the detection performance and the number of corresponding points of 3D landmark operators, we now analyze the localization accuracy. In this section, we consider the multi-step procedures for refined landmark

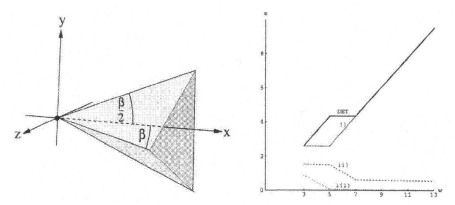

Figure 3.39.   Tetrahedron as a model of a sharp tip (left) and localization error e for a 3D detection operator (DET) as well as the 3D multi-step procedures i), ii), and iii) (right).

localization described in Section 2.5.7. These procedures combine landmark detection with additional steps for refined localization and yield subvoxel positions of 3D landmarks. As detection operators we utilize one of the operators $Op3$, $Op3'$, and $Op4$. Our study is based on 3D synthetic data as well as 3D MR images. We compare the results of the multi-step procedures with each other as well as with the result of the applied detection operator (Frantz et al. [176]–[179]).

First we investigate 3D synthetic data. To this end we have modelled a sharp tip by a tetrahedron as depicted in Figure 3.39 on the left. The tetrahedron is parameterized by an angle β both in the xy- and the xz-plane, and is a 3D generalization of the L-corner model described in Section 3.2.1 above (see also Figure 3.3). In Figure 3.39 on the right are the localization results for an aperture angle of $\beta = 90^o$, which corresponds to the corner of a cube. We have determined the localization errors e as a function of the window width w which specifies the volume over which the first order image derivatives are averaged. Window sizes of $3 \times 3 \times 3$ up to $13 \times 13 \times 13$ voxels have been used. As detection operator (DET) we have applied the operator $Op3'$. Note, that the operators $Op3$, $Op3'$, and $Op4$ yielded comparable localization results in our experiments. For DET as well as the multi-step procedure i) it can be seen that the localization error increases linearly with increasing the window width. Instead, for the multi-step procedures ii) and iii) (which include the differential edge intersection approach as described in Section 2.5.7), the error decreases with increasing window width and the localization accuracy is significantly better in comparison to that of DET and i). These results are analogous to the 2D case (see Section 3.2.1). We have also analyzed the localization accuracy for an ell ɔsoid, which is a model for a rounded tip. Also here, the performance of the ɔrocedures ii) and iii) is significantly better than that of DET and i).

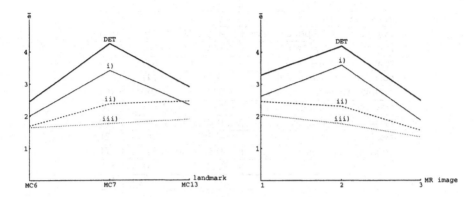

Figure 3.40. Mean localization errors $\bar{e}$ of the detection operator alone (DET) and the multi-step procedures i), ii), and iii) separately for each landmark (left) and for each MR image (right).

However, the accuracy of ii) and iii) depends more strongly on the chosen window width. For large window widths the localization error increases, since the approximation by tangent planes gets worse (see Section 2.5.7 above).

Next, we analyze the approaches for the case of 3D MR images of the human head. As landmarks we have used the tips of the frontal, occipital, and temporal horns of the ventricular system in three different MR datasets (see Figure 2.11 above). The localization accuracy has been plotted in Figure 3.40 separately for each landmark and for each MR image. We have computed the mean values $\bar{e}$ of the Euclidean distances (in voxel units) from the localized positions to manually specified positions, which we consider as ground truth. Note, that these reference positions have been determined in agreement of three to four persons to alleviate subjectivity. The mean values have been computed over all landmarks and datasets as well as for window widths $w = 3$ and $w = 5$. It can be seen that the multi-step procedures significantly improve the localization accuracy in comparison to applying a detection operator alone (DET). As detection operator we have used $Op3$. In the mean, the approaches i), ii) and iii) yield an improvement of $0.93vox$, $1.14vox$, and $1.52vox$ w.r.t. DET, respectively, where vox denotes spatial unity. An example of the localized positions in a 3D MR image has been provided in Figure 2.36 in Section 2.5.7 above.

3.3.6 Affine Registration Accuracy

In this section, we briefly describe an experiment, where we have used the semi-automatically localized landmarks as corresponding features for the registration of 3D MR and CT images of the human brain. In this experiment,

Landmark	$(\Delta x, \Delta y, \Delta z)$	e
4th ventricle roof	(1.73, 0.62, 0.42)	1.882
external occipital protuberance	(-0.63, 2.00, 0.45)	2.143
frontal ventricular horn, l	(0.44, -0.46, -0.40)	0.754
frontal ventricular horn, r	(-0.40, -0.47, 0.64)	0.887
occipital ventricular horn, l	(-0.12, -0.37, 0.14)	0.409
occipital ventricular horn, r	(-0.20, -0.12, -0.28)	0.364
temporal ventricular horn, r	(0.17, -2.04, -1.42)	2.490
zygomatic bone, l	(-0.28, 1.35, -0.59)	1.494
zygomatic bone, r	(-0.39, 2.20, 1.37)	2.621
processus mastoideus, l	(-0.31, -1.45, 0.52)	1.571
processus mastoideus, r	(0.00, -1.26, -0.84)	1.518
$\bar{e}$		1.467

Table 3.4.   Affine registration with 11 landmarks semi-automatically localized using $Op3$.

we have applied the operator $Op3$ and Gaussian derivative filters of $\sigma = 1.5$. The investigated MR dataset consists of 120 axial slices of 256×256 voxels resolution, and the CT dataset consists of 87 axial slices of 320×320 voxels resolution. The images represent the brain of the same person. We have used the following anatomical point landmarks: topmost concavity of fourth ventricle roof, external occipital protuberance, tip of frontal, occipital, and temporal ventricular horn, saddle point at zygomatic bone, as well as saddle point at processus mastoideus. The last five landmarks can be found in both hemispheres of the human brain. Note, that for the used CT dataset, the tip of the left temporal ventricular horn was significantly worse pronounced in comparison to the other landmarks, therefore we did not consider this landmark further. In total, we thus have a number of 11 homologous landmarks. To assess the registration accuracy on the basis of the localized landmarks we have applied an optimal affine transformation model. We hereby assume that an affine transformation model well approximates the true transformation. Note also, that the registration accuracy only checks the global consistency of the landmarks according to the applied transformation model. However, using 11 landmarks and an optimal affine transformation model we obtained a good registration result with a mean Euclidean error at the landmarks of $\bar{e} \approx 1.5$ voxels, where the individual errors at the landmarks varied between 0.4 and 2.6 voxels (see Table 3.4). Recently, we have performed a more systematic evaluation using a larger number of 3D MR and CT images and where different observers were involved (see Frantz et al. [181] as well as Section 3.4 below).

3.3.7   Projective Invariants

In the previous section, we have used the global consistency of localized 3D anatomical landmarks in two datasets under affine transformations as performance criterion. In this section, we analyze the consistency of localized 2D corners of 3D polyhedral objects. Thus, we now have to deal with projective transformations. We describe an approach to evaluate the performance of 2D corner operators which is based on *projective invariants* of 3D objects (Heyden and Rohr [242]). In comparison to our previous study on the localization accuracy for single points (L-corners) in Rohr [430] (Section 3.2.1), we here analyze sets of points. The considered points are corners of 3D polyhedral objects, e.g., L-, T-, Y-, and Arrow-corners. In comparison, Coelho et al. [98] applied projective invariants of planar (2D) objects (e.g., the cross ratio) to compare the performance of corner detectors. While they have considered three indirect corner detectors (which rely on prior extraction of edge points), we here investigate five direct schemes to corner extraction.

Our approach has the advantage that we do not need to know the true positions of the corners in the image, which is important since ground truth for real images is generally not available. Thus, the camera need not to be calibrated and the relative position and orientation between the camera and the considered 3D object need not to be known. Based on the used projective invariants we can determine consistency conditions, which the extracted point sets have to fulfill for a valid 3D interpretation. To assess the efficiency of the different corner extraction schemes we compute the variances (or standard deviations) w.r.t. the consistency conditions.

3.3.7.1 Investigated corner extraction schemes

We analyze the performance of five different direct schemes to corner extraction. The first scheme is manual selection of corners, which means that the corner positions are specified by hand. Second, we use the differential (local) corner operator of Kitchen and Rosenfeld [280], which consists of first and second order image derivatives (see also Section 2.5.1 above). As a third scheme we use the same operator but apply it to the nonlinearly diffused image instead of using the original image. Nonlinear diffusion approaches reduce the amount of noise, while at the same time try to preserve the systematic intensity variations. This reduces the noise sensitivity of the local operator. In our case, we apply the nonlinear diffusion approach of Schnörr [469]. As a fourth scheme, we apply the model-based approach of Rohr [425]-[427],[440], where a parametric corner model is directly fitted to the image (see also Section 2.6 above). The fifth scheme consists of applying this model fitting scheme to the nonlinearly diffused original image.

The effect of nonlinear diffusion on the result of the model fitting approach is demonstrated by Figures 3.41 and 3.42. In Figure 3.41 are given 3D plots of the fitted model (right) in comparison to the original intensities (left) for the top-left Arrow-corner in Figure 3.44. The nonlinear diffused image is shown in Figure 3.42 on the left, while the model fitted to the nonlinearly diffused

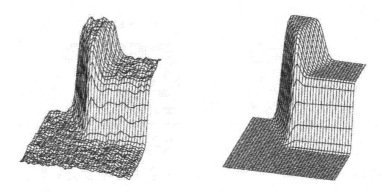

Figure 3.41.   3D plot of the Arrow-corner on the top-left in Fig. 3.44: original image (left) and fitted model (right).

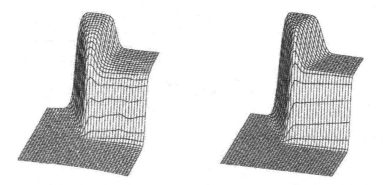

Figure 3.42.   3D plot of the Arrow-corner on the top-left in Fig. 3.44: nonlinear diffused image (left) and fitted model to the nonlinear diffused image (right).

image is shown on the right. It can be seen that the nonlinear diffused structure and the fitted model look very similar. However, the transitions of the fitted model are in both cases somewhat sharper than the transitions of the nonlinear diffused structure.

3.3.7.2 Approach

Depending on the a priori knowledge about objects in the scene, different invariants and thus different consistency conditions can be used. In our case, we consider the two objects depicted in Figures 3.43 and 3.44. For the truncated cube in Figure 3.43 we only assume that the four visible surfaces are planar. This condition can be formulated mathematically by the so called S-matrix (e.g., Heyden [241]). For the L-shaped object in Figure 3.44 we use two different

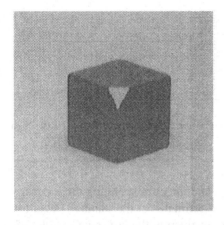

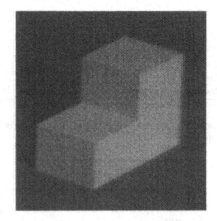

Figure 3.43. Image of a truncated cube.   *Figure 3.44.* Image of an L-shaped object.

levels of a priori knowledge. In the first case (I), we assume that the shape of the faces is known, for example, some faces are rectangular. In the second case (II), we use a complete model of the imaged object. As performance measure of the corner extraction schemes we compute the variances (or standard deviations) w.r.t. the different consistency conditions. For more details see Heyden and Rohr [242].

3.3.7.3 Results

All five corner extraction schemes have been applied to the images of the truncated cube and the L-shaped object in Figures 3.43 and 3.44. For the truncated cube image the estimated standard deviations of these schemes have been listed in Table 3.5. It turns out, that the best result is obtained with the model fitting approach followed by model fitting in conjunction with nonlinear diffusion, manual selection, local operator together with nonlinear diffusion, and local operator. It appears that nonlinear diffusion as a preprocessing step increases the accuracy of the local operator by a factor of three while the accuracy of the model fitting approach decreases slightly. In the case of the L-shaped object in Figure 3.44 we have applied two different consistency tests (denoted by I and II). The result is listed in Table 3.5. Also for this image and the two consistency tests the best result is obtained with the model fitting approach followed by model fitting in conjunction with nonlinear diffusion, manual selection, local operator together with nonlinear diffusion, and local operator. Nonlinear diffusion increases the accuracy of the local operator while the accuracy of the model fitting approach decreases slightly. For a more detailed discussion of the results see [242].

Type	Manually	Local op. (Kitchen/R.)	Local op. & nonlin. diff.	Model fitting (Rohr)	Model fitting & nonlin. diff.
Truncated cube	0.2571	1.5750	0.4564	0.1690	0.2486
L-shaped obj., I	0.7290	1.9395	1.7015	0.6057	0.6710
L-shaped obj., II	0.5869	1.6451	1.4799	0.4852	0.5587
Average	0.6493	1.7892	1.5624	0.5379	0.6060

Table 3.5. Estimated standard deviations (in pixels) for the five different corner extraction schemes.

Taking all estimates for the two images and the corresponding three consistency tests together, we obtain the averaged estimates of the standard deviation of the different corner extraction schemes as given in the last row of Table 3.5. For the model fitting approach the standard deviation turns out to be about 0.5 pixels. Model fitting in conjunction with nonlinear diffusion and manual selection are somewhat worse and the accuracy of the local operator is about three times worse than the model fitting approach.

3.4   Summary and Conclusion

We have described our studies on the validation and evaluation of 2D and 3D landmark operators. Central to our studies is the modelling of the signal structure of landmarks. We either have modelled the geometry of the contour of landmarks (surface of organs) or have established intensity models based on radiometric models. The models serve as a basis for the analytic studies and also for the experimental investigations, where we have used synthetic test data. Synthetic data is necessary, since here we have reliable ground truth in comparison to real image data.

In our analytic studies we have analyzed the localization accuracy of 2D corner operators and have also studied the minimal localization uncertainty under image noise for 2D and 3D image features (e.g., edges, lines, ridges, corners, rectangles, circular landmarks, blobs, boxes).

In the experimental studies, we have assessed the performance of the 3D differential landmark operators introduced in Chapter 2. On the basis of 3D synthetic data as well as 3D MR and CT images, we have carried out different studies employing different performance criteria and different performance measures. We have analyzed the detection performance, the number of corresponding points under elastic deformations and noise, the localization accuracy as well as the affine registration accuracy. Partly, the operators yielded significantly different results. We also saw that the performance depends on the specific landmark (e.g., frontal vs. temporal ventricular horn) as well as on the landmark type (e.g., tip or saddle). Overall, it turned out that the operators based on only first order image derivatives ($Op3$, $Op3'$, and $Op4$) yield the best results while $Op3$ and $Op4$ are superior among these three. Among the operators based on first and second order image derivatives the operator K^* (gradient-weighted Gaussian curvature) performs best. Generally, the Gaussian curvature based approach is superior to the mean curvature based approach. In another study [30], we have compared the performance of the operators based on the mean and Gaussian curvature with ridge-line based operators (e.g., [521]), which are computationally more expensive. There, the operator K^* yielded comparable results as the ridge-line based operators. Thus, we conclude that the operators based on only first order image derivatives are best among all existing 3D differential operators. We also demonstrated that 3D multi-step procedures can significantly improve the localization accuracy.

Finally, we have utilized projective invariants for performance characterization of 2D corner operators. There it turned out, that parametric approaches are superior to differential approaches.

Recently, we have performed a validation study to compare the performance of our semi-automatic procedure for landmark localization with manual landmark localization (Frantz et al. [181]). In this study, five different observers localized the landmarks for the purpose of intra-subject MR-CT registration (applying a rigid transformation). In the semi-automatic procedure we used the operator $Op3$ together with schemes for automatic ROI size selection and reduction of false detections (Frantz et al. [178],[180],[182]) as briefly mentioned in Sections 2.5.7 and 3.3.3 above. For the semi-automatic procedure in comparison to the manual procedure it turned out, that while the registration results have comparable quality, the elapsed time is significantly reduced and also the inter-observer variability in the landmark positions is smaller.

Chapter 4

Elastic Registration of Multimodality Images

Image registration (or image matching) denotes the task of finding an optimal *geometric transformation* between corresponding image data. A geometric transformation puts the images in spatial correspondence, i.e., we are searching a mapping that transforms all points of one image onto the (physically) corresponding points of another image. Note, that we are searching a spatial transformation, but not a mapping between the image intensities.

In this chapter, we are particularly interested in the registration of images from different modalities. These images are generally acquired from different sensors and represent different information of the same object or of different objects. Examples of *multimodality images* are shown in Figure 4.1, which all represent slices of the human brain (for details see below). The depicted images generally represent *complementary information* which can be accessed more easily and accurately if the images have been spatially aligned, i.e. have been put in one coordinate system for the purpose of *image fusion*. Whereas here we will focus on the registration of 2D and 3D tomographic images of the human brain, i.e., spatial images, the subsequently presented approach is also applicable to images from other domains as well as to images of arbitrary dimensions. Note, that the term image registration as defined above is very general and actually subsumes a number of classical tasks in computer vision, e.g., motion analysis, stereo-reconstruction, and structure-from-motion (e.g., [512]). There, typically 2D images of the *same* modality (monomodal images) are analyzed and a central task is to determine *image correspondences,* i.e., also there a geometric transformation has to be computed. Note also, that the finding of correspondences between multimodality images raises major difficulties in comparison to monomodal images, since multimodality images generally represent complementary structures and information.

179

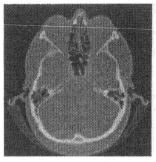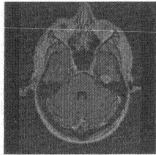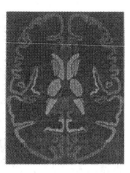

Figure 4.1.   Slices from 3D multimodality datasets of the human brain: CT (left), MR (middle), and digital atlas (right).

Generally, images to be registered have to be aligned globally as well as locally. This means that the mapping has to comprise a global rigid or affine transformation, for example, as well as a locally adaptive transformation which allows to cope with local differences (cf. Figure 4.2). In our case, we study a special class of locally adaptive nonlinear transformations, namely *elastic transformations*. These transformations are based on models from elasticity theory, which describe a continuous reversible deformation that preserves topology, e.g., cracks do not occur. Generally, we have an energy functional which has to be minimized (e.g., [268]). The central idea behind such type of approach is to consider images as continuous bodies and to model the geometric differences between images such that they have been caused by an elastic deformation. This approach has been pioneered by Bajcsy et al. [18],[20]. For earlier related approaches based on 'rubber sheets', which have been proposed for object recognition, see Fischler and Elschlager [153] and Widrow [560] (see also Section 1.5 above on deformable models). As an alternative to elastic models, models from fluid mechanics have been proposed by Christensen et al. [91]. Fluid models are much more flexible. However, the significantly larger flexibility is also a disadvantage since it is a problem to constrain the mapping. Speaking in physical terms, very large volumes of matter may stream through very small areas from one region to another, which is not the case with elastic transformations ([409]).

In this chapter, we describe a *model-based approach* to elastic image registration. In our context the meaning of model-based is twofold. Primarily, we present an elastic transformation model which is flexible enough to represent a sufficiently large variety of possible deformations occurring in practical applications, including particularly local deformations. The deformations describable by this *model-based registration* approach comprise deformations of a single brain as well as differences due to the variability between different

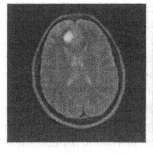 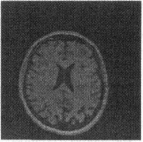 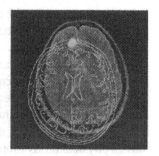

Figure 4.2. Registration problem: Human brain MR images of different persons with different imaging parameters (left and middle), and overlay of the first image with edges of the second image (right).

brains. Note, that the physical basis for these two cases principally differs. In the first case, the deformations are generally caused by the influence of forces and can be modelled by applying methods from elasticity theory. In the second case, however, a physically-based description of the occurring variability is rather unclear. While growth models could serve as a basis for a possible explanation, research in this direction is only at the beginning (e.g., Bro-Nielsen et al. [70]). In addition to these two principal cases of deformations, our elastic model can also be applied in the case of other geometric deformations, e.g., patient- and scanner-induced distortions. Thus, we consider our approach as a general tool for image registration whenever local adaptation is required. The model is *physically-motivated* and the general assumption is that the depicted objects have the same topological structure.

The second meaning of model-based in this chapter is related to a further main application of elastic image registration, namely the registration of images with digital atlases (e.g., Mazziotta et al. [336]). Here, we have a digital model of human anatomy, which has to be matched to the image of a patient. Such an approach can be considered as *model-based segmentation* since it allows to localize hardly visible or even non-visible anatomical structures in clinical images. The segmentation based on image-atlas registration either may be regarded as the final segmentation result or may also be the starting point for a subsequent improved data-driven segmentation. Note, that such a refinement step is only feasible in the case of visible structures.

For both of these main tasks of model-based registration and model-based segmentation, we suggest a *nonparametric* approach which uses corresponding point landmarks as image features (for a characterization of nonparametric schemes see Section 1.6 above). The approach is based on a minimizing functional for which a unique (exact) *analytic solution* can be stated. Actually, the solution consists of a *parametric* model, where the number of parameters depends on the number of the used landmarks. Approaches of this type are studied in the mathematical fields of calculus of variations and approximation theory (e.g., [545],[146],[323]). Since we have an analytic solution w.r.t. a minimizing functional our approach principally differs from those approaches to elastic registration that *numerically* solve a minimizing functional, for example, by applying finite differences (FD) or the finite element method (FEM) (e.g., Bajcsy and Kovačič [20], Christensen et al. [91], Davatzikos et al. [111], Peckar et al. [394]). Our approach uses certain splines, namely *thin-plate splines*, which have a physical motivation. The approach is embedded in a sound mathematical framework (Duchon [130], Wahba [545]) and the described extensions of the approach share the same basic properties. Also, the solution has a statistical interpretation as Bayes estimate. More practical advantages of the approach are computational efficiency, robustness, and generality w.r.t. different types and dimensions of images and atlases. Moreover, the approach is well-suited for user-interaction which in our opinion is important in clinical applications. Previously, thin-plate splines have been used in computer vision for surface reconstruction (e.g., Boult and Kender [56], Terzopoulos [517]). Medical image registration based on thin-plate splines has first been proposed by Bookstein [49]. Evans et al. [147], for example, applied such an approach to 3D images. Our main contribution is the incorporation of landmark localization errors, which is a step towards improved fault-tolerance in point-based elastic registration. This is important in practical applications, since landmark extraction is always prone to error. In our approach, we can cope with isotropic as well as anisotropic errors and we estimate the landmark localization uncertainty directly from the images. For a more detailed discussion of related work see particularly Section 4.9 below.

In the following, we first give some background and further motivation (Section 4.1). After that, we describe in more detail those clinical applications, which generally require the use of locally adaptive transformations (Section 4.2). Then, we introduce our approach to elastic image registration. We start with a description of the basic approach (Section 4.3) and relate it to elasticity theory (Section 4.4). Then, we introduce generalizations of the approach (Sections 4.5-4.7). Experimental results are presented for 2D as well as 3D multimodality images of the human brain. Finally, we briefly describe the problem of biomechanical modelling of brain deformations (Section 4.8), give a more detailed and comprehensive overview of related work (Section 4.9), and conclude the chapter with a summary and a description of future work (Section 4.10).

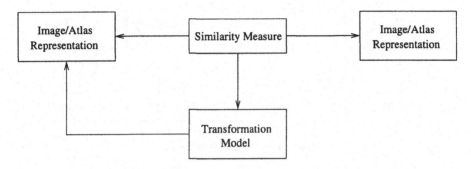

Figure 4.3.   General scheme for registration.

4.1 Background and Motivation

A key issue in medical applications is the registration of images from different modalities, e.g., MR (Magnetic Resonance), CT (X-ray Computed Tomography), and PET (Positron Emission Tomography) images, as well as the registration of images with digital atlas representations. The general task is to accurately match multimodality images such that the complementary information of the different datasets can be combined. In the case of atlases it is possible to exploit existing medical knowledge, which currently is mainly represented in textbook form. In either case, the central goal is to increase the accuracy of localizing anatomical structures in 3D space which is of fundamental importance in computer-assisted neurosurgery and radiotherapy. In this section, we give some further background and motivation w.r.t. image registration and also state the main characteristics of our point-based elastic registration scheme. For surveys on general registration methods or medical image registration, we refer to, e.g., Gerlot and Bizais [191], Brown [73], van den Elsen et al. [143], Maurer and Fitzpatrick [334], Verbeeck [538], Rohr [432],[439], Ayache [11], Viergever et al. [539], Lavallée [301], Mazziotta et al. [336], Glasbey and Mardia [196], Grenander and Miller [206], Maintz and Viergever [321], Lester and Arridge [308], Meijering et al. [338], and Toga [529]. For other surveys in medical image analysis, see also, e.g., Höhne [250],[253], Stiehl [501], Barillot et al. [23], Stytz et al. [504], Kuhn et al. [291],[31], Toennies [528], Grimson et al. [209],[210], Robb [421], Taylor et al. [516], Koslow and Huerta [288], Lehmann et al. [304], Lohmann [314], Shahidi et al. [481], Viergever [540], Handels [223], as well as Duncan and Ayache [134].

4.1.1 General Registration Scheme

A general scheme of medical image registration is depicted in Figure 4.3 (see also Rohr [432]). Generally, we want to register image or atlas representations with each other. While image-image registration has been investigated for a

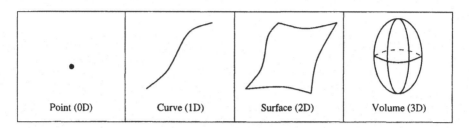

| Point (0D) | Curve (1D) | Surface (2D) | Volume (3D) |

Figure 4.4.   Types of landmarks.

longer time, the registration of images with atlases has only recently gained increased attention. If the development of different computerized atlases proceeds, it will also be important to register atlases with each other.

In each of these applications one has to decide which kind of *image/atlas information* should be used for registration and how this information should be represented. Often geometric features, denoted as landmarks, are used which can be represented by points (0D), curves (1D), surfaces (2D), or volumes (3D) (see Figure 4.4 as well as Chapter 2). Besides the location and the geometry, these features may also be characterized by additional attributes. For example, point features can additionally be specified by the direction of the intensity gradient. Alternatively to using landmarks, one can also directly exploit the image intensities or use a combination of landmarks and intensities.

Having specified the image/atlas information we next have to decide which class of *transformation* between the different representations should be used. If we apply a *rigid* transformation, then the accuracy of the resulting match often is not satisfactory w.r.t. clinical applications (see also Section 4.2 below). Rigid transformations preserve the distance between any two points x_1, x_2 of an object, i.e., $|u(x_2) - u(x_1)| = |x_2 - x_1|$, where u denotes the transformation. Thus, these transformations can only correct for translational and rotational differences:

$$u(x) = Rx + T, \qquad (4.1)$$

where R is an orthogonal matrix ($R^T = R^{-1}$) with $det R = 1$ and T is the translation vector. Rigid transformations are specified by 3 or 6 parameters in the 2D and 3D case, respectively. In general, however, *nonrigid* transformations are required to cope with the variations between datasets. With these transformations the distance between any two points of an object in general changes. A special class of general nonrigid transformations are *affine* transformations

$$u(x) = Ax + T, \qquad (4.2)$$

which consist of a *linear* transformation and a translation. They are specified by 6 or 12 parameters in the 2D and 3D case, respectively. Under affine

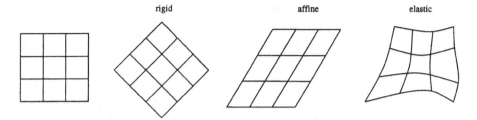

Figure 4.5.   Types of transformations.

transformations parallel lines remain parallel. The linear transformation can be decomposed into rotation, isotropic scaling, and an area-preserving pure shear. Thus, with affine transformations we can represent translation, rotation, scaling and shear between datasets. Note, that a translation is not a linear transformation, since $\mathbf{u}(\mathbf{x}_1 + \mathbf{x}_2) = \mathbf{A}\mathbf{x}_1 + \mathbf{A}\mathbf{x}_2 + \mathbf{T} \neq \mathbf{u}(\mathbf{x}_1) + \mathbf{u}(\mathbf{x}_2) = \mathbf{A}\mathbf{x}_1 + \mathbf{A}\mathbf{x}_2 + 2\mathbf{T}$. However, the entire affine transformation can be represented by a linear matrix transformation in the one dimension higher space. Rigid and affine transformations are special cases of general *polynomial (algebraic)* transformations. In the 2D case we have

$$
\mathbf{u}(\mathbf{x}) = \begin{pmatrix} a_{1,1} + a_{1,2}x + a_{1,3}y + a_{1,4}x^2 + a_{1,5}xy + a_{1,6}y^2 + \ldots \\ a_{2,1} + a_{2,2}x + a_{2,3}y + a_{2,4}x^2 + a_{2,5}xy + a_{2,6}y^2 + \ldots \end{pmatrix}
$$

$$
= \mathbf{T} + \mathbf{A}\mathbf{x} + \mathbf{x}^T\mathbf{B}\mathbf{x} + \ldots \tag{4.3}
$$

However, a problem with polynomials of higher order is that generally oscillations occur (e.g., [466],[199]). Another special class of nonrigid transformations are (model-based) *elastic* transformations. These transformations are based on models from elasticity theory, they are constrained to some kind of continuity or smoothness condition and generally minimize a certain energy measure. These transformations are more general than global rigid or affine transformations and allow to describe local deformations (see Figure 4.5). As an alternative to elastic models, models from fluid mechanics may be used. *Fluid models* are much more flexible, however, it is more difficult to constrain the mapping. So far, we have described *global* transformations, which act on the entire input data, possibly on the whole $\mathbb{R}^2$ or $\mathbb{R}^3$. A different class of mappings are *piecewise* or *local* transformations (e.g., [197]). Here, the data to be mapped is subdivided into regions and to each region a single transformation is applied (see Figure 4.6). Between adjacent regions generally some kind of continuity condition is imposed. It is obvious that local deformations can be represented by such a mapping. However, one problem with this approach is to find a suitable subdivision of the data. Note, that the general registration scheme in Figure 4.3 also applies to transformations which describe projections

Global Transformation

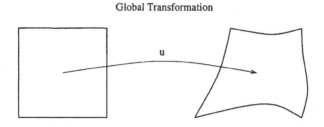

Piecewise (Local) Transformation

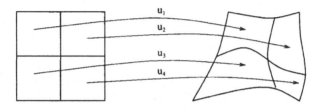

Figure 4.6.   Global vs. piecewise transformation.

of 3D objects onto the 2D image plane (3D-2D registration problem). In the field of computer vision, projections play a dominant role, since there the primary image type are video images. In this case, rigid transformations of a 3D object in general lead to nonrigid transformations of the object's projection. In the following, we will not consider further these types of transformations, but focus on mappings between image data of the same dimension. Furthermore note, that the term registration also includes the finding of correspondences between image data and *nonimage* data (e.g., the operation room, a surgical instrument or the current anatomy).

The third component of the general registration scheme in Figure 4.3 is a *similarity measure* which is used to compare the different representations with each other. On the one hand, a similarity measure is required to match the different representations, and on the other hand, we can employ a (possibly different) similarity measure to quantify the remaining registration error.

4.1.2 Point-Based Elastic Registration

One principal approach to elastic registration of medical image data is based on corresponding anatomical landmarks. Such a *landmark-based* approach comprises three steps: (1) extraction of landmarks in the different datasets, (2) establishing the correspondence between the landmarks, and (3) computing the transformation between the datasets using the information from (1) and (2). Among the different types of landmarks (points, curves, surfaces, and vol-

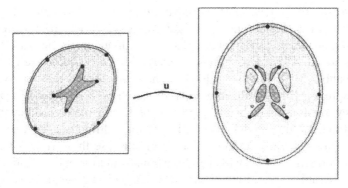

Figure 4.7. Point-based image registration.

umes) we here consider *point landmarks* (e.g., [49],[147]). Generally, we have a sparse set of points which are scattered over the image. Registration schemes based on other types of landmarks (curves, surfaces, volumes) take into account more information of the images. However, a disadvantage is that the segmentation, the representation of the segmented structures, as well as the finding of correspondences is more difficult. Note, that curve-based methods often are also denoted as line-based methods (e.g., [513],[115],[111],[524],[505]). *Intensity-based* (or *voxel-based*) approaches, on the other hand, rely on the intensities of the imaged objects, but generally not on geometric properties as in the case of landmark-based methods (e.g., [18],[20],[347],[188],[189],[91], [69],[474],[101],[184],[237],[456],[522]). Often, these approaches are based on the Navier equation in elasticity theory (e.g., [18],[20]) or employ a fluid model (e.g., [91],[69]). Generally, a global transformation has to be computed in a preprocessing step. A main advantage of intensity-based schemes is that an explicit segmentation of the images is not required. However, since the intensities are directly used to compute a similarity measure between images, these approaches generally depend rather strongly on the image modality and the chosen imaging parameters. A current trend to reduce this dependence is to use some kind of entropy measure as similarity measure (e.g., mutual information). It has been shown that approaches based such measures yield rather good results for rigid registration of multimodality images, see, for example, the evaluation study of West et al. [558]. For a more comprehensive overview of related work see Section 4.9 below.

Our scheme to elastic image registration uses point landmarks as image features (cf. Figure 4.7). Such schemes belong to the most efficient ones in image registration. Point landmarks may be either fiducial markers (e.g., points at a stereotactic frame, head screws, or skin markers) or anatomical point landmarks. The landmarks can be localized manually or by applying one of the operators proposed in Chapter 2. Anatomical point landmarks, in comparison to fiducial markers, have the advantage that they can directly be located within the relevant inner brain parts which generally increases the registration accuracy. Given landmarks, we compute an elastic transformation which is based on certain splines, namely *thin-plate splines* (e.g., Duchon [130], Wahba [545], Bookstein [49]). There are several reasons to use this kind of splines. First of all, thin-plate splines have a *physical interpretation* since they minimize the bending energy of a thin plate. Although a thin plate is a rather crude model to describe the local differences between images and atlases of generally different brains, in our case these splines serve as a flexible deformation model which yields a transformation of C^1-continuity with minimal curvature (see also Section 4.4). A *physically-motivated* approach generally leads to a more intuitive registration result, which is particularly important in clinical user-interaction scenaria. In such scenaria the clinician should have the possibility to control the result, while user-interaction is easier with such type of approach. A second advantage of thin-plate splines is that the *mathematical theory* is perfect understood (see Duchon [130], Meinguet [339], [340], Wahba [545]). Thin-plate splines result as the solution of an optimization problem which is well-posed, i.e., the solution exists, is unique, and depends continuously on the data. Moreover, the solution can be stated in closed form. In comparison to using polynomials of higher order for registration, a smaller number of transformation parameters and landmarks are needed, and generally no oscillations occur. Third, these splines have a *statistical interpretation*. Actually, thin-plate splines are Bayes estimates with a certain prior on the transformation. They are best linear unbiased estimates (BLUE) and there is a connection to the stochastic method of kriging (e.g., Kimeldorf and Wahba [279], Wahba [545], Cressie [107], Kent and Mardia [276]). Fourth, thin-plate splines can be implemented as *neural networks* with regularization properties, i.e., parallelization is directly possible (e.g., Broomhead and Lowe [72], Poggio and Girosi [403], Szeliski [511]). In this context, learning can be interpreted as fitting a function to a limited set of examples, while in our case the examples are the corresponding landmarks in the two images.

4.2 Clinical Applications

Principally, one can distinguish four main clinical application areas of computer-assisted image-guided medical applications: diagnosis, surgery planning (and simulation), intraoperative navigation, as well as robot-assisted interventions (e.g., Gerlot and Bizais [191], van den Elsen et al. [143], Maurer and Fitz-patrick [334], Lavallée [301], Taylor et al. [516]). In the case of *diagnosis*, the clinician uses images of the same patient to assess existence and severeness of pathologic processes. If two or even more images have been acquired, then judgement is easier and more accurate when the images have been registered and overlaid. For example, an overlay of MR and CT images helps to judge more precisely the position and shape of a tumor w.r.t. the bone. Note, that CT mainly represents bone which is not represented in MR, while the tumor may only be visible in the MR image (see Figure 4.1). In addition, the clinician may want to compare the image of a current person with the image of another person (e.g., which has the same disease) or with an atlas. Also here, accurately overlaying the image data helps the clinician. In *surgery planning* it is even more important to register different images and atlases. On the one hand, it is essential that operation targets (e.g., epilepsy centers) are accurately localized and treated, and on the other hand, it is important that healthy structures are not damaged and that surgical trauma is reduced. Particularly in brain surgery the latter requirement is difficult to meet, since due to the complexity of the 3D anatomical structures the risk of damaging healthy structures is relatively high. In the case of *intraoperative navigation* we have the additional problem that the surgeon has only a limited view of the brain structures, since generally only a small hole of the skull is opened (minimal-invasive surgery). Moreover, anatomical deformations occur during an intervention. For example, when opening the skull and the dura mater then liquor flows off, which generally leads to significant deformations, denoted as brain shift (e.g., Buchholz et al. [75], Hill et al. [246],[247], Dickhaus et al. [120], Reinges et al. [413]). Another example is the resection of a tumor. In either case, the preoperatively acquired image is no longer valid for navigation and has to be registered with the anatomy at hand in the operating theatre. For the fourth main application of *robot-assisted interventions*, it is even more important that anatomical structures have accurately been localized. In such a more automated procedure, a robot performs the intervention under the supervision of a surgeon.

Based on the above-mentioned four main application areas, we now give a more detailed classification of clinical applications and discuss in which cases the use of an elastic registration scheme, i.e., a locally adaptive transformation, is generally necessary (see also, e.g., [432],[443]). We distinguish applications, where we have no intraoperative deformations, from those, where we have to cope with such deformations. In the first case, we distinguish i) the registration of images of the same person, ii) image-atlas registration, and iii) the registration of images of different persons.

In the case of *registration of images of the same person* we have the same anatomy or also different anatomy (e.g., in the case of lesions) and monomodal or multimodal images. An example is MR-CT registration which is important for diagnosis and radiotherapy planning. Another example is the registration of MR images with functional images (e.g., PET). Although in these applications the images are from the same patient, generally elastic transformations should be applied even in the case of the same anatomy. The reason are scanner- as well as patient-induced distortions which can lead to significant distortions (e.g., Lüdeke et al. [318], Chang et al. [85], Sumanaweera et al. [507], Michiels et al. [345], Munck et al. [359]). Note, that scanner-induced distortions may be compensated through calibration, which, however, is not possible for patient-induced distortions, e.g., susceptibility distortions in MR images. In Section 4.5 below we show experiments with the latter type of distortions. Elastic transformations are certainly also needed in follow-up studies (i.e., images acquired at successive time instances) of metamorphic processes. In these studies generally monomodal images are used (e.g., MR images). With *image-atlas registration* we always have the problem of matching different anatomy, independently whether the applied atlas has been established on the basis of only one person or on the basis of several persons (e.g., Bajcsy et al. [19], Evans et al. [147], Höhne et al. [251], Roland and Zilles [451], Kikinis et al. [278], Mazziotta et al. [336], Nowinski et al. [386], Niemann et al. [379], Toga [529]). Additionally, atlases may carry probabilistic information about the different structures. In either case we have individual differences and thus elastic transformations are required. Examples for applications of image-atlas registration are trajectory planning for pain and epilepsy treatment, for a biopsy, or for the implantation of a deep electrode. Other examples are the segmentation of risk organs in radiotherapy planning or the labeling of the sulci. The case *registration of images of different persons* can be seen as a special case of image-atlas registration. Here, we also have different anatomy, but generally the same modality and no probabilistic information. One main application is atlas generation. Another application is a comparison of the brain anatomy of a current patient with that of another patient with similar disease. To improve the registration accuracy in this case, it may be advantageous to first retrieve a best matching brain with similar disease out of an image database and then match this brain. Note, that in the case of matching images of different anatomy, the topology may differ, while elastic transformations assume the same topology. However, in image registration this problem is often circumvented by only considering such features which represent the same topology. The other parts of the images are then transformed accordingly.

So far, we have discussed applications, where we have no intraoperative deformations. Such deformations may be due to skull opening or tumor resection, but may also occur in the case of different patient pose due to gravitational effects. It is obvious, that elastic transformations are necessary to cope with such deformations. One application is the registration of a preoperative image (of high resolution) with an intraoperative image of different modality or the same modality but lower resolution. Another example is the prediction of deformations based on sparse measurements (e.g., from an ultrasound device) or even without additional image-based measurements. Particularly in the latter case, a biomechanical model and knowledge of the material properties of the brain structures are necessary (see also Section 4.8 below).

4.3 Interpolating Thin-Plate Splines

In this section, we introduce the basic approach for point-based elastic image registration using *thin-plate splines*. Generalizations of this scheme are described subsequently in Sections 4.5-4.7. Originally, thin-plate splines have been introduced by Harder and Desmarais [228] in the context of aeroelastic calculations and have been termed *surface splines* there. Later, mathematicians have laid the theoretical foundations of this approach as well as have developed generalizations of it (Duchon [130],[131], Meinguet [339], Wahba [545]). Actually, thin-plate splines are a natural multidimensional generalization of the 1D splines of Schoenberg [472] and Reinsch [414]. The use of thin-plate splines for point-based registration of medical images has been proposed by Bookstein [49]. He considered *interpolating* thin-plate splines, where the landmarks are matched exactly, and applied this approach to 2D images, i.e. for computing mappings $\mathbf{u} : \mathbb{R}^2 \to \mathbb{R}^2$. Application to 3D images has been reported in Evans et al. [147], for example. Related approaches in computer vision dealing with the problem of surface interpolation, i.e. mappings $u : \mathbb{R}^2 \to \mathbb{R}$, given sparse scattered data have previously been described by Grimson [207],[208], Brady and Horn [60], Boult and Kender [56], and Terzopoulos [517]. While Bookstein [49] considered mappings $\mathbf{u} : \mathbb{R}^2 \to \mathbb{R}^2$, the following exposition describes the general case of $\mathbf{u} : \mathbb{R}^d \to \mathbb{R}^d$, i.e., we deal with the registration of images of arbitrary dimension d. Our approach is based on the mathematical work in Duchon [130] and Wahba [545]. Whereas the mathematical work studies mappings $u : \mathbb{R}^d \to \mathbb{R}$, in the following we describe a straightforward extension for mappings $\mathbf{u} : \mathbb{R}^d \to \mathbb{R}^d$ (Rohr et al. [443],[446], Sprengel et al. [496]).

Thin-plate spline interpolation can be stated as a multivariate interpolation problem: Given a number n of corresponding point landmarks $\mathbf{p}_i$ and $\mathbf{q}_i$, $i = 1, \ldots, n$ in two images of dimension d, find a continuous transformation $\mathbf{u} : \mathbb{R}^d \to \mathbb{R}^d$ within a suitable Hilbert space $\mathcal{H}$, which i) minimizes a given functional $J : \mathcal{H} \to \mathbb{R}$ and ii) fulfills the interpolation condition

$$\mathbf{q}_i = \mathbf{u}(\mathbf{p}_i), \qquad i = 1, \ldots, n, \tag{4.4}$$

i.e., the transformed landmarks of the first image $\mathbf{p}_i$ exactly match the landmarks $\mathbf{q}_i$ of the second image. The first and second image are also denoted as source and target image, respectively. It is assumed that landmark sets in two images as well as their correspondences are given and from this information we want to compute the correspondences for the whole image (cf. Figure 4.8). Actually, the input information can also be regarded as having available a set of landmarks in one image together with displacement vectors at these landmarks, and what we want to compute are the displacement vectors for all other points of this image. Thus, the task of point-based registration can also be seen as the task of

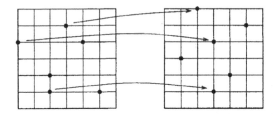
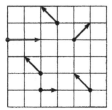

Figure 4.8.   Input to point-based elastic registration.   *Figure 4.9.*   Input to the interpolation of a displacement field.

interpolating a sparse set of displacement vectors (cf. Figure 4.9). With the 2D and 3D approaches in Bookstein [49] and Evans et al. [147], the minimizing functional represents the bending energy of a thin plate separately for each component $u_k, k = 1, \ldots, d$ of the transformation $\mathbf{u}$. Thus, the functional $J(\mathbf{u})$ can be separated into a sum of similar functionals each of which only depend on one component u_k of $\mathbf{u}$. Therefore, the problem of finding $\mathbf{u}$ can be decomposed into d problems.

In the case of d-dimensional images and for an arbitrary order m of derivatives in the functional we have

$$J_m^d(\mathbf{u}) = \sum_{k=1}^{d} J_m^d(u_k), \tag{4.5}$$

where the single functionals read as

$$J_m^d(u) = \sum_{\alpha_1 + \ldots + \alpha_d = m} \frac{m!}{\alpha_1! \cdots \alpha_d!} \int_{\mathbb{R}^d} \left(\frac{\partial^m u}{\partial x_1^{\alpha_1} \cdots \partial x_d^{\alpha_d}} \right)^2 d\mathbf{x} \tag{4.6}$$

according to Duchon [130], Wahba [545] with α_k being positive integers. The functional is invariant under similarity transformations (translation, rotation, and scaling). Note that, e.g., tensor product splines are not rotationally invariant. When choosing m and d, the condition

$$2m - d > 0 \tag{4.7}$$

has to be fulfilled. For the special case of $m = d = 2$ we have $2m - d = 2 > 0$ and we obtain from (4.6) the functional originally used in Bookstein [49]:

$$J_2^2(u) = \int_{-\infty}^{\infty} \int_{-\infty}^{\infty} u_{xx}^2 + 2u_{xy}^2 + u_{yy}^2 \, dx dy. \tag{4.8}$$

In the case of $m = 2$ and $d = 3$, i.e., $2m - d = 1 > 0$, we have the functional applied in Evans et al. [147]:

$$J_2^3(u) = \int\limits_{-\infty}^{\infty} \int\limits_{-\infty}^{\infty} \int\limits_{-\infty}^{\infty} u_{xx}^2 + u_{yy}^2 + u_{zz}^2 + 2(u_{xy}^2 + u_{xz}^2 + u_{yz}^2) \, dx dy dz. \quad (4.9)$$

Note, that the choice of second order derivatives $m = 2$ satisfies the above stated condition (4.7) for $d = 2$ as well as for $d = 3$. However, the choice $m = 2$ and $d = 4$, which would be interesting in the case of time-varying 3D images, does not satisfy this condition. Thus, in this case one has to choose a higher value of m.

Before stating the solution of the general functional in (4.6), we first consider its *nullspace*, i.e., the space of functions that are not measured by the functional. The nullspace of (4.6) are all polynomials in d variables up to order $m - 1$. Thus the functional can be interpreted as a semi-norm and the nullspace is necessary to obtain a complete Hilbert space. The dimension of the nullspace is given by

$$M = \binom{d + m - 1}{d} \quad (4.10)$$

and must be lower than the number of landmarks n, i.e., $M < n$. Thus, this condition determines the minimum number of landmarks by

$$n > \frac{(d + m - 1)!}{d!(m - 1)!}. \quad (4.11)$$

If $m = 2$, for example, we have the requirement $n > d + 1$. The M monomials of total degree up to order $m - 1$ that span the nullspace will be denoted by $\phi_1, ..., \phi_M$. For example, for $m = d = 2$ we have $M = 3$ and the nullspace is spanned by

$$\phi_1 = 1, \quad \phi_2 = x, \quad \phi_3 = y. \quad (4.12)$$

The minimal number of landmarks in this case is $n = 4$. For $m = 2$ and $d = 3$ we have $M = 4$. In this case, the minimal number of landmarks is $n = 5$ and the nullspace is spanned by

$$\phi_1 = 1, \quad \phi_2 = x, \quad \phi_3 = y, \quad \phi_4 = z. \quad (4.13)$$

Note, that for an optimal affine transformation in the least-squares sense, the minimal number of landmarks in the 2D case is $n = 3$ and in the 3D case it is $n = 4$. This means, that for thin-plate spline registration, we need at least one additional landmark in comparison to an optimal affine transformation.

The solution of minimizing the functional in (4.6) is unique under the very general condition that least-squares regression on the $\phi_1, ..., \phi_M$ is unique (Duchon [130], Wahba [545]). In the 2D and 3D case this means, that not all points may lie on a single line or plane, respectively. The solution can be stated analytically as

$$u(\mathbf{x}) = \sum_{\nu=1}^{M} a_\nu \phi_\nu(\mathbf{x}) + \sum_{i=1}^{n} w_i U(\mathbf{x}, \mathbf{p}_i) \tag{4.14}$$

with basis functions $U(\mathbf{x}, \mathbf{p}_i)$ depending on m, d, and the Hilbert space $\mathcal{H}$ of admissible functions. Note, that the basis functions span an n-dimensional space of functions that depend only on the landmarks $\mathbf{p}_i$ of the first image. Choosing the space of functions on $\mathbb{R}^d$ for which all partial derivatives of total order m are square integrable, i.e. are in $L_2(\mathbb{R}^d)^1$, results in the basis functions

$$U(r) = \begin{cases} \theta_{m,d} \, r^{2m-d} \ln r & \text{if } 2m - d \text{ an even integer,} \\ \theta_{m,d} \, r^{2m-d} & \text{otherwise,} \end{cases} \tag{4.15}$$

where

$$\theta_{m,d} = \begin{cases} \dfrac{(-1)^{d/2+1+m}}{2^{2m-1} \pi^{d/2} (m-1)!(m-d/2)!} & \text{if } 2m - d \text{ an even integer,} \\ \dfrac{\Gamma(d/2 - m)}{2^{2m} \pi^{d/2} (m-1)!} & \text{otherwise,} \end{cases} \tag{4.16}$$

with $\Gamma(x)$ denoting the Gamma function[2] and letting

$$r = |\mathbf{x} - \mathbf{p}| = \sqrt{\sum_{k=1}^{d} (x_k - p_k)^2} \tag{4.17}$$

we have

$$U(\mathbf{x}, \mathbf{p}) = U(|\mathbf{x} - \mathbf{p}|) = U(r). \tag{4.18}$$

As an example, for 2D images choosing $m = d = 2$ we obtain the well-known function $U(r) = 1/(8\pi)r^2 \ln r$. Since this basis function has a singularity at

---

[1]For $m = 2$, for example, this means that

$$|u|^2 = \int_{\mathbb{R}^d} \sum_{k,l=1}^{d} \left(\frac{\partial^2 u}{\partial x_k \partial x_l} \right)^2 dx < \infty.$$

[2]The Gamma function is defined by $\Gamma(x) = \int_0^\infty e^{-t} t^{x-1} dt$ for $x > 0$ and $\Gamma(x+1) = x\Gamma(x)$, $x \neq 0, -1, -2, ...$

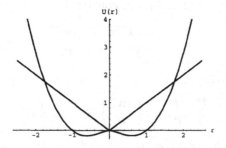

Figure 4.10. Thin-plate spline basis functions $U(r) = r^2 \ln r$ and $U(r) = r$ (disregarding constants).

	$d = 1$	$d = 2$	$d = 3$	$d = 4$
$m = 1$	$-\frac{1}{2}r$	–	–	–
$m = 2$	$\frac{1}{12}r^3$	$\frac{1}{8\pi}r^2 \ln r$	$-\frac{1}{8\pi}r$	–
$m = 3$	$-\frac{1}{240}r^5$	$-\frac{1}{128\pi}r^4 \ln r$	$\frac{1}{96\pi}r^3$	$\frac{1}{64\pi^2}r^2 \ln r$
$m = 4$	$\frac{1}{10080}r^7$	$\frac{1}{4608\pi}r^6 \ln r$	$-\frac{1}{2880\pi}r^5$	$-\frac{1}{1536\pi^2}r^4 \ln r$

Table 4.1. Thin-plate spline basis functions $U(r)$ for different orders m of derivatives in the functional and different image dimensions d.

$r = 0$ we define $U(0) = 0$. For 3D images, using $m = 2$ and $d = 3$, we obtain the function $U(r) = -1/(8\pi)r$. Figure 4.10 shows the graphs of these two functions. In Table 4.1 we have computed the thin-plate spline basis functions for different orders of derivatives m and different dimensions d. Due to the above stated condition in (4.7), which requires that $m > d/2$, the table has empty entries.

Note, that $U(r)$ is a *Green's function* for the m-iterated Laplacian, i.e., it solves the equation

$$\Delta^m U(r) = \delta(r), \qquad (4.19)$$

where $\delta(r)$ is the Dirac delta function[3].

The coefficients a_ν and w_i of the analytic solution (4.14) can be summarized by $\mathbf{a} = (a_1, \dots, a_M)^T$ and $\mathbf{w} = (w_1, \dots, w_n)^T$ and we can compute them by

---

[3]$\delta(r)$ has a singularity at $r = 0$ and is defined by

$$\delta(r) = 0, r \neq 0, \quad \int_{-\infty}^{\infty} \delta(r)dr = 1, \quad \int_{-\infty}^{\infty} f(r)\delta(r - r_0)dr = f(r_0). \qquad (4.20)$$

solving the following system of linear equations:

$$\mathbf{Pa + Kw} = \mathbf{v} \tag{4.21}$$
$$\mathbf{P}^T\mathbf{w} = \mathbf{0},$$

which can also be written as

$$\begin{pmatrix} \mathbf{P} & \mathbf{K} \\ \mathbf{0} & \mathbf{P}^T \end{pmatrix} \begin{pmatrix} \mathbf{a} \\ \mathbf{w} \end{pmatrix} = \begin{pmatrix} \mathbf{v} \\ \mathbf{0} \end{pmatrix}, \tag{4.22}$$

where $\mathbf{K} = (K_{ij})$, $K_{ij} = U(\mathbf{p}_i, \mathbf{p}_j)$, $\mathbf{P} = (P_{ij})$, $P_{ij} = \phi_j(\mathbf{p}_i)$, and $\mathbf{v}$ is the column vector of one component of the coordinates of the landmarks $\mathbf{q}_i$ of the second image, i.e., $\mathbf{v} = (q_{1,k}, ..., q_{n,k})^T$. The linear system of equations can be solved by standard routines, e.g., by applying lower-upper (LU) decomposition. The condition $\mathbf{P}^T\mathbf{w} = \mathbf{0}$ represents the *boundary condition* and ensures that the elastic part of the transformation is zero at infinity. For the case of $m = d = 2$ we have the conditions

$$\sum_{i=1}^{n} w_i = \sum_{i=1}^{n} w_i x_i = \sum_{i=1}^{n} w_i y_i = 0, \tag{4.23}$$

and for $m = 2$ and $d = 3$ we have

$$\sum_{i=1}^{n} w_i = \sum_{i=1}^{n} w_i x_i = \sum_{i=1}^{n} w_i y_i = \sum_{i=1}^{n} w_i z_i = 0. \tag{4.24}$$

For the condition $\mathbf{P}^T\mathbf{w} = \mathbf{0}$ there are also mathematical reasons (Wahba [545]). The problem is that the matrix $\mathbf{K}$ in (4.21) is not positive definite but only *conditionally positive definite* (positive definite up to the nullspace), a property, however, that turns out to be enough. This property is directly related to the notion of a generalized divided difference of order m. It is ensured that all polynomials of total order less than m are annihilated. From this follows that the functional in (4.6), which represents the bending energy, is always positive, i.e.,

$$J_m^d = \mathbf{w}^T\mathbf{Kw} > 0. \tag{4.25}$$

For general positions of the landmarks it is guaranteed that the system of linear equations is always solvable.

In the case of $m = 2$ the solution consists of an affine part as well as an elastic part. Note, that the solution for the affine part can be stated as

$$\mathbf{a} = (\mathbf{P}^T\mathbf{K}^{-1}\mathbf{P})^{-1}\mathbf{P}^T\mathbf{K}^{-1}\mathbf{v} \tag{4.26}$$

which is not the optimal affine part in the least-squares sense given by

$$\mathbf{a} = (\mathbf{P}^T\mathbf{P})^{-1}\mathbf{P}^T\mathbf{v} \tag{4.27}$$

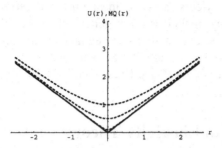

Figure 4.11. Comparison of the thin-plate spline basis function $U(r) = r$ (solid line) and the multiquadric function $MQ(r) = \sqrt{r^2 + c^2}$, for $c = 1, 0.5$, and 0.1 (dashed lines; from top to bottom).

(see also [545],[42],[497]). Actually, the affine part in the thin-plate spline approach can be regarded as a weighted least-squares solution with the weight matrix $\mathbf{K}^{-1}$.

We conclude this section by briefly relating the thin-plate spline approach to two other widely used scattered data interpolation methods, namely radial basis function approaches and the method of kriging (see also Myers [361], Little et al. [312]). Central to *thin-plate splines* is that they minimize a certain bending energy function. Thin-plate splines are radial symmetric and thus belong to the more general class of *radial basis functions (RBF)*. Generally, radial basis functions are used as interpolating functions without requiring certain minimization constraints (e.g., Micchelli [344], Alfeld [4], Hoschek and Lasser [256], Jackson [259], Buhmann [76], Nielsen [375], Arad et al. [13], Ruprecht et al. [457],[358], Schaback [462]). An interesting relation consists between thin-plate splines and the well-known multiquadric splines of Hardy [175],[229]. *Multiquadric splines* belong to the general class of radial basis functions and have been introduced mainly on the basis of heuristic arguments, although later mathematical properties have been proven. These splines yield quite good experimental results in surface interpolation. For both the 2D and 3D case multiquadric splines have the same basis function $MQ(r) = \sqrt{r^2 + c^2}$, where c is a constant, e.g., $c = 1$ or smaller. Actually, for $c = 0$ we have $MQ(r) = r$ which is identical to the basis function of thin-plate splines in the 3D case (using $m = 2$ and disregarding constants; see Table 4.1). For illustration we have plotted in Figure 4.11 the thin-plate spline basis function r in comparison to the multiquadric basis function $\sqrt{r^2 + c^2}$ choosing different values of $c = 1, 0.5$, and 0.1. It can be seen that for $c = 0.1$ the multiquadric function is already very close to the thin-plate spline function. *Kriging*, in comparison to thin-plate splines and general radial basis function approaches, is a stochastic method which minimizes the local mean-squared prediction error and yields the best linear unbiased estimate (BLUE) of the solution. The kriging method is more general than thin-plate splines. Under certain conditions, the two methods are equivalent to one another. It can be shown that thin-plate splines are Bayes estimates with a certain prior on the transformation (e.g., Wahba [545], Cressie [107], Kent and Mardia [276], and Mardia et al. [325]).

4.4   Relation to Elasticity Theory

Whereas the above exposition is purely mathematical, in this section we describe the embedding of thin-plate splines in elasticity theory and detail the physical assumptions behind this approach (see also, e.g., Courant and Hilbert [106], Grimson [207], Beskos [37], Ciarlet [96], Landau and Lifschitz [299], Eschenauer and Schnell [145], Binder et al. [42]).

4.4.1   Bending of a Thin Plate

In elasticity theory, the potential energy for bending a thin plate extended to infinity under perpendicular forces is given by (using $\mathbf{H}_u$ as the Hessian matrix of the function $u(x, y)$)

$$
\begin{aligned}
E &= \int_{-\infty}^{\infty} \int_{-\infty}^{\infty} \left((tr\mathbf{H}_u)^2 - 2(1-\nu)det\mathbf{H}_u \right) dxdy + \int_{-\infty}^{\infty} \int_{-\infty}^{\infty} f(x,y)u(x,y)dxdy \\
&= \int_{-\infty}^{\infty} \int_{-\infty}^{\infty} \left((u_{xx} + u_{yy})^2 - 2(1-\nu)(u_{xx}u_{yy} - u_{xy}^2) \right) dxdy \\
&\quad + \int_{-\infty}^{\infty} \int_{-\infty}^{\infty} f(x,y)u(x,y)dxdy,
\end{aligned}
\tag{4.28}
$$

where $f(x,y)$ denotes the applied force density (Courant and Hilbert [106]). The bending energy is related to the principal curvatures of the deformed plate. ν is a material parameter denoted as Poisson ratio and defines the ratio between transverse contraction and longitudinal dilation of a homogeneous material. It can be written as a function of the Lamé constants $\lambda, \mu > 0$ as

$$
\nu = \frac{\lambda}{2(\lambda + \mu)}.
\tag{4.29}
$$

The range of values of the Poisson ratio is $-1 \leq \nu \leq 0.5$, but for real materials we have $0 < \nu \leq 0.5$. Examples for different materials and their Poisson ratio are: iron ($\nu = 0.28$), aluminum ($\nu = 0.34$), gold ($\nu = 0.42$), and rubber ($\nu = 0.49$). For the human skull and brain different material values can be found in the literature. Typical values are $\nu = 0.21$ for skull bone and $\nu = 0.499$ for brain tissue (e.g., [543],[217],[220]).

If we set $\nu = 0$ in (4.28), which means that we assume no transverse contraction independent of a longitudinal dilation, and by disregarding the forces f for a moment, then we obtain the functional

$$J(u) = \int\limits_{-\infty}^{\infty} \int\limits_{-\infty}^{\infty} u_{xx}^2 + 2u_{xy}^2 + u_{yy}^2 \, dx dy. \tag{4.30}$$

This functional is actually the thin-plate spline functional in (4.8) above, which results from the general thin-plate spline functional (4.6) setting $m = d = 2$. In this case, the relation to the principal curvatures κ_1 and κ_2 of the plate is given by

$$\kappa_1^2 + \kappa_2^2 \approx u_{xx}^2 + 2u_{xy}^2 + u_{yy}^2, \tag{4.31}$$

while assuming that u_x and u_y are small. The relation can be derived by using the mean and Gaussian curvature $H = (\kappa_1 + \kappa_2)/2$ and $K = \kappa_1 \kappa_2$, which under the above assumption can be written as $H \approx (u_{xx} + u_{yy})/2$ and $K \approx u_{xx}u_{yy} - u_{xy}^2$. Then, we have $\kappa_1^2 + \kappa_2^2 = 4H^2 - 2K \approx (tr\mathbf{H}_u)^2 - 2det\mathbf{H}_u = tr\mathbf{H}_u^2 = u_{xx}^2 + 2u_{xy}^2 + u_{yy}^2$. Note, that the physical derivation of the bended thin plate assumes small deformations. Thus, only in this case the physical interpretation is valid. Minimizing the functional in (4.30) while considering the forces f leads to the following Euler-Lagrange differential equation (using the Laplacian $\Delta = \partial^2/\partial x^2 + \partial^2/\partial y^2$ and disregarding a negative sign for the forces)

$$\Delta^2 u = f \tag{4.32}$$

i.e.,

$$\left(\frac{\partial^4}{\partial x^4} + 2\frac{\partial^4}{\partial x^2 \partial y^2} + \frac{\partial^4}{\partial y^4} \right) u = f \tag{4.33}$$

with natural boundary conditions, since we did not require any other conditions. Up to some constant, this equation is known as the Kirchhoff plate equation. For $f = 0$ the equation is called the *biharmonic equation* (or bipotential equation):

$$\Delta^2 u = 0 \tag{4.34}$$

and Δ^2 is denoted biharmonic operator. Interestingly, there are other quadratic forms in the second derivatives of u which also lead to the biharmonic equation, e.g., the squared Laplacian

$$J(u) = \int\limits_{-\infty}^{\infty} \int\limits_{-\infty}^{\infty} (\Delta u)^2 \, dx dy = \int\limits_{-\infty}^{\infty} \int\limits_{-\infty}^{\infty} u_{xx}^2 + 2u_{xx}u_{yy} + u_{yy}^2 \, dx dy, \tag{4.35}$$

which is also rotationally symmetric and can be derived from the functional in (4.28) by setting $\nu = 1$. Actually, as shown by Brady and Horn [60], all rotationally symmetric quadratic forms in the second derivatives are linear combinations of the thin-plate spline quadratic form and the squared Laplacian, and lead to an identical Euler-Lagrange differential equation. However, the natural boundary conditions and the nullspace differ. In [60] it is stated, that w.r.t. these two criteria, the thin-plate spline quadratic form is superior to the other quadratic forms since it imposes tighter constraints. The relation to the principal curvatures of the plate in the case of the functional involving the squared Laplacian (4.35) is given by

$$(\kappa_1 + \kappa_2)^2 \approx (\Delta u)^2, \tag{4.36}$$

and represents the mean curvature (again assuming that u_x and u_y are small).

The *fundamental solution* to the biharmonic equation in (4.34), i.e., the solution to

$$\Delta^2 u = \delta, \tag{4.37}$$

where δ is the Dirac delta function, is given by $u^*(r) = 1/(8\pi)r^2 \ln r$, with r denoting the Euclidean distance. Note, that the fundamental solution u^* solves (4.37) without satisfying certain boundary conditions. In comparison, the *Green's function* to the problem (4.37) is given by $K = u^* + \gamma$ and includes a C^4-continuous function $\gamma(x, y)$ to satisfy certain boundary conditions (e.g., [106]). The fundamental solution (and also the Green's function) is of central importance since with u^* we also have the solution for arbitrary forces $f(x, y)$.

This is true for general inhomogeneous partial differential equations

$$Lu = f, \tag{4.38}$$

where $L = \sum_{|\alpha| \le k} c_\alpha D^\alpha$ is a linear differential operator of order k with constant coefficients as in our case of the biharmonic operator (e.g., [165]). If u^* is a fundamental solution of L, i.e., $Lu^* = \delta$, then the solution for arbitrary forces f can be stated as

$$u = u^* * f, \tag{4.39}$$

where the operation '$*$' means convolution. Thus, u^* represents the effect of a unit point force and we obtain the solution u by convolving the fundamental solution with the arbitrary force f. From the fundamental solution at the origin $r = 0$ we obtain the solution in an arbitrary point r_1 by

$$u_{r_1}^*(r) = u^*(r, r_1) = u^*(r - r_1). \tag{4.40}$$

Note, that u^* is symmetric, i.e., $u^*(r_1, r_2) = u^*(r_2, r_1)$. Superposition of shifted functions u^* corresponds to the second term of the analytic solution

(4.14) for the thin-plate spline functional (4.6). The fundamental solution is also denoted a weighting or influence function. Note, that δ is not a function in the classical sense but a distribution. Hence the notation of a fundamental solution can only satisfactorily be defined in the theory of distributions.

In summary, we have seen that the physical interpretation of the thin-plate spline functional assumes homogeneous material, no transverse contraction, and small deformations. We note, that the thin-plate spline formulation can also be considered in more general function spaces than considered here (Duchon [130],[131], Sprengel et al. [497]). With this approach it is possible to vary the smoothness properties of the solution introducing some parameter s:

$$U(r) = \begin{cases} c\, r^{2m-d+2s} \ln r & \text{if } 2m - d + 2s \text{ an even integer,} \\ c\, r^{2m-d+2s} & \text{otherwise,} \end{cases} \tag{4.41}$$

with constants c and requiring $2m - d + 2s > 0$. However, only in the case of $s = 0$, which is the case we considered here in Section 4.3 above, the solution u is the fundamental solution of the biharmonic equation (cf. (4.15)). Only in this case the physical interpretation is valid.

4.4.2   Relation to the Navier Equation

One main equation in elasticity theory is the *Navier equation,* which describes the deformation of homogeneous isotropic 3D bodies under applied forces. Assuming small deformations, which is the case in linear elasticity theory, we have for the (elastostatic) equilibrium

$$\mu\Delta\mathbf{u} + (\lambda + \mu)\nabla(\nabla \cdot \mathbf{u}) = \mathbf{f}, \tag{4.42}$$

where $\nabla = (\partial/\partial x, \partial/\partial y, \partial/\partial z)^T$ denotes the Nabla operator, $\nabla \cdot \mathbf{u} = div\ \mathbf{u} = u_{1,x} + u_{2,y} + u_{3,z}$ is the divergence of the displacement vector $\mathbf{u} = (u_1, u_2, u_3)$, and $\mathbf{f} = (f_1, f_2, f_3)$ is a vector of force density. The Navier equation has been introduced for elastic image registration by Bajcsy et al. [18],[20]. We directly see from (4.42), that the Navier equation includes the Lamé constants $\lambda, \mu > 0$, which describe material properties, whereas the biharmonic equation in (4.34), which corresponds to thin-plate splines, does not include material parameters. Also, the Navier equation is based on partial derivatives of order two, while the biharmonic equation incorporates partial derivatives of order four. A more direct relation between the Navier and the biharmonic equation in the case of 3D deformation can be seen if we set $\lambda = -\mu$. Note, however, that this choice of material constants is physically not possible. With this parameter setting we obtain three decoupled differential equations, one equation for each component of the displacement vector **u**,

$$\Delta u_1 = \frac{1}{\mu} f_1$$

$$\Delta u_2 = \frac{1}{\mu} f_2 \qquad (4.43)$$

$$\Delta u_3 = \frac{1}{\mu} f_3$$

which correspond to the well-known membrane model (e.g., [106],[517],[46]). These equations can be compared with the thin-plate spline equations in the 3D case:

$$\Delta^2 u_1 = f_1$$
$$\Delta^2 u_2 = f_2 \qquad (4.44)$$
$$\Delta^2 u_3 = f_3.$$

While the membrane splines have a C^0-continuity, i.e., the first partial derivatives need not be continuous and thus kinks may occur, thin-plate splines have a C^1-continuity (e.g., [517]). Besides the remaining material parameter μ, which only scales the forces, and besides the different power of the Laplacian operator, the above equations have the same structure. Both systems of equations are decoupled, i.e., a change in one coordinate direction does not influence the result in other coordinate directions. In the case of thin-plate splines this effect is a direct consequence of extending this approach from mappings $u : \mathbb{R}^3 \rightarrow \mathbb{R}$ to mappings $\mathbf{u} : \mathbb{R}^3 \rightarrow \mathbb{R}^3$, while associating bending energies to each component of **u** separately (see also Section 4.3 above). Thus, in comparison to real elastic material we here have no interconnection between the components of **u**. This behavior may be a disadvantage when dealing with real deformations of tissues (e.g., brain tissue), but may be an advantage when matching images of different brains. In the latter case, we have to cope with individual differences, and a coupling between the components may lead to unwanted effects. Another example is tumor growth and resection, where material expands or shrinks. Also in this case, a coupling between the components of **u** as in the Navier equation may lead to undesired effects.

A different way to derive a special case of the Navier equation in (4.42) is to set $\mathbf{u} = (0, 0, u_3(x, y))$ and $\mathbf{f} = (0, 0, f_3)$. This means, that we assume forces and displacements only in z-direction, while the z-coordinate of **u** only depends on x and y. This setting corresponds to the thin-plate spline problem in 2D, where we have perpendicular forces acting on the material. Actually, in this case we obtain

$$\Delta u_3 = \frac{1}{\mu} f_3, \qquad (4.45)$$

where $\Delta u_3 = u_{3,xx} + u_{3,yy}$ is the 2D Laplacian of u_3. Thus, we arrive at the 2D harmonic equation involving partial derivatives of the second order which corresponds to the membrane model.

Another relation between the Navier equation in (4.42) and the thin-plate spline approach can be obtained, when we assume that the force vector field can be derived from a harmonic potential (e.g., [90])

$$\mathbf{f} = \nabla\phi, \qquad \nabla \cdot \mathbf{f} = \Delta\phi = 0, \tag{4.46}$$

where ϕ is the force potential field. If we apply the divergence operator to the Navier equation, then we obtain the relation $\Delta(\nabla \cdot \mathbf{u}) = 0$. If we now apply the Laplacian to the Navier equation then we yield

$$\mu\Delta^2\mathbf{u} + (\lambda + \mu)\nabla\Delta(\nabla \cdot \mathbf{u}) = \nabla\Delta\phi, \tag{4.47}$$

and therefore

$$\Delta^2\mathbf{u} = \mathbf{0}. \tag{4.48}$$

This means, that the displacement vector field that satisfies the Navier equation must solve the biharmonic equation. Another method to relate the Navier equation to the thin plate formulation is known as Galerkin vector method (e.g., [90]).

For the Navier equation in (4.42) no general analytic solution exists ([145]). However, by imposing certain explicit forces while assuming certain boundary conditions, analytic solutions can be obtained. Such an approach has recently been introduced by Davis et al. [113] and the resulting splines have been termed elastic body splines (EBS). The authors argue that point forces as represented by the Dirac function δ are not appropriate since the solution contains a singularity at the center. Instead, one should choose forces such that the deformation is smooth. They argue further, that one way to obtain smooth deformations is to have a smooth force field given by

$$\mathbf{f} = \mathbf{c}\,r, \tag{4.49}$$

where $\mathbf{c} = (c_1, c_2, c_3)$ is a constant vector. Under these forces an analytic solution to the Navier equation (4.42) can be obtained via the Galerkin vector method. Interestingly, the used forces (not the displacements!) minimize the thin-plate spline functional in 3D. However, the physical interpretation of these forces is not quite clear, since they are zero at the origin and increase with the distance to the origin. The solution under these forces can be stated as

$$\mathbf{u} = r(\alpha r^2 \mathbf{I} - 3\mathbf{x}\mathbf{x}^T)\mathbf{c}, \tag{4.50}$$

where $\alpha = 12(1 - \nu) - 1$, ν is the Poisson ratio, $\mathbf{I}$ is the 3×3 identity matrix, and $\mathbf{x} = (x, y, z)$. In this case, the components of $\mathbf{u}$ are coupled. For another choice of the forces

$$f = c\frac{1}{r}, \tag{4.51}$$

the analytic solution

$$u = (\beta r I - xx^T \frac{1}{r})c \tag{4.52}$$

results, where $\beta = 8(1 - \nu) - 1$. In this case, we have a direct relation to the thin-plate spline solution which in the 3D case can be written as

$$u = rIc. \tag{4.53}$$

In comparison to (4.52) there is no interconnection between the components of u. Also, elastic body splines include one material parameter ν, while thin-plate splines include no such parameter. In addition to the solutions (4.50) and (4.52) Davis et al. [113] add an affine transformation for use in medical image registration, which is analogous to the thin-plate spline approach. However, whereas for thin-plate splines the addition of an affine transformation is mathematically well-motivated (see Section 4.3 above), for elastic body splines this choice seems to be arbitrary.

As a summary of this section, we compare the thin-plate spline approach with the other principal approach to elastic image registration based on the Navier equation, which is usually solved numerically by applying finite differences (FD) or the finite element method (FEM) (e.g., Bajcsy and Kovačič [20], Davatzikos et al. [111], Peckar et al. [394]). The main properties have been listed in Table 4.2 (see also Boult and Kender [56] as well as Terzopoulos [517] for a comparison of analytic and numeric methods for solving functionals corresponding to thin plates). The main advantages of thin-plate splines are that we have a unique analytic solution, that the approach is computationally efficient, and that the overall transformation (global and elastic) can be computed in one step. Approaches that numerically solve the Navier equation generally use more image information (e.g., intensity or edge information) and model the real physical 2D or 3D deformation. More image information generally leads to a better registration result, however, depending on the type of image information, the solution may not be unique or the input data may be more difficult to determine (e.g., computation of forces from images or finding dense correspondences for curved surfaces). The modelling of real physical deformations is advantageous in case of matching images, where the geometric differences have been caused by physical deformation processes. However, in the case of matching the anatomy of different patients there is no advantage over thin-plate splines. Also, when using the Navier equation, we have to compute the global transformation (e.g., rigid or affine) in a separate step from the elastic transformation (2-step procedure). We also point out, that the indicated numeric

	Thin-plate splines	Navier equation
Image features	sparse point sets (scattered data)	image intensities, edgeness, or dense point sets (e.g., contours)
Physical interpretation	physically-motivated (physical deformation for each coordinate)	physically-based (physical deformation for the whole body)
Assumption	small deformations	small deformations
Transformation properties	C^1-continuous (no kinks)	C^0-continuous (may have kinks)
Free parameters	none	Lamé constants
Procedure type	1-step (affine and elastic in one step)	2-step (separate global transformation)
Solution	unique	often not unique (depends on the features)
Solution type	in closed form	numeric approximation (FD, FEM)
Basis functions	global support	local/compact support
Number of basis functions	number of landmarks n, small	depends on fineness of tessellation, large
Matrix of LSE	dense (num. problems for $n > 100$)	sparse
Computation time	low	high

Table 4.2. Elastic image registration: Comparison between thin-plate splines and numeric approaches based on the Navier equation.

problems with thin-plate splines in Table 4.2 for landmark numbers $n > 100$ (in each of the datasets), e.g., [256], are actually not a practical problem. In our case of manual or semi-automatic landmark localization the number of landmarks is usually $n < 50$, since the specification of more landmarks would be too tedious and time-consuming, particularly in clinical routine. Additionally note, that the numeric problems can significantly be reduced if we extend the thin-plate spline approach from an interpolation to an approximation scheme as described below in Sections 4.5 and 4.6.

4.5 Approximating Thin-Plate Splines with Isotropic Landmark Errors

So far, we have considered *interpolating* thin-plate splines for elastic image registration. With this approach corresponding landmarks are forced to match exactly. The underlying (implicit) assumption is that the landmark positions are known exactly. However, in practical applications landmark localization is always prone to error. This is true for manual, semi-automatic as well as fully automatic landmark localization. To take into account landmark localization errors, we now introduce a generalization of the above described interpolation

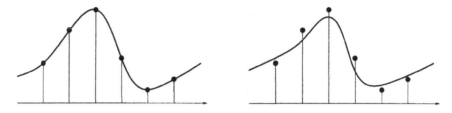

Figure 4.12.   Interpolation vs. approximation.

scheme (Rohr et al. [443]), which is based on the mathematical work in Duchon [130] and Wahba [545]. We relax the interpolation condition (4.4) by

$$\mathbf{q}_i \approx \mathbf{u}(\mathbf{p}_i), \qquad i = 1, \dots, n, \tag{4.54}$$

which states that the transformed landmarks of the first image $\mathbf{p}_i$ approximately match the landmarks $\mathbf{q}_i$ of the second image. To model this *approximation* behavior an additional term is introduced in the functional (4.5). See Figure 4.12 for the fundamental difference between interpolation and approximation. With our approximation approach it is possible to individually weight the landmarks according to their localization errors and thus to control the influence of the landmarks on the registration result. It turns out, that we generally obtain a more accurate and robust registration result.

4.5.1   Theory

For the components of the transformation $\mathbf{u}$ given the landmarks $\mathbf{p}_i$ and $\mathbf{q}_i$ in the first and second image, respectively, we assume the following model

$$q_i = u(\mathbf{p}_i) + n_i, \qquad i = 1, ..., n, \tag{4.55}$$

with q_i denoting one component of $\mathbf{q}_i$, and additive zero-mean Gaussian random errors $\mathbf{n} = (n_1, ..., n_n)^T \sim \mathcal{N}(\mathbf{0}, \sigma_i^2 \mathbf{I})$, where $\sigma_i^2 \mathbf{I} = \text{diag}\{\sigma_1^2, \dots, \sigma_n^2\}$ is a diagonal matrix representing the variances σ_i^2. The functional to be minimized now reads

$$J_\lambda(\mathbf{u}) = \frac{1}{n} \sum_{i=1}^{n} \frac{|\mathbf{q}_i - \mathbf{u}(\mathbf{p}_i)|^2}{\sigma_i^2} + \lambda J_m^d(\mathbf{u}), \tag{4.56}$$

where $|\cdot|$ denotes the Euclidean distance and J_m^d is the smoothness term as a function of the image dimension d and the order m of derivatives according to (4.5),(4.6) in Section 4.3 above.

Within the field of computer vision variational problems of this type have previously been considered for the reconstruction of surfaces from sparse depth data, i.e., for finding a mapping $u : \mathbb{R}^2 \to \mathbb{R}$ (e.g., Grimson [208], Boult and

Kender [56], Terzopoulos [517]). Such variational problems can be formulated in the mathematical framework of regularization theory for solving inverse problems, which are often ill-posed (e.g., Tikhonov and Arsenin [527], Poggio et al. [404], Terzopoulos [517], Bertero et al. [34], Szeliski [511]). The key idea in regularization is to restrict the range of possible solutions, which is usually done by incorporating a priori knowledge in form of smoothness constraints. Inverse problems typically arise in low-level computer vision. Arad et al. [12] used a 2D approximation approach as in (4.56) to represent and modify facial expressions. In the literature, typically equal weights $\sigma_i = 1$ are used.

In the case of medical image registration, Bookstein [51] has proposed a different approach to relax the interpolation condition. In comparison to our scheme, the approach in [51] has not been related to a minimizing functional w.r.t. the searched transformation, but combines different metrics based on a technique called curve décolletage (Leamer [302]). Generally, it is not clear whether all solutions in the whole function space are obtained this way. The approach has been described for the 2D case and experimental results have been reported for 2D synthetic data ('simulated PET images') only. Recently, Christensen et al. [93] introduced a hierarchical approach to image registration based on a different minimizing functional and where different splines have been used (see also [206]). In Gee et al. [188] isotropic landmark errors have been integrated within an intensity-based elastic registration scheme. This approach, however, is not based on an analytic solution of the underlying functional but solves it numerically by applying the finite element method (FEM), which is computationally much more expensive. For work on the inclusion of uncertainties in rigid or affine registration of medical images, see, e.g., Collignon et al. [100], Meyer et al. [342], Pennec and Thirion [398], and Maurer et al. [335].

In our case, the first term of the functional in (4.56), the so-called *data term*, measures the sum of the squared Euclidean distances between the transformed landmarks $\mathbf{p}_i$ and the landmarks $\mathbf{q}_i$. Each distance can be weighted by the variances σ_i^2 representing isotropic landmark localization errors. If, for example, the localization of a landmark is very uncertain, then the variance is high and the contribution to the first term is low. Figure 4.13 sketches two sets of landmarks with isotropic errors indicated by the circles of different size. Note, that we have only one parameter to represent the localization uncertainties of two corresponding landmarks. Thus, we have to combine the variances of corresponding landmarks to end up with one parameter. In our case, we use the sum of both variances, i.e., $\sigma_i^2 = \sigma_{i,p}^2 + \sigma_{i,q}^2$, where $\sigma_{i,p}^2$ and $\sigma_{i,q}^2$ are the variances associated with the landmarks $\mathbf{p}_i$ and $\mathbf{q}_i$, respectively. In Section 4.6.3 below we discuss this combination in more detail.

The second term in (4.56) represents the *bending energy* and measures the *smoothness* of the resulting transformation. Thus, with this functional there is

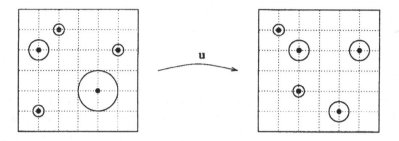

Figure 4.13.   Point landmarks in two images and corresponding isotropic errors.

a tradeoff between fidelity to the data and smoothness of the solution. The relative weight of the two terms is determined by the parameter $\lambda > 0$. Since the formulation of the approximation problem in (4.56) above is identical to problems in regularization theory (e.g., [527],[404],[34],[511]), λ is often denoted as *regularization parameter.* If λ is small, then the resulting transformation is well adapted to the local structure of the deformations between the two images, whereas if λ is large, then we obtain a very smooth transformation with little adaption to the deformations. There are two limiting cases: For $\lambda \to 0$ we obtain the original interpolating thin-plate spline transformation described above, while for $\lambda \to \infty$ we have a global polynomial of order up to $m - 1$, which has no bending energy at all. Choosing $m = 2$ in the latter case results in an affine transformation. Thus, for $m = 2$ and arbitrary values of $\lambda > 0$ we obtain an approximating elastic transformation the behavior of which lies in the range between the two extremes of an interpolating thin-plate spline transformation and an approximating affine transformation. Therefore, interpolating thin-plate splines and affine transformations are special cases of approximating thin-plate splines.

The functional in (4.56) can also be written as

$$
J_\lambda(\mathbf{u}) = \frac{1}{n} \sum_{i=1}^{n} \left(\frac{\sum_{k=1}^{d} (q_{i,k} - u_k(\mathbf{p}_i))^2}{\sigma_i^2} \right) + \lambda \sum_{k=1}^{d} J_m^d(u_k) \quad (4.57)
$$

$$
= \sum_{k=1}^{d} \left(\frac{1}{n} \sum_{i=1}^{n} \frac{(q_{i,k} - u_k(\mathbf{p}_i))^2}{\sigma_i^2} + \lambda J_m^d(u_k) \right) \quad (4.58)
$$

and, by introducing

$$
S(u_k) = \frac{1}{n} \sum_{i=1}^{n} \frac{(q_{i,k} - u_k(\mathbf{p}_i))^2}{\sigma_i^2}, \quad (4.59)
$$

we have

$$J_\lambda(\mathbf{u}) = \sum_{k=1}^{d} \left(S(u_k) + \lambda J_m^d(u_k) \right)$$

$$= \sum_{k=1}^{d} J_\lambda(u_k). \tag{4.60}$$

Thus, we see that the functional can be decomposed into functionals which depend only on one component of the transformation $\mathbf{u}$.

The interesting fact is that the solution to the approximation problem (4.56) exists, is unique, and can be stated analytically for the single components as

$$u(\mathbf{x}) = \sum_{\nu=1}^{M} a_\nu \phi_\nu(\mathbf{x}) + \sum_{i=1}^{n} w_i U(\mathbf{x}, \mathbf{p}_i) \tag{4.61}$$

with the same basis functions as in the case of interpolation (Duchon [130], Wahba et al. [547],[135],[545]; see also Section 4.3). The computational scheme to compute the coefficients of the transformation $\mathbf{u}$ is nearly the same:

$$\begin{aligned} \mathbf{Pa} + (\mathbf{K} + n\lambda\mathbf{W}^{-1})\mathbf{w} &= \mathbf{v} \\ \mathbf{P}^T\mathbf{w} &= \mathbf{0}, \end{aligned} \tag{4.62}$$

or, equivalently,

$$\begin{pmatrix} \mathbf{P} & \mathbf{K} + n\lambda\mathbf{W}^{-1} \\ \mathbf{0} & \mathbf{P}^T \end{pmatrix} \begin{pmatrix} \mathbf{a} \\ \mathbf{w} \end{pmatrix} = \begin{pmatrix} \mathbf{v} \\ \mathbf{0} \end{pmatrix}, \tag{4.63}$$

where

$$\mathbf{W}^{-1} = \begin{pmatrix} \sigma_1^2 & & 0 \\ & \ddots & \\ 0 & & \sigma_n^2 \end{pmatrix} \tag{4.64}$$

In comparison to the interpolation case we only have to add $n\lambda\mathbf{W}^{-1}$ to the matrix $\mathbf{K}$, which in fact means that we have to add $n\lambda\sigma_i^2$ to the diagonal elements of $\mathbf{K}$. As a by-product, this results in a better conditioned linear system of equations which allows a more robust numeric solution. To refer to these splines resulting from the stated approximation problem, we here use the term *approximating thin-plate splines*. Note, that in the mathematical literature generally the term *thin-plate smoothing splines* is used (e.g., [545]).

The transformation behavior of the thin-plate spline approximation scheme can be visualized by deforming a regular 2D grid. Figure 4.14 shows an

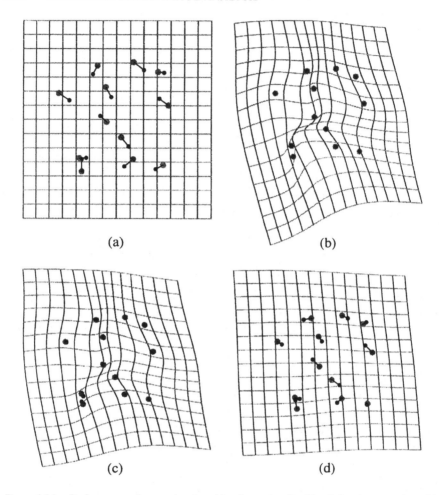

Figure 4.14. Performance of approximating thin-plates visualized by deforming a regular grid: (a) Two different landmark sets represented by the small black dots and the larger grey dots, (b) interpolation ($\lambda = 0$), (c) approximation (intermediate value of λ), and (d) nearly affine approximation (large value of λ).

example for different values of λ while setting $m = d = 2$ and assuming equal weights $\sigma_i = 1$. In (a) are shown the landmarks of the first and second image, which have been marked on a regular grid by the small black dots and the larger grey dots, respectively. In (b) the transformation result is shown for $\lambda = 0$, which is the case of thin-plate spline interpolation, where the landmarks match exactly. For an intermediate value of $\lambda = 0.001$ we obtain an approximation behavior with generally smaller local deformations (c). A much larger value of $\lambda = 0.1$ yields a nearly pure affine transformation with hardly any local deformations, as can be seen in (d).

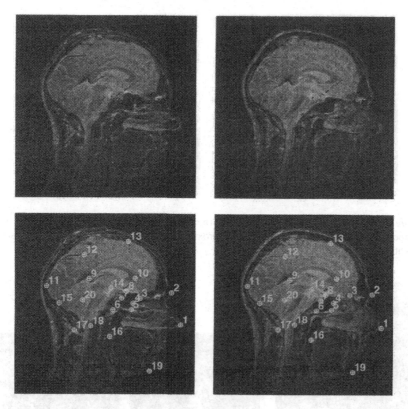

Figure 4.15. 2D MR images of the same patient: First, low-gradient image (left), and second, high-gradient image (right) with marked landmarks (bottom row).

4.5.2 Experimental Results

We now present experimental results of applying the approximating thin-plate spline registration scheme to tomographic images. Within the clinical application of MR-CT registration as described above in Section 4.2 we here consider the important application of correcting patient-induced susceptibility distortions of MR images (see also Rohr et al. [443]). Two sagittal MR brain images with typical susceptibility distortions of a healthy human volunteer have been acquired. In our experiment we use a high-gradient MR image as ground truth (instead of a clinically common CT image) to avoid exposure of the volunteer to radiation. Both turbo-spin echo images have consecutively been acquired using a modified Philips $1.5T$ MR scanner with a slice thickness of $4mm$ without repositioning. Therefore, we are sure that we actually have identical slicing in space. Using a gradient of $1mT/m$ and $6mT/m$ for the first and second image, respectively, then leads to a shift of ca. $7.5...10mm$ and ca. $1.3...1.7mm$, respectively. The original images are shown in Figure 4.15 at

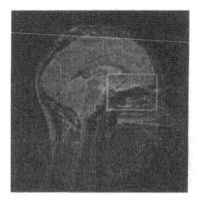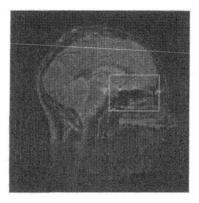

Figure 4.16. 2D registration result (transformed first image) for the images in Fig. 4.15: Interpolating thin-plate splines (left) and approximating thin-plate splines using equal scalar weights (right).

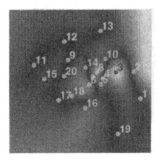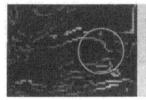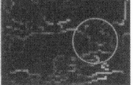

Figure 4.17. Difference between the two registration results in Fig. 4.16.

Figure 4.18. Registration errors for the marked image parts in Fig. 4.16: Interpolating thin-plate splines (left) and approximating thin-plate splines using equal scalar weights (right).

the top. It can be seen that the local deformations caused by different imaging parameters are significant. Particularly, this can be seen in the area of the sinus sphenoidalis (the dark region in the middle of the image). Within each of the two images we have manually specified 20 point landmarks. To simulate large landmark localization errors, one of the landmarks in the second image (Nr. 3) has been shifted about 15 pixels away from its true position (Figure 4.15 at the bottom). This large shift has been chosen for demonstration purposes. Note, however, that manual localization can actually be prone to relatively large errors. Figure 4.16 shows the results of interpolating thin-plate splines (left) vs. approximating thin-plate splines while setting $m = d = 2$ and using equal scalar weights $\sigma_i = 1$ (right). For the regularization parameter we have used a value of $\lambda = 50$. Note, that for a comparison of this value with the values used in the synthetic experiment in Figure 4.14 above one has to keep in mind that there a (normalized) image dimension of 1×1 pixels has been used. Thus, we have to normalize the regularization parameter to the current image dimension. Doing this, we obtain $\lambda_{norm} = 50/(256^2) \approx 0.0008$, which is close to the intermediate value of λ in Figure 4.14 ($\lambda = 0.001$). Each result represents the transformed first image. It can be seen that the interpolation scheme yields a rather unrealistic deformation since it forces all landmark pairs, including the pair with the simulated localization error, to exactly match each other. Using the approximation scheme instead yields a more accurate registration result. In the difference image of the two results in Figure 4.17, we see that the largest differences occur at the shifted landmark Nr. 3 which is what we expect. The increased accuracy of the approximation scheme can also be demonstrated by computing the distance between the grey-value edges of the transformed images and those of the second image. In our case, we applied a distance transformation [391] to detected grey-value edges [79]. The results for the marked rectangular image parts in Figure 4.16 can be seen in Figure 4.18. Here, the intensities represent the registration error, i.e., the brighter the larger is the error. In particular within the marked circular areas, which indicate the grey-value edges perpendicular to the simulated shift, we see that the registration accuracy has increased significantly.

To analyze the sensitivity w.r.t. the regularization parameter we have also computed the registration result for different values of λ. In Figure 4.19 the results are shown for values of $\lambda = 0, 1, 10, 50, 100, 10000$ which correspond to normalized values of $\lambda_{norm} \approx 0, 0.000015, 0.00015, 0.0008, 0.0015, 0.15$ (from top-left to bottom-right). The corresponding deformed regular grids have been overlaid. It can be seen, that the registration result varies smoothly between the two extremes of an interpolating transformation ($\lambda_{norm} = 0$) and an affine transformation ($\lambda_{norm} \approx 0.15$). Thus, the approach obeys the important principle of graceful degradation as advocated by Marr [328]. Clearly, an important topic for future research is the automatic determination of an optimal value of λ, e.g., by applying the method of general cross validation of Wahba [545].

We also show experimental results of applying the approximating thin-plate spline approach to 3D atlas data (Sprengel et al. [497], Rohr et al. [445]). In our experiment we have simulated nonlinear deformations of the digital SAMMIE atlas [257]. This 3D human brain atlas consists of 110 slices each of 270×346 voxels resolution. One slice is shown in Figure 4.20 on the left. Different anatomical structures are labeled with different grey values. The deformed atlas with overlaid contours from the original atlas is shown on the right. It can be seen that the deformations are relatively large (see also the enlarged sections in Figure 4.21). For the deformation we used a nonlinear function that depends on the angle between the top-left and the bottom-right diagonal of the image, with

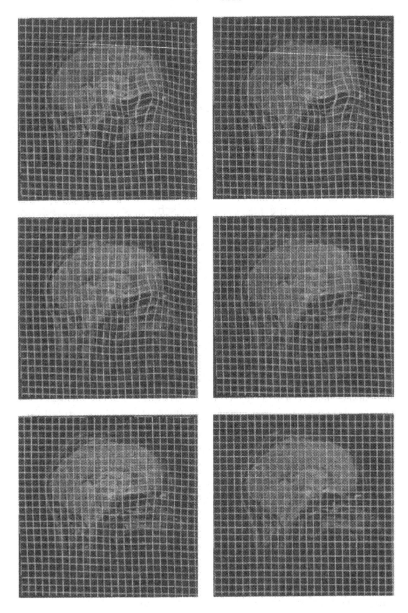

Figure 4.19.   Registration results as a function of λ with overlaid deformed regular grid.

the largest deformation in the direction of the bottom-left diagonal of the image. Note, that the simulated nonlinear deformation does not lie within the function space of thin-plate splines or polynomials. To register the deformed atlas with the original atlas, we have manually specified 34 homologous landmarks and

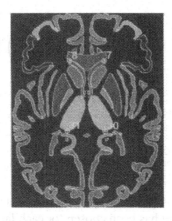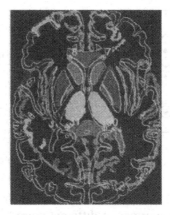

Figure 4.20.   Original (left) and analytically deformed (right) 3D human brain atlas (slice 45 of the SAMMIE atlas).

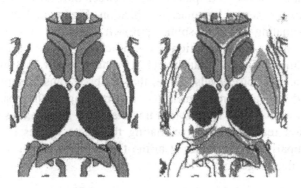

Figure 4.21.   Sections of the 3D human brain atlas: Original (left) and deformed (right).

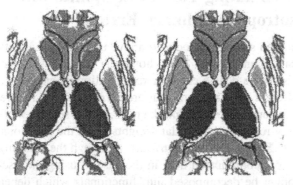

Figure 4.22.   3D registration result using individual scalar weights: Optimal affine approximation (left) and thin-plate spline approximation (right).

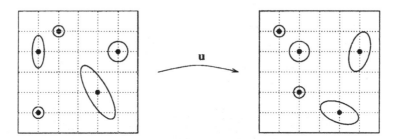

Figure 4.23.   Anisotropic errors at point landmarks.

have added Gaussian noise to the landmark positions such as to simulate typical localization errors. A different noise level has been chosen for each landmark, with standard deviations $\sigma_{n,i}$ in the range between 0.5 and 3.5 voxels. For our experiment, this resulted in displacements between 0.5 and 7 voxels which are to be expected for manual landmark localization. Figure 4.22 shows the result of the approximating thin-plate spline approach ($m = 2$, $d = 3$) in comparison to an optimal affine transformation (limiting case $\lambda \to \infty$ of approximating thin-plate splines). For the scalar weights we have used values in accordance with the simulated noise levels. Note, that for both transformation functions we have used the same input information consisting of the positions of the landmarks as well as their localization uncertainties. However, as can be seen, the registration result with approximating thin-plate splines is significantly better in comparison to an optimal affine transformation, particularly in the lower part of the image.

4.6   Approximating Thin-Plate Splines with Anisotropic Landmark Errors

The approximation scheme introduced above uses scalar weights to represent landmark localization errors. This, however, implies isotropic localization errors which is only a coarse error characterization. Generally, the errors are different in different directions and thus are *anisotropic* (cf. Figure 4.23). To be able to cope with anisotropic landmark errors, in this section we further extend our approach by replacing the scalar weights σ_i^2 in the functional (4.56) with *weight matrices* Σ_i *(covariance matrices)*. Although the resulting minimizing functional is more complicated than in the case of using only scalar weights, and can no longer be decomposed into functionals which depend only on a single component of the transformation $\mathbf{u}$, we still obtain an analytic solution the parameters of which can efficiently be computed by solving an analogous linear system of equations. Besides the handling of error information, another advantage of the generalization is that we can now include different types of landmarks. In addition to 'normal' point landmarks, which have a unique position in all directions, it is now possible to include *quasi-landmarks* which are not uniquely definable in all directions, e.g., arbitrary edge points. The latter landmark type is used, for example, in the reference system of Talairach [514] to define the 3D bounding box of the human brain. Note, that this reference system is applied in clinical practice. The incorporation of quasi-landmarks is important since it is often hard to define a larger number of corresponding normal point landmarks, particularly at the outer parts of the human head. Having extended the thin-plate spline approach, we then consider the problem of specifying landmark localization uncertainties in practical applications. We here propose a statistical approach which allows to estimate the covariance matrices directly from the image data. In our case, these matrices represent the minimal localization uncertainty at landmark points (Cramér-Rao bound) and we use theses estimates as additional input to the generalized approximating thin-plate spline approach. Our experiments for 2D and 3D tomographic images of the human brain show that the incorporation of quasi-landmarks together with the estimation of the covariance matrices significantly improves the registration result (Rohr et al. [446], Rohr [436]).

4.6.1 Incorporation of Weight Matrices

We consider the multiresponse model

$$q_{i,k} = u_k(\mathbf{p}_i) + n_{i,k}, \qquad k = 1, ..., d; \ i = 1, ..., n, \qquad (4.65)$$

where $q_{i,k}$ is the k-th component of the target landmark $\mathbf{q}_i$ and u_k is the k-th component of the transformation $\mathbf{u}$. We assume additive zero-mean Gaussian correlated random errors $n_{i,k}$ with variances $\sigma^2_{ii,kk}$ and covariances $\sigma_{ij,kl}, i \neq j, k \neq l$. The significant difference to the approximating thin-plate spline approach with scalar weights is that we now have to deal with *correlated errors*. In the mathematical literature on spline smoothing almost all of the work is based on the assumption that the random errors are independent, and only recently the topic of correlated errors has gained increased attention (Wang [551]). Note, that the mathematical work treats the case of general correlations. In (medical) image registration, however, the errors for a single landmark, $i = 1, ..., n$, are generally correlated, but one can well assume that there is no correlation between *different* landmarks. In this case, the minimizing functional can be stated as

$$J_\lambda(\mathbf{u}) = \frac{1}{n} \sum_{i=1}^{n} (\mathbf{q}_i - \mathbf{u}(\mathbf{p}_i))^T \Sigma_i^{-1} (\mathbf{q}_i - \mathbf{u}(\mathbf{p}_i)) + \lambda J_m^d(\mathbf{u}), \qquad (4.66)$$

with the covariance matrices

$$\Sigma_i = \begin{pmatrix} \sigma^2_{i,11} & \cdots & \sigma_{i,1d} \\ \vdots & \ddots & \vdots \\ \sigma_{i,d1} & \cdots & \sigma^2_{i,dd} \end{pmatrix}. \tag{4.67}$$

The functional can be written more compactly if we combine all covariance matrices Σ_i in the block-diagonal matrix

$$\mathbf{W}^{-1} = \begin{pmatrix} \Sigma_1 & & \mathbf{0} \\ & \ddots & \\ \mathbf{0} & & \Sigma_n \end{pmatrix}, \tag{4.68}$$

and denote all landmark coordinates of the second image by $\mathbf{Q} = (\mathbf{Q}_1^T, ..., \mathbf{Q}_n^T)^T$, $\mathbf{Q}_i^T = (q_{i,1}, ..., q_{i,d})$, and all transformed landmarks of the first image by $\mathbf{U} = (\mathbf{U}_1^T, ..., \mathbf{U}_n^T)^T$, $\mathbf{U}_i^T = (u_1(\mathbf{p}_i), ..., u_d(\mathbf{p}_i))$. Then we can write

$$J_\lambda(\mathbf{u}) = \frac{1}{n}(\mathbf{Q} - \mathbf{U})^T \mathbf{W}(\mathbf{Q} - \mathbf{U}) + \lambda J_m^d(\mathbf{u}) \tag{4.69}$$

with random errors $\mathbf{n} \sim \mathcal{N}(\mathbf{0}, \mathbf{W}^{-1})$, $\mathbf{n} = (\mathbf{n}_1^T, ..., \mathbf{n}_n^T)^T$, $\mathbf{n}_i^T = (n_{i,1}, ..., n_{i,d})$. The generalized functional can no longer be separated into the components of $\mathbf{u}$ and has to be treated as a *vector-valued problem*. However, it can be shown that the solution to minimizing this functional exists and is unique, and can be stated analytically as

$$u_k(\mathbf{x}) = \sum_{\nu=1}^M a_{k,\nu}\phi_\nu(\mathbf{x}) + \sum_{i=1}^n w_{k,i}U(\mathbf{x}, \mathbf{p}_i), \quad k = 1, ..., d, \tag{4.70}$$

with monomials ϕ_ν up to order $m - 1$ and the same radial basis functions $U(\mathbf{x}, \mathbf{p})$ as in the case of interpolation (see Wahba [546] and Wang [551], [552]).

The computational scheme to compute the coefficients $\mathbf{a}$ and $\mathbf{w}$ of the transformation $\mathbf{u}$ has the same structure as in the case of approximating thin-plate splines with scalar weights (4.62). However, since here a separation into the components u_k of the transformation $\mathbf{u}$ is no longer possible, we do not have a linear system of equations for each component u_k. Instead, the resulting system of equations comprises all components of $\mathbf{u}$ and thus is d-times larger. As in (4.62) we have

$$\mathbf{Pa} + (\mathbf{K} + n\lambda\mathbf{W}^{-1})\mathbf{w} = \mathbf{Q} \tag{4.71}$$
$$\mathbf{P}^T\mathbf{w} = \mathbf{0},$$

which can also be written as

$$\begin{pmatrix} \mathbf{P} & \mathbf{K}+n\lambda\mathbf{W}^{-1} \\ 0 & \mathbf{P}^T \end{pmatrix} \begin{pmatrix} \mathbf{a} \\ \mathbf{w} \end{pmatrix} = \begin{pmatrix} \mathbf{Q} \\ 0 \end{pmatrix}, \tag{4.72}$$

but now the coefficient vectors represent the coefficients for all components of $\mathbf{u}$ by $\mathbf{a} = (\mathbf{a}_1^T, ..., \mathbf{a}_M^T)^T$, $\mathbf{a}_i^T = (a_{1,i}, ..., a_{d,i})$, and $\mathbf{w} = (\mathbf{w}_1^T, ..., \mathbf{w}_n^T)^T$, $\mathbf{w}_i^T = (w_{1,i}, ..., w_{d,i})$. The matrices $\mathbf{P}$ and $\mathbf{K}$ are given by

$$\mathbf{P} = \begin{pmatrix} \phi_1(\mathbf{p}_1)\mathbf{I}_d & \cdots & \phi_M(\mathbf{p}_1)\mathbf{I}_d \\ \vdots & \ddots & \vdots \\ \phi_1(\mathbf{p}_n)\mathbf{I}_d & \cdots & \phi_M(\mathbf{p}_n)\mathbf{I}_d \end{pmatrix} \tag{4.73}$$

and

$$\mathbf{K} = \begin{pmatrix} U(\mathbf{p}_1,\mathbf{p}_1)\mathbf{I}_d & \cdots & U(\mathbf{p}_1,\mathbf{p}_n)\mathbf{I}_d \\ \vdots & \ddots & \vdots \\ U(\mathbf{p}_n,\mathbf{p}_1)\mathbf{I}_d & \cdots & U(\mathbf{p}_n,\mathbf{p}_n)\mathbf{I}_d \end{pmatrix}, \tag{4.74}$$

respectively, with $\mathbf{I}_d$ being the $d \times d$ identity matrix. We also have $\mathbf{Q} = (\mathbf{Q}_1^T, ..., \mathbf{Q}_n^T)^T$, $\mathbf{Q}_i^T = (q_{i,1}, ..., q_{i,d})$ as used in (4.69) and $\mathbf{W}$ as defined in (4.68) above.

From the stated approximating thin-plate spline approach in (4.66), which is valid for arbitrary image dimensions d and arbitrary orders of derivatives m in the functional (provided that the criterion $2m - d > 0$ in (4.7) is fulfilled), we can deduce special cases. First assume, that we have no correlations for single landmarks, i.e., $\sigma_{i,kl} = 0, k \neq l$ and let $\sigma_{i,kk}^2 = \sigma_{i,k}^2$. Then, for the weight matrix in (4.68) we have

$$\mathbf{W}^{-1} = \begin{pmatrix} \sigma_{1,1}^2 & & & & & \\ & \ddots & & & 0 & \\ & & \sigma_{1,d}^2 & & & \\ & & & \ddots & & \\ & & & & \sigma_{n,1}^2 & \\ & 0 & & & & \ddots \\ & & & & & \sigma_{n,d}^2 \end{pmatrix}. \tag{4.75}$$

The variances are generally different for the landmarks as well as for the different coordinates $k = 1, ..., d$ of the landmarks. In this case, we can represent anisotropic landmark errors, but anisotropy is allowed only along the coordinate axes. Thus, all error ellipses or error ellipsoids associated with the landmarks are aligned with the coordinate axes. Only in special practical applications such a requirement is met. Note, however that in this special case we have no interconnections between the components u_k of the transformation **u**, since we can write the minimizing functional in (4.66) as the superposition of functionals that depend only on the components of **u**:

$$J_\lambda(\mathbf{u}) = \frac{1}{n}\sum_{i=1}^{n}\left(\sum_{k=1}^{d}\frac{(q_{i,k}-u_k(\mathbf{p}_i))^2}{\sigma_{i,k}^2}\right) + \lambda\sum_{k=1}^{d}J_m^d(u_k) \quad (4.76)$$

$$= \sum_{k=1}^{d}\left(\frac{1}{n}\sum_{i=1}^{n}\frac{(q_{i,k}-u_k(\mathbf{p}_i))^2}{\sigma_{i,k}^2} + \lambda J_m^d(u_k)\right) \quad (4.77)$$

$$= \sum_{k=1}^{d}J_\lambda(u_k). \quad (4.78)$$

Thus, the problem can be separated into d minimization problems for each component while different variances can be used for the components. Note, that throughout this chapter we consider the smoothing term J_m^d to be decomposable into functionals that depend only on the components. If we further assume for the weight matrix in (4.75), that the variances are constant for the different components, i.e., $\sigma_{i,k}^2 = \sigma_i^2$, then we can write the functional as

$$J_\lambda(\mathbf{u}) = \frac{1}{n}\sum_{i=1}^{n}\frac{|\mathbf{q}_i - \mathbf{u}(\mathbf{p}_i)|^2}{\sigma_i^2} + \lambda J_m^d(\mathbf{u}), \quad (4.79)$$

which actually represents the approximating thin-plate spline approach with scalar weights as introduced in Section 4.5 above. In this case we can only include isotropic landmark errors.

An interesting and important aspect of the generalized approximation scheme is that it is now possible to include different types of point landmarks, e.g., 'normal' point landmarks as well as quasi-landmarks. *Normal* point landmarks have a unique position and low localization uncertainties in all directions. An example of *quasi-landmarks* are arbitrary edge points. Such points are not uniquely definable in all directions, and they are used, for example, in the clinically applied reference system of Talairach [514] to define the 3D bounding box of the human brain. The incorporation of such landmarks is important since normal point landmarks are hard to define, for example, at the outer parts of the human head. Below in Section 4.6.4 we give a more detailed discussion on the different types of landmarks. There, we also describe an approach for directly estimating the weight matrices from the image data. A separate issue results from the fact that with our thin-plate spline formulation we have only a single weight matrix for two corresponding landmarks, although we determine the localization errors of all landmarks (i.e. in both images). Thus, to end up with one weight matrix for two corresponding landmarks, we have to combine two weight matrices. This topic will be addressed separately in Section 4.6.3 below. Prior to that, in Section 4.6.2 we detail our approach for the practically most relevant cases of registering 2D and 3D datasets. Note, that our approximation scheme using weight matrices is also a generalization of the recent work of Bookstein [53],[54], where the interpolation problem is considered while the landmarks are allowed to slip along straight lines within a 2D image. Actually, this is a special case of our approximation scheme, since for straight lines the variance in one direction is zero whereas in the perpendicular direction it is infinite.

4.6.2 Special Cases of 2D and 3D Images

We now detail our general approach described above for the practically most relevant cases of 2D and 3D datasets ($d = 2$ and $d = 3$). We choose second order derivatives of **u** in the minimizing functional ($m = 2$).

4.6.2.1 2D Images

In the case of 2D images, we have as input data n corresponding landmarks in two images as well as associated 2×2 covariance matrices which can be represented by error ellipses (see also Figure 4.23 above). The smoothness term, i.e. the bending energy, consists of

$$J_2^2(\mathbf{u}) = J_2^2(u_1) + J_2^2(u_2), \tag{4.80}$$

where

$$J_2^2(u_k) = \int\limits_{-\infty}^{\infty} \int\limits_{-\infty}^{\infty} u_{k,xx}^2 + 2u_{k,xy}^2 + u_{k,yy}^2 \, dx dy. \tag{4.81}$$

The optimal transformation $\mathbf{u} : \mathbb{R}^2 \to \mathbb{R}^2$ as the solution to the minimizing functional for anisotropic landmark errors in (4.66) is given by

$$u_1(x, y) = a_{1,1} + a_{1,2}x + a_{1,3}y + \sum_{i=1}^{n} w_{1,i} U(\mathbf{x}, \mathbf{p}_i) \tag{4.82}$$

$$u_2(x, y) = a_{2,1} + a_{2,2}x + a_{2,3}y + \sum_{i=1}^{n} w_{2,i} U(\mathbf{x}, \mathbf{p}_i), \tag{4.83}$$

where

$$U(\mathbf{x}, \mathbf{p}_i) = \frac{1}{8\pi} r_i^2 \ln r_i \tag{4.84}$$

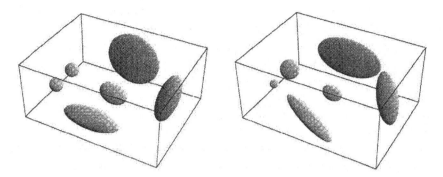

Figure 4.24.   Point landmarks and associated error ellipsoids in two images.

and $r_i = |\mathbf{x} - \mathbf{p}_i| = \sqrt{(x - p_{i,1})^2 + (y - p_{i,2})^2}$. The transformation consists of a 2D affine transformation and a superposition of radial basis functions representing the elastic part. Note, that the constant factor $1/8\pi$ of the basis function can be integrated into the weights $w_{k,i}$. The linear system of equations (4.71) to compute the coefficient vectors

$$\mathbf{a} = (a_{1,1}, a_{2,1}, a_{1,2}, a_{2,2}, a_{1,3}, a_{2,3})^T, \tag{4.85}$$

$$\mathbf{w} = (w_{1,1}, w_{2,1}, ..., w_{1,n}, w_{2,n})^T \tag{4.86}$$

is two times larger than in the case of approximating thin-plate splines with scalar weights. The matrix $\mathbf{P}$ can be stated as

$$\mathbf{P} = \begin{pmatrix} 1 & 0 & x_1 & 0 & y_1 & 0 \\ 0 & 1 & 0 & x_1 & 0 & y_1 \\ & & & \vdots & & \\ 1 & 0 & x_n & 0 & y_n & 0 \\ 0 & 1 & 0 & x_n & 0 & y_n \end{pmatrix}, \tag{4.87}$$

where we have used the abbreviations $x_i = p_{i,1}$ and $y_i = p_{i,2}$. The matrices $\mathbf{K}$ and $\mathbf{W}^{-1}$ are given as in (4.74) and (4.68), respectively, while setting $d = 2$.

4.6.2.2 3D Images

In the 3D case, the input data consists of n corresponding landmarks as well as associated 3×3 covariance matrices which can be represented by error ellipsoids as visualized in Figure 4.24. The smoothness term can be written as

$$J_2^3(\mathbf{u}) = J_2^3(u_1) + J_2^3(u_2) + J_2^3(u_3), \tag{4.88}$$

where

$$J_2^3(u_k) = \int\limits_{-\infty}^{\infty} \int\limits_{-\infty}^{\infty} \int\limits_{-\infty}^{\infty} u_{k,xx}^2 + u_{k,yy}^2 + u_{k,zz}^2 + 2(u_{k,xy}^2 + u_{k,xz}^2 + u_{k,yz}^2)\, dx dy dz.$$

(4.89)

The analytic solution for the transformation $\mathbf{u} : \mathbb{R}^3 \to \mathbb{R}^3$ is given by

$$u_1(x, y, z) \;=\; a_{1,1} + a_{1,2}x + a_{1,3}y + a_{1,4}z + \sum_{i=1}^{n} w_{1,i}\, U(\mathbf{x}, \mathbf{p}_i) \quad (4.90)$$

$$u_2(x, y, z) \;=\; a_{2,1} + a_{2,2}x + a_{2,3}y + a_{2,4}z + \sum_{i=1}^{n} w_{2,i}\, U(\mathbf{x}, \mathbf{p}_i) \quad (4.91)$$

$$u_3(x, y, z) \;=\; a_{3,1} + a_{3,2}x + a_{3,3}y + a_{3,4}z + \sum_{i=1}^{n} w_{3,i}\, U(\mathbf{x}, \mathbf{p}_i), \quad (4.92)$$

where

$$U(\mathbf{x}, \mathbf{p}_i) = -\frac{1}{8\pi} r_i,$$

(4.93)

and $r_i = \sqrt{(x - p_{i,1})^2 + (y - p_{i,2})^2 + (z - p_{i,3})^2}$. Thus, we have a 3D affine transformation together with an elastic part. The coefficient vectors are

$$\mathbf{a} \;=\; (a_{1,1}, a_{2,1}, a_{3,1}, a_{1,2}, a_{2,2}, a_{3,2}, a_{1,3}, a_{2,3}, a_{3,3}, a_{1,4}, a_{2,4}, a_{3,4})^T, \quad (4.94)$$
$$\mathbf{w} \;=\; (w_{1,1}, w_{2,1}, w_{3,1}, ..., w_{1,n}, w_{2,n}, w_{3,n})^T, \quad (4.95)$$

and can be computed through solving the linear system of equations (4.71), where

$$\mathbf{P} = \begin{pmatrix} 1 & 0 & 0 & x_1 & 0 & 0 & y_1 & 0 & 0 & z_1 & 0 & 0 \\ 0 & 1 & 0 & 0 & x_1 & 0 & 0 & y_1 & 0 & 0 & z_1 & 0 \\ 0 & 0 & 1 & 0 & 0 & x_1 & 0 & 0 & y_1 & 0 & 0 & z_1 \\ & & & & & \vdots & & & & & & \\ 0 & 0 & 1 & 0 & 0 & x_n & 0 & 0 & y_n & 0 & 0 & z_n \end{pmatrix}, \quad (4.96)$$

with $x_i = p_{i,1}$, $y_i = p_{i,2}$, $z_i = p_{i,3}$, while $\mathbf{K}$ and $\mathbf{W}^{-1}$ are given as in (4.74) and (4.68), respectively, setting $d = 3$. The linear system of equations is a factor of three larger than in the case of approximating thin-plate splines with scalar weights. Note, that the constant factor $1/(8\pi)$ of the basis function in (4.93) can be integrated into the weights $w_{k,i}$, while the negative sign cannot. Thus, it is important to use the correct sign of the basis function. Otherwise the bending energy would be negative, and then a negative regularization parameter

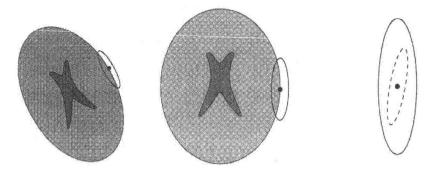

Figure 4.25.   Corresponding landmarks and error ellipses in two images (left and middle) and transformed ellipses (right).

λ would be required to compensate this, although it has been defined that $\lambda > 0$. To see this, recall from (4.25) that the bending energy can be expressed as $J_m^d = \mathbf{w}^T \mathbf{K} \mathbf{w} > 0$, while $\mathbf{K}$ consists of the elements $U(|\mathbf{p}_i - \mathbf{p}_j|)$ which in our case are negative or equal to zero. Thus, to ensure that the bending energy remains positive we can only integrate constants into $\mathbf{w}$ leading to $J_m^d = (\mathbf{w}^*)^T \mathbf{K} \mathbf{w}^*$, where $\mathbf{w}^* = (1/\sqrt{8\pi})\mathbf{w}$, but integrating the negative sign is not possible.

4.6.3   Combination of Weight Matrices

We already mentioned that the approximating thin-plate spline functional with anisotropic landmark errors in (4.66) includes only one covariance matrix $\boldsymbol{\Sigma}_i$ for two corresponding landmarks. Generally, however, we have covariance matrices for each of the landmarks in both images. Thus, to apply our approach, we have to combine the covariance matrices of corresponding landmarks. Since we deal with elastic image registration, it is generally necessary to apply an elastic transformation for correct combination of the matrices to ensure that both matrices refer to the same coordinate system. Finding the elastic transformation is, however, the general goal of our work. Thus, we have a 'chicken-and-egg' problem. A way out of this problem is to take into account the fact that the covariance matrices describe the localization errors at a certain point, i.e., these matrices are very local descriptions. Thus, it is reasonable to assume that the two covariance matrices depend only slightly on the elastic part of the transformation. In this case, we can combine two matrices by applying a linear transformation (rotation, scaling) to one of the matrices followed by adding them (see also Figure 4.25). Below, we describe in more detail the combination of covariance matrices for one landmark pair (see also the work concerning error propagation in, e.g., Förstner [169], Smith et al. [489], Haralick [225], Pennec and Thirion [398]).

For the noise model in (4.65) we have assumed additive zero-mean Gaussian stochastic errors, which are correlated for single landmarks but are uncorrelated otherwise, i.e. uncorrelated for other landmarks of the same or a different image. Now, suppose that both corresponding landmarks $\mathbf{p}$ and $\mathbf{q}$ in the first and second image are corrupted by noise $\mathbf{n_p} = (n_{p,1}, ..., n_{p,d})^T$ and $\mathbf{n_q} = (n_{q,1}, ..., n_{q,d})^T$, respectively. Then, we can state

$$\mathbf{q} = \mathbf{u}(\mathbf{p} + \mathbf{n_p}) + \mathbf{n_q} \qquad (4.97)$$

and for the corresponding mean values and covariance matrices we have

$$\bar{\mathbf{n}}_p = E\{\mathbf{n_p}\} = \mathbf{0}, \qquad \Sigma_p = E\{\mathbf{n_p}\mathbf{n_p^T}\}, \qquad (4.98)$$

$$\bar{\mathbf{n}}_q = E\{\mathbf{n_q}\} = \mathbf{0}, \qquad \Sigma_q = E\{\mathbf{n_q}\mathbf{n_q^T}\}, \qquad (4.99)$$

where $E\{\cdot\}$ denotes the expectation operation.

Let us first assume that the errors have been measured in the same coordinate system, i.e., $\mathbf{u}(\mathbf{p} + \mathbf{n_p}) = \mathbf{p} + \mathbf{n_p}$. Then, we have $\mathbf{q} = \mathbf{p} + \mathbf{n}$, where $\mathbf{n} = \mathbf{n_p} + \mathbf{n_q}$, and the corresponding covariance matrix is

$$
\begin{aligned}
\Sigma &= E\{\mathbf{n}\mathbf{n^T}\} \\
&= E\{(\mathbf{n_p} + \mathbf{n_q})(\mathbf{n_p} + \mathbf{n_q})^T\} \\
&= E\{\mathbf{n_p}\mathbf{n_p^T}\} + E\{\mathbf{n_q}\mathbf{n_p^T}\} + E\{\mathbf{n_p}\mathbf{n_q^T}\} + E\{\mathbf{n_q}\mathbf{n_q^T}\} \\
&= \Sigma_p + \Sigma_q, \qquad (4.100)
\end{aligned}
$$

since above we assumed $E\{\mathbf{n_q}\mathbf{n_p^T}\} = E\{\mathbf{n_p}\mathbf{n_q^T}\} = \mathbf{0}$. Thus, the combined covariance matrix is obtained by just adding the two covariance matrices.

Now, we consider the case when the matrices have been measured in different coordinate systems while both coordinate systems are related by an affine transformation

$$\mathbf{q} = \mathbf{A}\mathbf{p} + \mathbf{T}. \qquad (4.101)$$

Then, disregarding the noise influence $\mathbf{n_q}$, the expected value of $\mathbf{q}$ is $\bar{\mathbf{q}} = \mathbf{A}\bar{\mathbf{p}} + \mathbf{T}$ and the covariance matrix of $\mathbf{q}$ calculates to

$$
\begin{aligned}
\Sigma_q' &= E\{(\mathbf{q} - \bar{\mathbf{q}})(\mathbf{q} - \bar{\mathbf{q}})^T\} \\
&= E\{(\mathbf{A}(\mathbf{p} - \bar{\mathbf{p}}))(\mathbf{A}(\mathbf{p} - \bar{\mathbf{p}}))^T\} \\
&= \mathbf{A}E\{(\mathbf{p} - \bar{\mathbf{p}})(\mathbf{p} - \bar{\mathbf{p}})^T\}\mathbf{A^T} \\
&= \mathbf{A}\Sigma_p\mathbf{A^T}. \qquad (4.102)
\end{aligned}
$$

In summary, taking the results in (4.100) and (4.102) together, we have the following formula for combining two corresponding covariance matrices of the first and second image:

$$\Sigma = \mathbf{A}\Sigma_p\mathbf{A^T} + \Sigma_q. \qquad (4.103)$$

Thus, we have to apply a linear transformation to $\Sigma_{\mathbf{p}}$ followed by adding $\Sigma_{\mathbf{q}}$ to the result. Within our approach for elastic registration this formula can be applied as follows: (i) determine the linear transformation $\mathbf{A}$, e.g., by computing an optimal affine transformation using all landmarks of the two images, (ii) use $\mathbf{A}$ and (4.103) to calculate the combined matrices Σ for all landmark pairs $i = 1, ..., n$, and (iii) include the combined matrices for computing the elastic transformation, again using all landmarks of the two images. Note, that in the case when the two images have approximately the same orientation and scaling, then step (i) is not necessary and we can simply add the two covariance matrices:

$$\Sigma = \Sigma_{\mathbf{p}} + \Sigma_{\mathbf{q}}. \qquad (4.104)$$

Simplifying this further for the case of isotropic errors, then for one component we obtain

$$\sigma^2 = \sigma_{\mathbf{p}}^2 + \sigma_{\mathbf{q}}^2, \qquad (4.105)$$

which is just the addition of the variances.

To illustrate the effects of combining different covariance matrices, we show in Figure 4.26 some examples for the 2D case visualized by the corresponding error ellipses. For two isotropic ellipses, i.e. circles, we again have an isotropic result (first row). Combining ellipses which are elongated in the same direction maintains this direction, but combining ellipses with different principal directions gives an intermediate direction (second and third row). If the principal directions of two otherwise equal ellipses are orthogonal, then we obtain a circle as combination result (fourth row). Note, that correlated errors are represented by ellipses whose principal directions are different from the coordinate axes. In the 3D case, i.e. for 3×3 covariance matrices, we obtain analogous combination results (see Figure 4.27).

4.6.4   Estimation of Landmark Localization Uncertainties

Above, we have developed an elastic registration scheme which allows to integrate anisotropic landmark errors. However, so far we have not considered the problem of specifying these errors. One possibility is to use error information derived from anatomical studies concerning the variability of brain structures. However, currently we are not aware that such anatomical knowledge is available. Alternatively, a user in a certain registration application may provide confidence levels representing the degree of localization uncertainty for single landmarks (e.g., high, middle, low confidence) as well as may specify certain directions in which the uncertainty is observed to be extremal. A disadvantage of such a procedure is, however, that it is tedious and time-consuming.

Instead, we here propose a different approach which allows to estimate landmark localization uncertainties directly from the image data (Rohr [436]).

First image   Second image   Combination

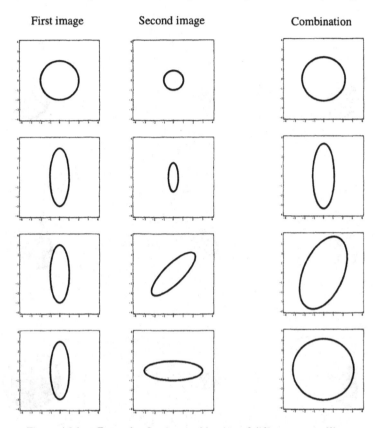

Figure 4.26.   Examples for the combination of different error ellipses.

With this approach we exploit the *minimal stochastic localization error* due to the intensity variations in the neighborhood of a landmark. The minimal error is determined by the *Cramér-Rao bound* (e.g., van Trees [533]) which we have already introduced above. In Sections 3.2.2 and 3.2.3 we have used this bound to derive closed-form expressions for analytically given intensity structures. In Section 2.5.5 we have used the Cramér-Rao bound as basis for a statistical interpretation of 3D operators for detecting anatomical point landmark. Here, we apply the discrete version of the Cramér-Rao bound to estimate the minimal localization uncertainty for 2D and 3D point landmarks from real image data. The Cramér-Rao bound in the discrete case for arbitrary image dimensions d can be stated as

$$\Sigma_g = \frac{\sigma_n^2}{m} \mathbf{C}_g^{-1}, \tag{4.106}$$

where σ_n^2 denotes the variance of additive white Gaussian image noise, m is the number of image points in a local neighborhood of the considered point

First image   Second image   Combination

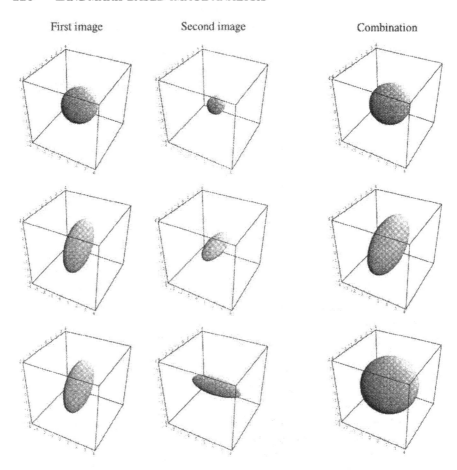

Figure 4.27.   Examples for the combination of different error ellipsoids.

landmark, and $\mathbf{C}_g = \overline{\nabla g \, (\nabla g)^T}$ is the averaged dyadic product of the image gradient with $g(\mathbf{x})$ denoting the image function. Thus, the bound depends on the local variation of the image gradient, the image noise, and the size of the local neighborhood. $\mathbf{C}_g$ and thus $\boldsymbol{\Sigma}_g$ can directly be computed from the image data. The required first order image derivatives in (4.106) in our case are computed by applying either Gaussian derivative filters or Beaudet filters [28]. Averaging is generally performed in a 5×5 or $5 \times 5 \times 5$ neighborhood, respectively. Having computed $\boldsymbol{\Sigma}_g$ we can derive, for example, the 3D error ellipsoid of the position estimate with semi-axes σ_x, σ_y, and σ_z. Note, that in the case if we have no Gaussian image noise, we consider (4.106) as an approximation. However, investigations on the error statistics of medical image data have shown the validity of the Gaussian model (Barrett and Swindell [27], Abbey et al. [1]).

	σ_x	σ_y
normal landmark	≈ 0	≈ 0
quasi-landmark	≈ 0	$+$
homogeneous region	$+$	$+$

Table 4.3. Classification of landmarks in 2D images on the basis of the semi-axes σ_x, σ_y of the minimal error ellipse according to the Cramér-Rao bound.

Although for many imaging modalities the image data follow Poisson counting statistics, the statistics are well approximated by a Gaussian at count levels typical for clinical imaging. On the other hand, it has recently been argued in [1] that for large signal-to-noise ratios the dependence of the noise on the signal should be taken into account. In our approach, however, we assume that this dependence can be neglected. Note also, that since we use a lower bound our procedure is applicable to any point within an image, independently of how this point has been localized (manually or automatically). Dealing with stochastic errors, we hereby assume that we have the same systematic errors for each landmark pair. On the other hand, if we knew the systematic errors we could compensate them prior to application of our scheme.

Based on the covariance matrix Σ_g of the Cramér-Rao bound in (4.106) we can distinguish different types of points in 2D and 3D images. Landmarks with locally high intensity variations in all directions, i.e. strongly curved intensity surfaces, have low localization uncertainties in all directions and we refer to them as *normal point landmarks*. Points, where the localization uncertainty is high in a least one principal direction of the minimal error ellipsoid (but not in all directions) will be denoted as *quasi-landmarks,* since these points are not uniquely definable in all directions. An example are arbitrary points on image edges, where we have low localization uncertainties perpendicular to the edge but high localization uncertainties along the edge (e.g., the 3D bounding box landmarks of Talairach [514]). Note, that edges in 3D images are generally surfaces whereas in 2D they are curves. Another example for quasi-landmarks are arbitrary points on curve and surface structures. Finally, normal landmarks and quasi-landmarks can be distinguished from *points in homogeneous regions* where we have high localization uncertainties in all directions. In Table 4.3 we have listed the classification of landmarks in 2D images on the basis of the semi-axes σ_x, σ_y of the minimal error ellipse according to the Cramér-Rao bound. Note, that the semi-axes have been arranged such that $\sigma_y \geq \sigma_x$ without loss of generality. We have used the following symbols: '$\approx$' for values approximately zero and '$+$' for values significantly larger than zero. In the 2D case we have three different types of landmarks: normal landmarks, quasi-landmarks (edge and curve points), and points in homogeneous regions (see also Figure 4.28). Note, that for edge and curve points (line points) we have

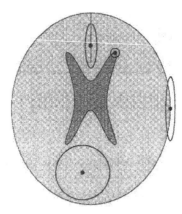

Figure 4.28.   Different types of 2D landmarks and corresponding uncertainty ellipses.

the same form of the uncertainty ellipse. It should also be mentioned, that, e.g., points in homogeneous regions should ideally have infinite uncertainties in all directions. However, since we here deal with real images which are always corrupted by noise and other effects, the uncertainty ellipses are finite. The classification for 3D images has been listed in Table 4.4, where the semi-axes of the minimal error ellipsoid have been arranged such that $\sigma_z \geq \sigma_y \geq \sigma_x$. In the 3D case we have four different types of points: normal point landmark, quasi-landmark 1 (curve, edge or surface point; low uncertainty in two principal directions), quasi-landmark 2 (edge or surface point; low uncertainty in one principal direction), and point in homogeneous region (see also Figure 4.29).

Analogous classifications have been reported for 2D images by Förstner [168],[171], Rohr [424], as well as Harris and Stephens [230], for example. The classification in [168],[171] as well as the one here is based on a statistical interpretation of the position estimate. Other classifications including spatio-temporal grey-value structures and 3D images are based on the geometric concept of local orientation. There the matrix $\mathbf{C}_g = \overline{\nabla g\,(\nabla g)^T}$ from (4.106) above is employed, which essentially is the inverse of $\mathbf{\Sigma}_g$. The matrix $\mathbf{C}_g$ is generally known as *orientation tensor* or *structure tensor* and is used, e.g., for feature extraction, optic flow estimation, shape-adapted smoothing, and feature tracking (see also, e.g., Lucas and Kanade [317], Knutsson [282], Bigün and Granlund [41], Nitzberg and Shiota [382], Jähne et al. [260],[238], Shi and Tomasi [483], Weickert [555],[556], Kang et al. [273], Lindeberg and Gårding [310], Westin et al. [559], as well as Section 2.5 above). Note, that the classification in this section is also related to the classification of the intensity structure based on differential geometry as described in Section 2.3.1 above. A difference is that there the involved principal curvatures may have positive as well as negative values, while the semi-axes $\sigma_x, \sigma_y, \sigma_z$ are always larger or

	σ_x	σ_y	σ_z
normal landmark	≈ 0	≈ 0	≈ 0
quasi-landmark 1	≈ 0	≈ 0	$+$
quasi-landmark 2	≈ 0	$+$	$+$
homogeneous region	$+$	$+$	$+$

Table 4.4. Classification of landmarks in 3D images on the basis of the semi-axes $\sigma_x, \sigma_y, \sigma_z$ of the minimal error ellipsoid according to the Cramér-Rao bound.

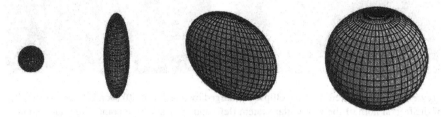

Figure 4.29. Different types of 3D image points characterized by their uncertainty ellipsoids (from left to right): Normal point landmark, curve point or edge point (quasi-landmark 1), edge point (quasi-landmark 2), and point in homogeneous region.

equal to zero. The reason for this is that the matrix Σ_g is positive semidefinite (see also Section 2.5.5 above). A consequence is that saddle structures cannot be distinguished.

The error characterization described in this section is based on the minimal errors, which are generally different from the errors obtained by an anatomical study or specified by a user. However, in either case we suspect that the localization errors depend on the geometry of the landmark, e.g., for an edge point we have large uncertainties along the edge but low uncertainties perpendicular to the edge. Also, all approaches to error characterization should share the property that increasing the image noise generally leads to larger localization errors, which is the case with our scheme.

We now show some examples of applying our approach to 2D and 3D medical image data. In Figure 4.30 are depicted the estimated error ellipses (68.3% probability corresponding to 1σ regions) for the tip of the frontal horn of the ventricular system as well as for an arbitrary edge point at the outer contour of the head within a 2D MR dataset. The selected points are examples for normal landmarks and quasi-landmarks. The image sections are of size 51×51 pixels. The local neighborhood is 5×5 pixels large and $\sigma_n^2 = 25$ has been used for the variance of the image noise. Note, that the error ellipses have been enlarged by a factor of 30 for visualization purposes. It can be seen that the error ellipse of the tip is small and close to a circle which means that the localization uncertainty for this point is low in arbitrary directions. For the edge point, however, the error ellipse is largely elongated and indicates a large

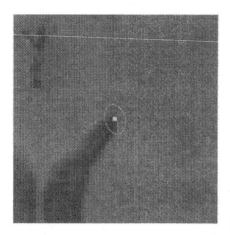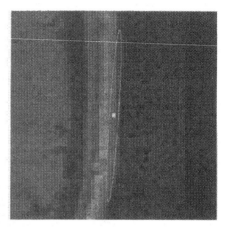

Figure 4.30.   Estimated 2D error ellipses (enlarged by a factor of 30) for a 2D MR dataset: Tip of the frontal horn of the ventricular system (left) and arbitrary edge point at the outer contour of the head (right).

localization uncertainty along the contour and a low localization uncertainty perpendicular to the contour. This is what we expect from the local intensity structure at the considered points.

In Figure 4.31 we show the estimated 3D error ellipsoid for the landmark 'genu of corpus callosum' within a 3D MR dataset of the human brain. The 3D error ellipsoid has been displayed by three orthogonal views (sagittal, axial, coronal) and corresponds to 1σ confidence regions. Note, that the ellipsoid has been enlarged by a factor of 30 for visualization purposes. The section of the image, i.e. the region-of-interest (ROI), is of size $21 \times 21 \times 21$ voxels and has been centered around the landmark. The landmark position has automatically been detected using the 3D differential operator $Op3$ as introduced in Section 2.5 above. We have used a local neighborhood of $5 \times 5 \times 5$ voxels and $\sigma_n^2 = 25$ for the variance of the image noise. In Figure 4.31 we see within the sagittal plane that the localization uncertainty along the edge is much larger than the localization uncertainty perpendicular to the edge. The axial and coronal views of the 3D error ellipsoid indicate an approximately isotropic localization uncertainty, where the uncertainty within the coronal plane is larger than within the axial plane. Another example is given in Figure 4.32 which shows the estimated 3D error ellipsoid for the landmark 'lower cusp between pons and medulla oblongata'.

4.6.5   Experimental Results

We now present experimental results of applying the approximating thin-plate spline registration scheme using anisotropic landmark errors while estimating

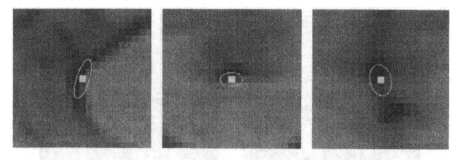

Figure 4.31. Estimated 3D error ellipsoid (enlarged by a factor of 30) for the landmark 'genu of corpus callosum' within a 3D MR dataset of the human brain (orthogonal views: sagittal (left), axial (middle), coronal (right)).

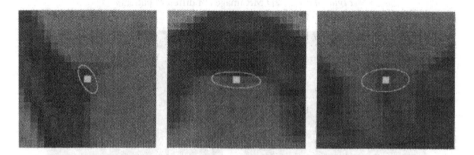

Figure 4.32. Same as Fig. 4.31 but for the landmark 'lower cusp between pons and medulla oblongata'.

the covariance matrices directly from the image data. We have investigated 2D as well as 3D datasets.

We first consider the registration of 2D MR head images of different patients as shown in Figure 4.33. Although the images are of the same modality they are rather different since different imaging parameters have been used (T_1- vs. T_2-weighting). For many anatomical structures this leads to an inversion of the intensities. Thus, intensity-based approaches which directly match the intensities would probably have problems in comparison to landmark-based approaches. Also note that the shape of the two heads is rather different. For this 2D example we have manually selected seven normal landmarks in the inner parts of the brain (numbers 1-6 and 8; see Figure 4.34 top) as well as four quasi-landmarks at the outer contour of the head (numbers 9-12; see Figure 4.34 bottom). For all landmarks we have automatically estimated the error ellipses at these points with the approach described in Section 4.6.4 and have drawn them in Figure 4.35. Note, that the ellipses have been enlarged by a factor of 7 for visualization purposes. We see, that for the normal landmarks the ellipses are small and more or less isotropic while for the quasi-landmarks the ellipses

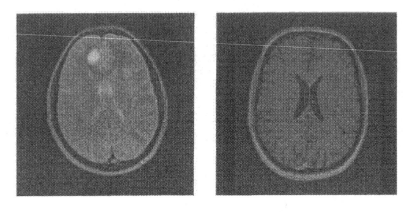

Figure 4.33.   2D MR images of different patients.

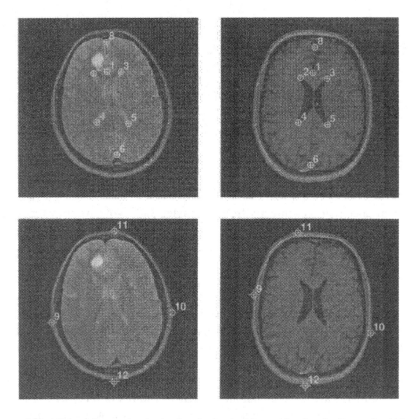

Figure 4.34.   Selected normal point landmarks (top) and quasi-landmarks (bottom) within the images of Fig. 4.33.

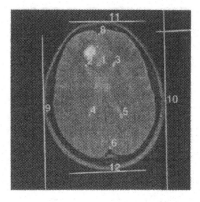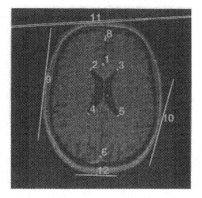

Figure 4.35. 2D MR datasets of different patients: Normal landmarks, quasi-landmarks, and estimated error ellipses (enlarged by a factor of 7).

are strongly elongated along the edges. Given this input data we have applied different approaches to elastic registration. Figure 4.36 on the left shows the registration result when applying interpolating thin-plate splines while using all landmarks. The edges of the second image have been overlaid onto the transformed first image. We see that an unrealistic deformation towards the top left is obtained since corresponding landmarks are forced to match exactly although they are generally not homologous points (i.e., they do not correspond physically). Note, that since we selected the landmarks manually in this 2D example, it would be possible to specify improved corresponding positions for the quasi-landmarks and thus to reduce the effect of the unrealistic deformation. However, the basic problem would remain. By this example we wanted to simulate automatic determination of quasi-landmarks, e.g., by searching for the most frontal point or by fitting a bounding box to the brain. In either case, the localization of quasi-landmarks would be rather sensitive w.r.t. the shape of the head as well as the image orientation. Thus, we generally expect larger localization errors which are comparable to the simulated errors of this experiment. Using approximating thin-plate splines with equal scalar weights ($m = d = 2$ in (4.56)) instead of interpolating thin-plate splines, the registration result is improved but it is still not satisfactory (Figure 4.36 on the right). A further improvement is obtained if we apply this procedure only to the normal landmarks (Figure 4.37 on the left). However, the best result is achieved if we use both the normal landmarks and the quasi-landmarks together with the estimated ellipses, and apply approximating thin-plate splines with anisotropic errors ($m = d = 2$ in (4.66)). From the result in Figure 4.37 on the right it can be seen, that the combination of both types of landmarks significantly improves the registration accuracy, particularly at the outer parts of the head.

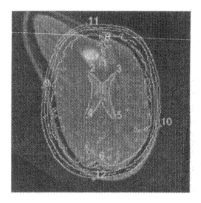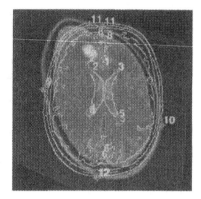

Figure 4.36. Registration result: Thin-plate spline interpolation (left), and thin-plate spline approximation with equal scalar weights (right) using normal landmarks and quasi-landmarks.

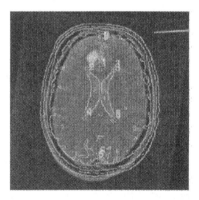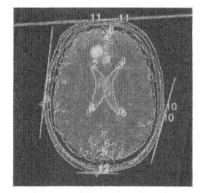

Figure 4.37. Registration result: Thin-plate spline approximation using normal landmarks and equal scalar weights (left), and using normal landmarks, quasi-landmarks and estimated error ellipses (right).

We have also applied our approach to the registration of 3D MR and CT images. The MR dataset consists of 120 axial slices of 256×256 voxels each and the CT dataset consists of 87 axial slices of 320×320 voxels each. The images have been acquired from the same patient (see Figure 4.38 for slices 34 and 38 of the original images, respectively). In this example, the landmarks have semi-automatically been localized using the 3D differential operator $Op4 = det\mathbf{C}_g$ described in Section 2.5. For registration, we have applied the approximating thin-plate spline approach with incorporated weight matrices in (4.66) using $m = 2$ and $d = 3$. The 3×3 weight matrices have automatically been estimated. For the current example of 3D MR-CT registration we have used only normal landmarks since this choice already leads to an

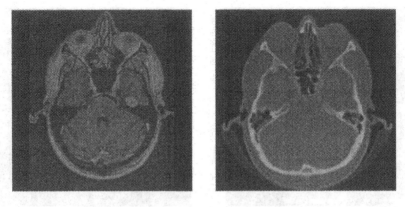

Figure 4.38. 3D MR and CT datasets of the same patient (slices 34 and 38, respectively).

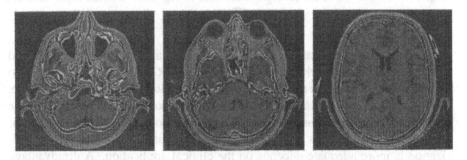

Figure 4.39. 3D registration result using approximating thin-plate splines and estimated 3D weight matrices (slices 21, 38, and 84).

accurate registration result. Note, that we here deal with images of the same patient. Figure 4.39 shows the registration result by superimposing the 3D edges of the CT image onto the transformed MR image. The edges have been computed using a 3D extension of the approach of Canny [79]. It can be seen that the registration accuracy is rather good. For these datasets it turned out that the registration accuracy is nearly independent of the parameter λ. Thus, in the case of MR-CT registration of the same patient, and when the distortions of the MR image can be assumed to be small, an optimal affine transformation (which is a limiting case of our approach) seems to be sufficient. Note, that in the MR image a tumor is visible which is not represented in the CT image (see the bright region in about the middle of the MR image). Using the integrated image allows a better diagnosis, e.g., the location and shape of the tumor w.r.t. the bone is now easier to assess in comparison to observing the images separately. To see this more clearly, we have enlarged slice 38 of the 3D registration result (Figure 4.40 on the left). Another visualization of the combination result is shown in Figure 4.40 on the right. Here, we have per-

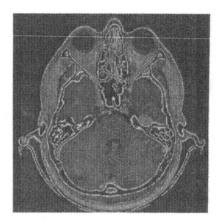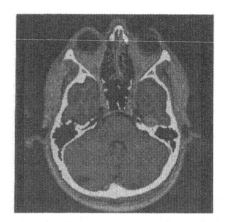

Figure 4.40.   Slice 38 of the 3D registration result in Fig. 4.39: Overlaid edges (left) and overlaid region segmentation (right) of the CT image.

formed a region segmentation of the CT image by applying a simple threshold operation and have overlaid the result onto the MR image. This example also demonstrates that image registration and combination of registered images, i.e. image fusion, are separate problems. Certainly, also other visualizations of the combined images are possible, e.g., 3D visualizations with different values of transparency parameters for the anatomical structures. Which type of visualization is more adequate depends on the clinical application. A disadvantage of 3D visualizations is that generally a full segmentation of the 3D datasets including a labeling of the anatomical structures is necessary. Such a region (or volume) segmentation can generally not be achieved automatically, which is a disadvantage in comparison to computing 'only' image edges.

With the next example, we demonstrate the application of the approximating thin-plate spline approach with weight matrices to the registration of 3D MR images of different patients. The datasets consist of $179 \times 236 \times 165$ voxels and $177 \times 245 \times 114$ voxels, respectively (see Figure 4.41 for slices 57 and 41 of the original images). We have used ten normal landmarks as well as eight quasi-landmarks while setting $m = 2$ and $d = 3$ in (4.66). The normal point landmarks have been localized semi-automatically using the 3D differential operator $Op4 = det\mathbf{C}_g$. As quasi-landmarks we have used the 3D bounding box landmarks of the brain (Talairach [514]) as well as two landmarks at the top of the ventricular system. The six bounding box landmarks in [514] are the uppermost point of the parietal cortex, the lowest point of the temporal cortex, the most anterior point of the frontal cortex, the most posterior point of the occipital cortex, the most lateral point of the left parieto-temporal cortex, and the most lateral point of the right parieto-temporal cortex. The quasi-landmarks have been localized manually. For all landmarks the weight matrices have

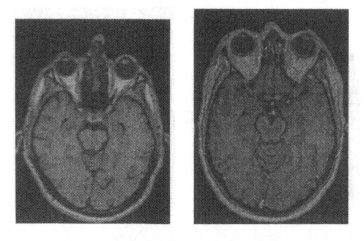

Figure 4.41. 3D MR datasets of different patients (slices 57 and 41, respectively).

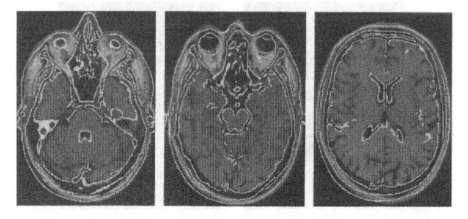

Figure 4.42. 3D registration result using approximating thin-plate splines, normal landmarks, quasi-landmarks and estimated 3D weight matrices (slices 29, 41, and 67).

automatically been estimated directly from the image data as described above. Figure 4.42 shows that we generally obtain a good registration result (see slices 29, 41, and 67), while some deviations can be observed at the bottom left of the slices 41 and 67.

The last example shows an application of our registration scheme to image-atlas registration. We have chosen two corresponding slices of an MR image and the SAMMIE atlas [257], see Figure 4.43. In both images ten landmarks (six normal landmarks and four quasi-landmarks) have manually been selected and the error ellipses have been determined. In the atlas the ellipses have been specified manually, since the atlas is not an intensity image but a segmented and

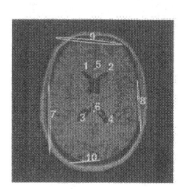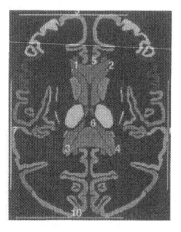

Figure 4.43.   MR image and digital atlas (SAMMIE).

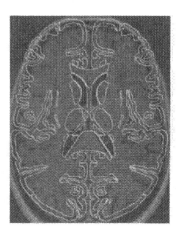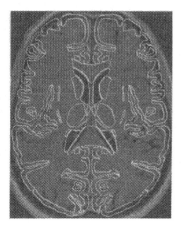

Figure 4.44.   Registration result with interpolating thin-plate splines using normal landmarks (left) and approximating thin-plate splines using normal landmarks and quasi-landmarks (right).

labeled representation. Note, however, that the assignment of error information for an atlas has to be done only once, and then this information can be used in all further registration applications involving this atlas. The error ellipses for the MR data have been computed directly from the image. The registration result is shown in Figure 4.44. We have applied interpolating thin-plate splines using only normal landmarks (left) and approximating thin-plate splines using normal landmarks and quasi-landmarks (right). It can be seen that the approximation approach yields a significantly better registration result. However, for the gyri structures (see the outer parts of the brain) deviations can be observed. On the other hand, note that the registration accuracy for these structures is difficult to assess, since there seem to be differences in the topology for the used slices. With this example of image-atlas registration we also demonstrate the potential of our registration scheme for model-based segmentation. Here the atlas is taken as geometric model which is elastically matched to the actual MR patient data. In this way it is possible to segment anatomical structures which are hardly visible in the MR image. It is even possible to predict the location of *invisible* structures, which is particularly important in surgical interventions. Note, however, that particular in the latter case a validation is rather difficult and generally requires the use of histological sections.

4.7 Orientation Attributes at Landmarks

Starting out from the original interpolating thin-plate spline approach, we have introduced above an approximation scheme which allows to incorporate land-mark localization uncertainties. The input data to this elastic image registration scheme consists not only of the landmarks' positions, but we can also include additional attributes at the landmarks in form of weight matrices which represent error ellipses or error ellipsoids. On the one hand, this approach allows to incorporate additional knowledge in image registration. On the other hand, we can include a more general class of landmarks, namely quasi-landmarks. This is important since finding homologous point landmarks particularly at the outer parts of the human brain is difficult.

In this section, we briefly describe a further extension of our scheme which allows to incorporate additional attributes at landmarks. As attributes we here consider *orientations* at point landmarks in both images to be mapped onto each other. Generally, these attributes characterize the local orientation of the contours at the landmarks (Fornefett et al. [158]–[160], Rohr et al. [448]). With this extended approach it is possible to integrate localization uncertainties as well as orientations at point landmarks. Thus, we can integrate *statistical* as well as *geometric* information as additional knowledge in elastic image registration. The general aim of incorporating orientations is to improve the registration accuracy without the necessity of selecting further landmarks. Previous work by Bookstein and Green [55] use a finite difference approach and approximate orientations by two landmarks. Mardia et al. [324],[325] have proposed an exact solution based on the stochastic method of kriging. They described an interpolation approach where the orientation vectors are required to be unit vectors. In comparison to that, our approach is based on a minimizing functional which also has an exact analytic solution. However, we treat the interpolation as well as the approximation case. In the case of interpolation the lengths of orientation vectors are not required to be unit vectors. The approach is suitable for images of arbitrary dimension d and yields a linear system of equations analogously to that of our previous approach described above. While in [158]–[160] we have treated the case of isotropic landmark errors together with orientation attributes, in [448] we have extended this scheme for inclusion of anisotropic errors.

At corresponding landmarks we assume to have orientations which we want to match (note, that these landmarks are generally a subset of all landmarks). We denote those landmarks in the first and second image by $\mathbf{p}_{\theta_i}$ and $\mathbf{q}_{\theta_i}$ and the corresponding orientations by $\mathbf{d}_i$ and $\mathbf{e}_i$, respectively. To define a matching criterion between the orientations, we need the transformed vector of $\mathbf{d}_i$. This vector can be stated as $(\mathbf{d}_i^T \nabla) \mathbf{u}(\mathbf{p}_{\theta_i})$. Now we require that this transformed vector is perpendicular to $\mathbf{e}_{i,k}^{\perp}$, which are the k-th orthogonal vectors to the orientation vector $\mathbf{e}_i$ in the second image. In this case, the scalar product between the vectors is zero, otherwise it is different from zero. Note, that this is analogous to the case of matching the positions of landmarks in the functional (4.66) from above, i.e., if the landmarks match exactly the contribution is zero, otherwise it is different from zero. Choosing vectors from the orthogonal space has the advantage that the corresponding scalar product is zero independently of the length of the vectors. Note, however, that the property of length independence only holds in the case of interpolation, but not for approximation. In general we have $d - 1$ perpendicular orientations $\mathbf{e}_{i,k}^{\perp}$ which constrain the transformed orientation vector of the first image to lie on a line. If the number of perpendicular orientations is smaller, i.e., the number of constraints is lower, then the transformed orientation vector is not constrained w.r.t. a line, but w.r.t. a plane, for example (see also [158]).

Having defined the matching criterion between orientations we can now state the generalized minimizing functional:

$$J_\lambda(\mathbf{u}) = \frac{1}{n} \sum_{i=1}^{n} (\mathbf{q}_i - \mathbf{u}(\mathbf{p}_i))^T \boldsymbol{\Sigma}_i^{-1} (\mathbf{q}_i - \mathbf{u}(\mathbf{p}_i))$$

$$+ \frac{c}{n_2} \sum_{i=1}^{n_\theta} \sum_{k=1}^{d-1} \left((\mathbf{d}_i^T \nabla) \mathbf{u}^T (\mathbf{p}_{\theta_i}) \mathbf{e}_{i,k}^{\perp} \right)^2 + \lambda J_m^d(\mathbf{u}), \quad (4.107)$$

where $n_2 = n_\theta(d-1)$. In comparison to the functional for anisotropic landmark errors (4.66) from above we here have an additional term that incorporates the orientation constraints. n_θ is the total number of orientations in each of the images. The parameter $c > 0$ weights the orientation term w.r.t. the term representing the landmark positions and also determines (besides λ) whether we interpolate or approximate the orientations. Note, that we can incorporate an arbitrary number of orientations at each landmark. As described above, the orientation constraints are incorporated by scalar products between the transformed orientations of the first image and orientations perpendicular to the orientations in the second image. The solution to the functional in (4.107) can be stated as

$$\mathbf{u}(\mathbf{x}) \;=\; \sum_{\nu=1}^{M}\sum_{k=1}^{d} a_{k,\nu}\phi_{\nu}(\mathbf{x})\varepsilon_{k}$$

$$+\sum_{i=1}^{n}\sum_{k=1}^{d} w_{1,k,i}U(\mathbf{x},\mathbf{p}_{i})\varepsilon_{k}$$

$$-\sum_{i=1}^{n_{\theta}}\sum_{k=1}^{d-1} w_{2,k,i}(\mathbf{d}_{i}^{T}\nabla)U(\mathbf{x},\mathbf{p}_{\theta_{i}})\mathbf{e}_{i,k}^{\perp}, \qquad (4.108)$$

with monomials ϕ up to order $m-1$ and radial basis functions U as above. ε_{k}, $k = 1\ldots d$, are the canonical basis vectors of the $\mathrm{I\!R}^{d}$. The solution is analogous to (4.70) from above, but additionally we have a term that represents the constraints due to the orientation information. Note, that in order to obtain bounded functionals the used function space has to be constrained. Choosing $m = 2$ for the order of derivatives of the smoothness term, then for both cases of 2D and 3D images ($d = 2, 3$) incorporating orientations, we have the basis function $U(r) = r^{3}$. Note, that we have to choose different values of $s = 1/2$ and $s = 1$, respectively, in (4.41) above, while the parameter s defines the chosen function space.

   In particular, our approach can be applied in cases, where it is important to preserve rigid parts within otherwise elastically deformed material. Rigid parts such as bone should be prevented from elastic deformations since they undergo only rigid transformations. Application tasks are the registration of brain images or images of the spine. With Figure 4.45 we illustrate the basic idea of our approach. The square represents a rigid structure which is embedded in an otherwise elastic material. The source and target images simulate a rotation of the square for about 45° degrees. For these images we have first selected four landmarks at the corner of the square as well as four landmarks at the corners of the image and we have used this information for applying interpolating thin-plate splines (Figure 4.46 on the left). It can be seen, that the whole image including the rigid structure is elastically deformed. If we additionally incorporate orientations at the landmarks of the square, then we can significantly improve the registration result, i.e., the shape of the square is well preserved (Figure 4.46 on the right). In this example, we have added two orientations at each of the landmarks of the square and these orientations have been aligned with the contours of the square. We have used $c = 1$ and $m = 2$ for the functional in (4.107) and assumed no landmark errors. Previously, Little et al. [312] have considered the problem of preserving rigid structures within elastic material (see also Müller and Ruprecht [358]). However, in their approach a full segmentation of the rigid structures is necessary. In comparison to that, with our scheme we neither need a full segmentation nor do we need

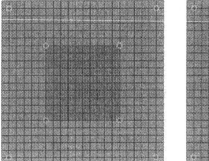
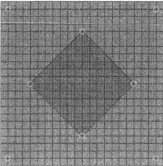

Figure 4.45.   2D synthetic images simulating the rotation of a rigid structure in an otherwise elastic material.

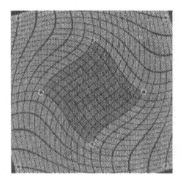
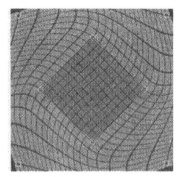

Figure 4.46.   Registration result: Interpolating thin-plate splines using only point landmarks (left) and incorporation of orientations at landmarks (right).

additional point landmarks. We have just included a few additional orientations at existing landmarks to end up with a very good registration result.

In the second example we treat the case of several rigid structures embedded in elastic material. Figure 4.47 shows two synthetic images that simulate the bending of a spine which is represented by five rigid components (see also [312]). The registration result in Figure 4.48 on the left is obtained if we apply interpolating thin-plate splines while using four landmarks for each rigid component as well as four image border landmarks. In Figure 4.48 in the middle, the result is shown if we include two orientations at each landmark of the rigid components, while still applying an interpolation scheme. It can be seen that the shape of the rigid structures is better preserved, particularly the outer contours of the rigid components are not curved as in the case of using point landmarks only. A further improvement is achieved if we use both the point landmarks and the orientations but apply an approximation scheme (Figure 4.48 on the right). Here we have used equal isotropic landmarks errors

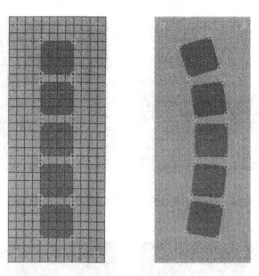

Figure 4.47. Synthetic images simulating a spine that is bended.

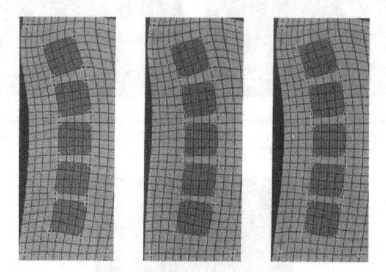

Figure 4.48. Registration results: Interpolating thin-plate splines using only point landmarks (left), integration of two orientations at each object landmark (middle), and approximating thin-plate splines using point landmarks and orientations (right).

in the functional in (4.107). From the result it can be seen that the contours of the rigid components are straight and now also the gridlines within the rigid components are nearly straight. Thus the shape of the rigid structures is better preserved.

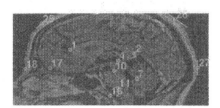

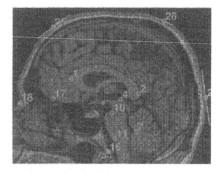

Figure 4.49. MR images of different patients: Normal landmarks, quasi-landmarks, and estimated error ellipses.

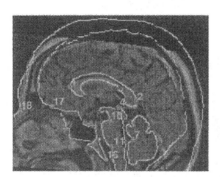

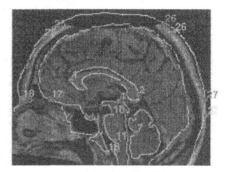

Figure 4.50. Registration results: Interpolating thin-plate splines using normal landmarks (left), and approximating thin-plate splines using normal landmarks, quasi-landmarks and estimated covariance matrices (right).

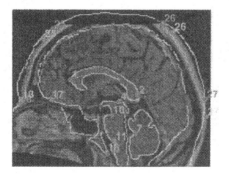

Figure 4.51. Registration result: Approximating thin-plate splines using normal landmarks, quasi-landmarks, estimated covariance matrices, and orientations.

With the third example we show an application where we have integrated both anisotropic landmark errors and orientation attributes at landmarks. In Figure 4.49 two MR images of different patients are shown. We have selected normal point landmarks, quasi-landmarks, and have estimated the error ellipses directly from the image data. If we use only the normal landmarks (9 landmarks; Nr. 1,2,4,7,10,11,16,17,18) and apply interpolating thin-plate splines, then we obtain the result shown in Figure 4.50 on the left. Deviations can be observed in the regions where no landmarks have been specified, particularly at the upper part of the brain and at the corpus callosum. Next, we have used the normal landmarks from above together with three quasi-landmarks at the skin contour (landmarks Nr. 25,26,27). For all landmarks we have automatically estimated the covariance matrices and we have applied the approximating thin-plate spline approach incorporating anisotropic errors, i.e. we have used full covariance matrices Σ_i. From Figure 4.50 on the right it can be seen that the registration accuracy at the upper part of the brain is now much better while at the corpus callosum there is still a larger deviation. We can further improve the registration accuracy in this region if we additionally integrate orientations at landmarks. In this example, we have included one orientation at landmark Nr. 1 (genu of corpus callosum). In both images this orientation points to the top of the corpus callosum. From Figure 4.51 we see, that we now obtain a significantly better registration accuracy of the whole corpus callosum.

For additional experimental results including the 3D case, see [158]–[160], [448]. One problem with this type of approach is that the influence of incorporated orientations is rather global, i.e., image parts far away from landmarks with added orientations are generally strongly affected, which is often not desired. This observation has also been made in Mardia et al. [324],[325]. Thus, in future work, means have to be found to constrain this global influence, e.g., by using alternative radial basis functions, which have a more local influence. An example are the radial basis functions of Wendland [557], which have a similar shape as the Gaussian function but have compact support. Thus, they have a well-defined local influence. Moreover, solvability of the resulting system of linear equations is always guaranteed since the basis functions are positive definite, and the computational scheme is efficient. Recently, the basis functions of Wendland [557] have been applied to simulate facial expressions in video coding applications (Soligon et al. [492]). In Fornefett et al. [161], [164] we have introduced these basis functions for elastic image registration.

4.8 Biomechanical Modelling of Brain Deformations

Above in Section 4.7 we have demonstrated that our approach is to some extend suited to deal with different kinds of tissues, namely rigid and elastic anatomical structures. A main advantage of this spline-based approach is computational efficiency. Recently, in medical image registration there is a also trend to model biomechanical properties of anatomical structures more precisely using computationally more expensive *biomechanical models*. A central topic there is to deal with general *nonhomogeneous* tissue properties. In the case of the human head one basically has to distinguish between rigid (e.g., bone), elastic (e.g., brain tissue), and fluid parts (e.g., the ventricular system). The relevant physical theory is continuum mechanics comprising elasticity theory and fluid mechanics. For biomechanical models of the human head, there are a number of potential applications, e.g., in surgery simulation and intraoperative navigation. Image-guided intraoperative navigation, as mentioned in Section 4.2 above, relies on preoperatively acquired image data. During an operation, however, generally brain deformations occur. For example, opening the skull and the dura mater leads to a *brain shift* since liquor flows off, and also the resection of a tumor leads to brain deformations, e.g., Buchholz et al. [75], Hill et al. [246], [247], Dickhaus et al. [120], Reinges et al. [413] (see Figure 4.52). For accurate localization of brain structures it is then necessary to correct the preoperative image by registering it with the current anatomical situation. If a further image can be acquired intraoperatively (e.g., a CT image by a portable CT scanner), then we could apply our spline-based elastic registration scheme, provided that enough corresponding landmarks can be found in the surgical relevant regions. If the intraoperatively acquired data is not as detailed as with CT or MR images (e.g., images from an ultrasound device or other measurements) or even if we have no additional image information, then generally the incorporation of a biomechanical model is required to predict the occurring deformations.

Approaches for *intraoperative image correction* have been reported by Buchholz et al. [75], who applied a mass-spring system incorporating linear elastic materials, and Edwards et al. [138],[139] who combined different energy terms. Both models have been described for the 2D case while real physical material parameters have not been included. Thus, reliable prediction of brain deformations can be questioned. Approaches dealing with nonhomogeneous tissues based on elasticity theory which incorporate real physical material parameters and apply thefinite element method (FEM), have been proposed by Kyriacou et al. [292],[293], Hagemann et al. [217],[220], and Miga et al. [346]. For work on other applications dealing with nonhomogeneous tissue properties, see Davatzikos et al. [112], Lester et al. [307], Martin et al. [332]. In other work on intraoperative brain shift correction, homogeneous material is assumed or deformations are restricted by imposing certain boundary conditions (e.g., Škrinjar et al. [488], Hata et al. [237], Peckar et al. [396], Ferrant et al. [151], Rezk-Salama et al. [415]). Biomechanical brain models for simulation purposes but not for registration have been described, for example, in Schill et al. [467], Hartmann and Kruggel [236] (see also Section 4.9 below).

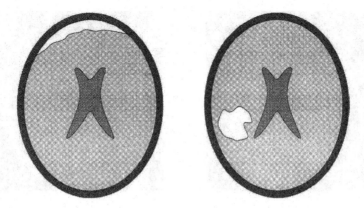

Figure 4.52. Sketch of intraoperative brain deformations: Brain shift due to skull opening (left) and tumor resection (right).

Besides treating nonhomogeneous material properties, a central problem in intraoperative image correction is to cope with large deformations. To illustrate the complexity of the task, we show in Figure 4.53 pre- and postoperative MR images, which were routinely acquired in conjunction with the planning and verification of a tumor resection. Instead of an intraoperative image we here use a postoperative image for demonstration purposes. Registration of these two images is difficult because we have large deformations due to tumor resection as well as a brain shift as can be seen at the top of the image. Our approach described in Hagemann et al. [216]–[220] is based on the Navier equation (4.42) which is solved numerically using the *finite element method (FEM)*. Using the pre- and postoperative MR images in Figure 4.53 first corresponding tumor contours were manually specified by a medical expert and landmark correspondences have been determined using a snake algorithm (see also Peckar et al. [396]). Then, based on a coarse segmentation of the images into combined skin/skull region, brain, ventricular system (CSF), and surrounding air (using an interactive watershed algorithm; Tieck et al. [526]) as well as associating corresponding material parameter values we were able to well predict the occurring deformations in the area around the tumor. The material parameter values for tissues of the human head have been obtained through a comprehensive literature study [216],[220].

So far, we have modelled different material properties based on *one* physical model, in this case a purely elastic model. Recently, we have introduced for the first time an approach for intraoperative image correction, where different physical models have been coupled, namely an elastic model based on the Navier equation and a fluid model based on the Stokes equation. This extension allows to model deformations of *combined elastic/fluid* parts more accurately [221].

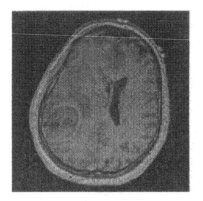 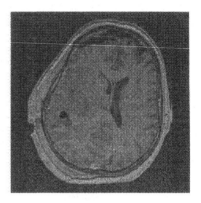

Figure 4.53.   Preoperative (left) and postoperative image (right) of a tumor resection.

4.9   Related Work

Thin-plate splines have first been introduced in 1972 for *surface interpolation* by Harder and Desmarais [228], while the mathematical foundations have been laid later by Duchon [130],[131] and Meinguet [339] (see Wahba [545]). Actually, thin-plate splines are a natural multidimensional generalization of the 1D splines of Schoenberg [472] and Reinsch [414]. In the field of computer vision, thin-plate functionals have been proposed for surface reconstruction, particularly for interpolation of depth maps (e.g., Grimson [207],[208], Brady and Horn [60], Boult and Kender [56], Terzopoulos [517], Blake and Zisserman [46], Bertero et al. [34], Szeliski [510],[511], Bolle and Vemuri [48]). Surface fitting given sparse scattered data is also a topic in the fields of computer graphics or computer-aided geometric design. Here, thin-plate splines as well as other radial basis functions have been investigated (e.g., [175],[298],[344], [157],[4],[256],[259],[229],[200],[375]). Related approaches have also been used in computer animation, particularly for image warping and morphing, as well as for image coding and compression (e.g., Wolberg [568],[569], Beier and Neely [29], Arad et al. [12],[13], Ruprecht et al. [457],[358], Soligon et al. [492]).

In the context of morphometrics and medical image analysis, Bookstein [49] first proposed the use of thin-plate splines for point-based *elastic image registration.* He considered the interpolation case and applied this approach to 2D images. Application for 3D image registration has been reported by Evans et al. [147],[148], for example. Interpolating thin-plate splines have also been applied in other fields, e.g., in photogrammetry for the registration of 2D aerial images (e.g., Goshtasby [198], Flusser [156], Wiemker et al. [561]). Our approach of approximating thin-plate splines using scalar weights is based on the mathematical work in Duchon [130] and Wahba [545] and has first been introduced for medical image registration in Rohr et al. [443],[497]. There, the scheme allowed to deal with isotropic errors and it has been applied to the registration of 2D tomographic images of the human brain. In Rohr et al. [446], [436] we have generalized this approach for inclusion of anisotropic errors and have applied this scheme to 2D as well as 3D tomographic images. The anatomical landmarks have been localized semi-automatically using differential operators and landmark localization uncertainties have directly been estimated from the image data based on the Cramér-Rao bound (Rohr [436]). Our generalization allows to include additional types of landmarks, e.g., quasi-landmarks. From the theoretical point of view, this generalization requires to deal with correlated errors and vector splines (see the mathematical work of Wahba [546] and Wang [551],[552]). A different approach to relax the interpolation condition has been proposed by Bookstein [51]. The basis of this approach is a linear regression model and the technique is referred to as curve décolletage (Leamer [302]). With this approach different energy terms are combined and it is possible to incorporate isotropic as well as anisotropic errors. However, since this approach has not been related to a minimizing functional w.r.t. the searched transformation it is generally not clear whether all solutions in the whole function space are obtained. The approach has been described for 2D datasets and experimental results have been reported for 2D synthetic data. The landmarks as well as the corresponding errors have been specified manually.

Other work on the *integration of error information* for point features has focused on rigid, similarity, or affine transformations. In medical image analysis the inclusion of uncertainties for rigid or affine image registration has been described by Collignon et al. [100], Meyer et al. [342], Pennec and Thirion [398], and Maurer et al. [335]. In Gee et al. [188] isotropic landmark errors have been integrated within an intensity-based elastic registration scheme. This approach, however, is not based on an analytic solution of the underlying functional but solves it numerically by applying the finite element method (FEM), which is computationally much more expensive. Recently, Christensen et al. [93] described a spline-based approach involving the linear elasticity operator, where isotropic landmark errors have been included (see below for a more detailed description). Related tasks in computer vision and photogrammetry where error information has been integrated are the determination of absolute orientation (e.g., [255],[243]) or model-based object recognition (e.g., [459], [405]), see also [169],[225]. Handling of error information is also relevant in the field of robotics for estimating spatial relationships (e.g., [489]).

Incorporation of orientations at point landmarks has been proposed by Bookstein and Green [55]. There, a finite difference approach has been applied where orientations are approximated by two landmarks. Mardia et al. [324], [325] have proposed an exact analytic solution based on the stochastic method of kriging. It is required that the orientation vectors are unit vectors. They also proposed to incorporate curvature attributes at landmarks. Both approaches in [55] and [324],[325] deal with interpolating transformations. In comparison to these schemes, our approach for incorporating orientations in Fornefett et al. [158]–[160] and Rohr et al. [448] is based on a minimizing functional within the framework of thin-plate splines. We have an exact analytic solution and we treated interpolating as well as approximating transformations, while in the interpolation case the requirement of unit orientation vectors is not necessary. Whereas in [158]–[160] we have treated the case of isotropic landmark errors together with orientation attributes, in [448] we have extended this scheme for inclusion of anisotropic errors. Note, that approximating transformations can also be treated within the framework of kriging, however, application to image registration has not yet been reported. With our approach in [158]–[160] we have shown that it is possible to preserve rigid structures in otherwise elastic material. Previously, Little et al. [312] have also considered this problem. Their approach incorporates additional weighting functions and requires a full segmentation of the rigid structures which is not necessary with our approach.

Another main direction towards generalization of point-based elastic registration is to include *more general types of landmarks,* e.g., curves or surfaces. Such an approach has recently been proposed by Bookstein [53],[54]. There, 2D contours are represented by quasi-landmarks and straight line segments. While solving the interpolation thin-plate spline problem, the quasi-landmarks are allowed to slip along straight lines. The approach has been applied to 2D image data. Actually, this approach is a special case of our approximation scheme incorporating anisotropic errors (Rohr et al. [446],[436]), since for straight lines the variance in one direction is zero whereas in the perpendicular direction it is infinite. Other approaches dealing with the incorporation of contour information have been reported by Cutting et al. [109],[110], Green [204],[205], Joshi et al. [265], Gabrani and Tretiak [183], as well as Fornefett et al. [163]. While in contour-based approaches more information of the images is taken into account than with point-based approaches, a disadvantage is that the segmentation, the representation of the segmented structures, as well as the finding of correspondences is generally more difficult. Related to the above-mentioned contour-based approaches are curve- or surface-based methods for elastic image registration (e.g., Moshfeghi [356],[357], Szeliski and Lavallée [513], Declerck et al. [115], Davatzikos et al. [111], Subsol et al. [505], Peckar et al. [397], Amini et al. [7]). Note, that curve-based methods often are also denoted as line-based methods. These approaches are related to deformable models in computer vision (see the survey of McInerney and Terzopoulos [337] and the literature therein as well as Boult et al. [57]). Generally, these approaches are not based on an analytic solution but solve the underlying elasticity equations numerically, e.g., by applying finite differences (FD) or the finite element method (FEM), therefore the computation time is generally higher. For application of the boundary elements method (BEM), see Gladilin et al. [195]. A promising research direction seems to be the combination of deformations based on physical models as described above with experimental (or statistical) deformations which are based on training examples. In the latter case, deformations of the model are only allowed in accordance with the training data (e.g., Martin et al. [332], Nastar et al. [365], Cootes and Taylor [102]).

Recent work on spline-based medical image registration has been done on combining thin-plate splines with mutual information as similarity measure for refinement of initially coarsely specified landmarks (Meyer et al. [343]). For an application of thin-plate splines in the context of 3D-2D registration see Guéziec et al. [211]. Thin-plate splines have also been applied for analysis of spatio-temporal medical images (cardiac images), e.g., Rueckert et al. [455], Kerwin and Prince [277]. A different spline-based approach has been introduced by Davis et al. [113]. These authors do not use thin-plate splines but propose analytic solutions to the Navier equation as a basis of their registration scheme. The resulting splines have been termed elastic body splines (EBS) and the intention is to model the physical behavior more adequately. Note, however, that the derived analytic solutions to the Navier equation are only valid under the assumption of certain forces, the physical interpretation of which is not quite clear (see also Section 4.4 above). Recently, Christensen et al. [93] introduced a hierarchical approach to image registration combining a landmark-based scheme with an intensity-based approach using a fluid model (see also Grenander and Miller [206]). The landmark-based scheme employs the linear elasticity operator and the applied splines are different from thin-plate splines. Another difference to our approach in [446],[436] is that the nonaffine part of the transformation is separated from the affine part in their functional. While the stated functional allows to treat anisotropic errors in one of the two images to be registered, in their application only isotropic errors have been included. Since no further details have been given on how the errors have been determined, it seems that equal isotropic errors have been used. Splines with tension, where derivatives of all orders are involved in the minimizing functional, have been used for the reconstruction of 3D ultrasound images by Rohling et al. [423]. Splines with compact support (Wendland functions), which are particularly suited to increase the local influence in elastic registration, have recently been introduced in Fornefett et al. [161],[164].

Besides landmark-based approaches, also *intensity-based schemes* have been proposed for elastic registration of medical images. Intensity-based (or voxel-based) schemes rely on the intensities of the imaged objects, but generally not on geometric properties (e.g., Bajcsy et al. [18],[20], Gee et al. [188], Christensen et al. [91], Bro-Nielsen and Gramkow [69], Schormann et al. [474], Feldmar et al. [150], Collins et al. [101], Gaens et al. [184], Hata et al. [237], Rueckert et al. [456], Thirion [522]). Partly, intensity information is combined with geometric information (e.g., using some kind of edgeness measure), but generally explicit image segmentation is not required. In a preprocessing step often a global transformation has to be computed. Since the intensities are directly used to compute a similarity measure between images, often by computing the sum of the squared differences, these approaches generally depend rather strongly on the image modality and the chosen imaging parameters. To reduce this dependence, entropy measures have recently been used for elastic registration (e.g., Gaens et al. [184], Hata et al. [237], Rueckert et al. [456]). The most prominent entropy measure is mutual information, a concept from information theory, which has successfully been applied earlier for rigid registration (Maes et al. [319], Viola and Wells [541]; see also the evaluation study of West et al. [558]). With intensity-based approaches there exists a close relation to optic flow estimation (motion estimation) algorithms in computer vision, where typically monomodal 2D video images are analyzed (e.g., Szeliski and Coughlan [512], Thirion [522], Vemuri et al. [537], Warfield et al. [553], [554]). *Hybrid* approaches, which combine landmark-based and intensity-based schemes, have been suggested, for example, in Gee et al. [188], Meyer et al. [343], Christensen et al. [93], Collins et al. [101], and Cootes et al. [104].

Most intensity-based as well as landmark-based approaches to elastic image registration are based on linear elasticity theory and thus assume small deformations. However, in clinical applications this assumption is often violated. To cope with *large deformations*, Christensen et al. [91],[92] proposed a fluid model. A problem with this approach is to constrain the significantly larger flexibility of the model (Rabitt el al. [409]). Since the approach is rather time-consuming, an acceleration has been proposed by Bro-Nielsen and Gramkow [69]. A hyperelastic model to deal with large deformations has been introduced by Rabitt el al. [409]. Grenander and Miller [206] have described a landmark-based approach for large deformation maps. A landmark-based approach using an incremental elastic approach to cope with large deformations has been introduced by Peckar et al. [395]–[397] (see [393] for further details). Criteria to distinguish between small and large deformations have been proposed by Binder et al. [42] and Peckar et al. [396].

Recently, work has been reported on modelling the biomechanical properties of the human head more accurately (see also Section 4.8 above). An important application for such *biomechanical models* is the prediction of brain deformations for intraoperative navigation tasks (e.g., Buchholz et al. [75], Edwards et al. [138],[139], Kyriacou et al. [292],[293], Hagemann et al. [217],[220], Miga et al. [346]). A central topic here is to deal with nonhomogeneous material properties (see also, e.g., Davatzikos et al. [112], Lester et al. [307], Martin et al. [332]). In other work on intraoperative brain shift correction, homogeneous material is assumed or deformations are restricted by imposing certain boundary conditions (e.g., Škrinjar et al. [488], Hata et al. [237], Peckar et al. [396], Ferrant et al. [151], Rezk-Salama et al. [415]). Particularly the issue of modelling soft tissue deformations is challenging, which is also a recent topic in computer graphics. Most work, however, is devoted to surgery simulation for educational and training purposes, where real-time performance is the main objective and where model accuracy does not play a dominant role as it does in the case of intraoperative navigation (e.g., Kuhn et al. [290], Cotin et al. [105], Schill et al. [467], Bro-Nielsen [68], Delingette [116], Hartmann and Kruggel [236], Gibson et al. [193], Maurel et al. [333], Schiemann and Höhne [465]).

4.10 Conclusion and Future Work

In this chapter, we have described a model-based approach to elastic registration of multimodality images. The approach is based on anatomical point landmarks and thin-plate splines. Thin-plate splines have a physical motivation and are a flexible model to represent a rich class of possible deformations between two images. An important feature is that these splines result as a unique solution w.r.t. a minimizing functional, i.e., we have a mathematically well-founded optimization criterion. Moreover, the solution can be stated in closed form. The approach has been described for images of arbitrary dimension as well as for different smoothness properties of the transformation (determined by the order of the derivatives in the functional). The mathematical theory of thin-plate splines is well understood. Concerning practicability, the approach is computationally efficient, robust, general w.r.t. different types of images as well as atlases, and is well-suited for user-interaction, e.g., it has few controllable parameters. Central to our approach is the incorporation of localization errors of landmarks. In comparison to an interpolation scheme, the landmarks are not forced to match exactly. With our approximation scheme, the errors can be represented either by scalar weights or by weight matrices. In the latter case, we can cope with general anisotropic errors. Moreover, optimal affine transformations and interpolating thin-plate splines are special cases of our scheme. The required anatomical landmarks are localized semi-automatically by applying 3D differential operators, and the localization uncertainties of the landmarks are estimated directly from the image data. The localization uncertainties represent the minimal stochastic errors given by the Cramér-Rao bound. An important property is that we can integrate different types of landmarks, e.g., uniquely defined point landmarks and also quasi-landmarks which are not uniquely defined in all directions, e.g., arbitrary edge points. The performance of our scheme has been demonstrated for the case of 2D as well as 3D tomographic images of the human brain. We have also shown that further

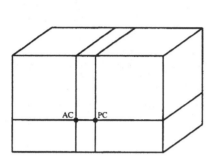

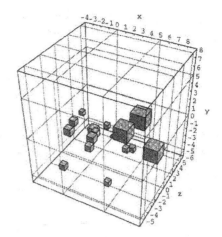

Figure 4.54. Talairach reference system for one hemisphere of the human brain.

Figure 4.55. Computed region-of-interests for landmarks within the Talairach reference system.

generalizations are possible within the same mathematical framework, e.g., the incorporation of orientation attributes at landmarks.

A topic for future work is to further improve and automate the semi-automatic procedure for localizing anatomical point landmarks. For example, prior to elastic registration one could use a coarse registration scheme to predict the region-of-interests (ROIs) of the landmarks in which a 3D differential operator is applied. As coarse registration scheme one can employ the Talairach reference scheme [514] which is used in clinical practice. This reference scheme subdivides each hemisphere of the brain into six cuboids on the basis of the dimensions of the brain as well as by using the anatomical structures anterior commissure (AC) and posterior commissure (PC) (see Figure 4.54). The sketched approach for predicting ROIs is closely related to the procedure in [148], where the Talairach reference scheme has been used to verify the positions of landmarks specified manually in images of different subjects. Our first investigations show that ROI prediction for the semi-automatic landmark localization procedure is possible, at least for those landmarks which exhibit small anatomical variability. To this end, we have localized anatomical landmarks in three different MR datasets on the basis of the Talairach reference scheme and have computed the means as well as the standard deviations of the positions. The result is shown in Figure 4.55, where the ROIs are represented by cubes. While certain landmarks have a relatively large ROI, the ROIs of other landmarks seem to be well suited for our purpose. Clearly, we have to evaluate this procedure on a much larger number of 3D images. A disadvantage of the procedure is that we have to apply the Talairach registration scheme beforehand to predict the landmark positions.

Another topic for future research is the choice of an optimal value of the regularization parameter λ which weights the smoothness term relative to the data term in the minimizing functional. Here, one possibility is to apply the method of general cross validation [545]. First experimental results with our scheme show that this seems to be a useful estimate. Provided a real-time implementation, as an alternative one should also consider a user-driven setting of λ on the basis of an appropriate visual feedback for assessment of the registration result. Further work should also be devoted to incorporation of additional knowledge in elastic registration. Besides orientation attributes at landmarks one could also consider to include curvature information analogously to [324], [325].

General Statements

We conclude this chapter by making some general statements concerning elastic registration. As already indicated above, a main characteristic is certainly that the spectrum of applications for elastic registration is very broad. In the medical area this comprises diagnosis, surgery planning and simulation, intraoperative navigation as well as robot-assisted interventions. Other application areas are, for example, morphometrics, remote sensing, cartography, geographic information systems, geology, computer graphics, and virtual reality. In addition, the spectrum of imaging modalities particularly in medicine is very large (comprising anatomical and functional data) and also the range of tasks is very large. While here we mainly considered images of the human head, elastic registration is also important for other organs, e.g., human liver, kidney, breast, and heart. Given that the spectrum of applications, imaging modalities, and tasks is rather large, it is thus questionable that one general elastic registration approach will be found which satisfies all needs. Instead, in the opinion of the author the aim should be the development of a certain number of principal approaches for which the range of applications, the imaging modalities, and the tasks can safely be stated.

As can be learned from the literature, the work on elastic and nonrigid registration has increased tremendously in recent years. Currently, it is very hard to keep track of all different approaches. Most importantly, it is currently not possible to judge which approaches perform better than others. A systematic evaluation study as in the case of rigid registration [558] has not yet been performed. However, one has to note, that performance characterization of elastic schemes and quantification of the registration accuracy is also very difficult. On the one hand, a prerequisite would be the quantification of typical deformations of anatomical structures as well as the provision of ground truth. On the other hand, one should note, that elastic registration of multimodality images is still a relatively young research field, and the current focus is on exploring fundamental models and approaches. Actually, the task of elastic registration is rather difficult, and the mathematical level for understanding existing work or developing new approaches is generally rather high. Nevertheless, theoretical soundness is important to guarantee required properties and to end up with algorithms of predictable performance.

Important general topics for further research are, for example, the integration of more physics in form of biomechanical models, the combination of physical and statistical deformation models, the combination of landmark-based and intensity-based schemes, the treatment of large deformations, the integration of uncertainties and error information, the investigation of similarity measures between images, as well as the development of computational efficient schemes. In comparison to traditional monomodal 2D image analysis, a clear challenge is the analysis of multimodality 3D or higher-dimensional image data.

Bibliography

[1] C.K. Abbey, E. Clarkson, H.H. Barrett, S.P. Müller, and F.J. Rybicki, "A method for approximating the density of maximum-likelihood and maximum *a posteriori* estimates under a Gaussian noise model", *Medical Image Analysis* 2:4 (1998) 395-403

[2] M. Abramowitz and I.A. Stegun, *Handbook of Mathematical Functions*, Dover Publications New York 1965

[3] J.K. Aggarwal, Q. Cai, W. Liao, and B. Sabata, "Nonrigid Motion Analysis: Articulated and Elastic Motion", *Computer Vision and Image Understanding* 70:2 (1998) 142-156

[4] P. Alfeld, "Scattered Data Interpolation in Three or More Variables", *Mathematical Methods in CAGD*, T. Lyche and L.L. Schumaker (Eds.), Academic Press 1989, 1-33

[5] Y. Aloimonos (Ed.), *Active Perception*, Lawrence Erlbaum Assoc., Hillsdale New Jersey 1993

[6] L. Alvarez and F. Morales, "Affine Morphological Multiscale Analysis of Corners and Multiple Junctions", *Int. J. of Computer Vision* 25:2 (1997) 95-107

[7] A.A. Amini, Y. Chen, and D. Abendschein, "Comparison of Land-Mark-Based and Curve-Based Thin-Plate Warps for Analysis of Left-Ventricular Motion from Tagged MRI", *Proc. Second Internat. Conf. on Medical Image Computing and Computer-Assisted Intervention (MICCAI'99)*, Cambridge, England, Sept. 19-22, 1999, *Lecture Notes in Computer Science* 1679, C.J. Taylor and A. Colchester (Eds.), Springer-Verlag Berlin Heidelberg 1999, 498-507

[8] H.C. Andrews and B.R. Hunt, *Digital Image Restoration*, Prentice-Hall Englewood Cliffs, New Jersey 1977

[9] N. Ansari and E.J. Delp, "Partial shape recognition: a landmark-based approach", *IEEE Trans. on Pattern Anal. and Machine Intell.* 12:5 (1990) 470-483

[10] F. Arman and J.K. Aggarwal, "Model-Based Object Recognition in Dense-Range Images – A Review", *ACM Computing Surveys* 25:1 (1993) 5-43

[11] N. Ayache, "Medical computer vision, virtual reality and robotics", *Image and Vision Computing* 13:4 (1995) 295-313

[12] N. Arad, N. Dyn, D. Reisfeld, and Y. Yeshurun, "Image warping by radial basis functions: Application to facial expressions", *Computer Vision, Graphics, and Image Processing* 56:2 (1994) 161-172

259

[13] N. Arad and D. Reisfeld, "Image Warping Using Few Anchor Points and Radial Functions", *Computer Graphics forum* 14:1 (1995) 35-46

[14] H. Asada and M. Brady, "The Curvature Primal Sketch", *IEEE Trans. on Pattern Anal. and Machine Intell.* 8:1 (1986) 2-14

[15] P. Astheimer, K. Böhm, W. Felger, M. Göbel, and S. Müller, "Die Virtuelle Umgebung – Eine neue Epoche in der Mensch-Maschine-Kommunikation ", Part I and II, *Informatik Spektrum* 17 (1994) 281-290 and 357-367

[16] S. Back, H. Neumann, and H.S. Stiehl, "On Scale-Space Edge Detection in Computed Tomograms", *11. DAGM - Symposium Mustererkennung,* 2.-4. Okt. 1989, Hamburg, *Informatik-Fachberichte* 219, H. Burkhardt, K.H. Höhne, and B. Neumann (Eds.), Springer-Verlag Berlin Heidelberg 1989, 216-223

[17] R. Bajcsy, "Active Perception", *Proc. of the IEEE* 76:8 (1988) 996-1005

[18] R. Bajcsy and C. Broit, "Matching of Deformed Images", *Proc. 6th Internat. Conf. on Pattern Recognition,* 1982, München/FRG, 351-353

[19] R. Bajcsy, R. Lieberson, and M. Reivich, "A Computerized System for the Elastic Matching of Deformed Radiographic Images to Idealized Atlas Images", *J. of Computer Assisted Tomography* 7:4 (1983) 618-625

[20] R. Bajcsy and S. Kovačič, "Multiresolution Elastic Matching", *Computer Vision, Graphics, and Image Processing* 46 (1989) 1-21

[21] S. Baker, S.K. Nayar, and H. Murase, "Parametric Feature Detection", *Int. J. of Computer Vision* 27:1 (1998) 27-50

[22] D.H. Ballard and C.M. Brown, *Computer Vision,* Prentice Hall London 1982

[23] C. Barillot, B. Gibaud, O. Lis, L.L. Min, A. Bouliou, G. Le Certen, R. Collorec, and J.L. Coatrieux, "Computer Graphics in Medicine: A Survey", *CRC Critical Reviews in Biomedical Engineering* 15:4 (1988) 269-307

[24] S.T. Barnard and W.B. Thompson, "Disparity analysis of images", *IEEE Trans. on Pattern Anal. and Machine Intell.* 2:4 (1980) 333-340

[25] A.H. Barr, "Superquadrics and Angle-Preserving Transformations", *IEEE Computer Graphics & Appl.* 1:1 (1981) 11-23

[26] A.H. Barr, "Global and local deformations of solid primitives", *Computer Graphics* 18:3 (1984) 21-30

[27] H.H. Barrett and W. Swindell, *Radiological Imaging,* Vols. 1 and 2, Academic Press New York London 1981

[28] P.R. Beaudet, "Rotationally invariant image operators", *Proc. Int. Joint Conf. on Pattern Recognition,* Kyoto/Japan, Nov. 7-10, 1978, 579-583

[29] T. Beier and S. Neely, "Feature-Based Image Metamorphosis", *Computer Graphics* 26:2 (1992) 35-42

[30] W. Beil, K. Rohr, and H.S. Stiehl, "Investigation of Approaches for the Localization of Anatomical Landmarks in 3D Medical Images", *Proc. Computer Assisted Radiology and Surgery (CAR'97)*, Berlin, Germany, June 25-28, 1997, H.U. Lemke, M.W. Vannier, and K. Inamura (Eds.), Elsevier Amsterdam Lausanne 1997, 265-270

[31] L. Beolchi and M.H. Kuhn (Eds.), *"Medical Imaging – Analysis of Multimodality 2D/3D Images"*, *Studies in Health Technology and Informatics Vol. 19*, IOS Press Amsterdam Oxford 1994

[32] F. Bergholm, "Edge Focusing", *IEEE Trans. on Pattern Anal. and Machine Intell.* 9 (1987) 726-741

[33] F. Bergholm and K. Rohr, "A Comparison between Two Approaches Applied for Estimating Diffuseness and Height of Step Edges", Techn. Report TRITA-NA-P9105, CVAP 83, Dept. of Num. Analysis and Computing Science, Royal Institute of Technology, Stockholm/Sweden, March 1991

[34] M. Bertero, T.A. Poggio, and V. Torre, "Ill–Posed Problems in Early Vision", *Proc. of the IEEE* 76:8 (1988) 869-889

[35] R. Bertolini and G. Leutert, *Atlas der Anatomie des Menschen, Band 3: Kopf und Hals, Gehirn, Rückenmark und Sinnesorgane*, Springer-Verlag Berlin Heidelberg 1982

[36] V. Berzins, "Accuracy of Laplacian Edge Detectors", *Computer Vision, Graphics, and Image Processing* 27 (1984) 195-210

[37] D.E. Beskos, *Boundary Element Methods in Mechanics*, Vol. 3 of *Computational Methods in Mechanics*, T. Belytschko and K.J. Bathe (Eds.), North-Holland Amsterdam New York 1987

[38] P.J. Besl, "Geometric Modeling and Computer Vision", *Proc. of the IEEE* 76:8 (1988) 936-958

[39] P.J. Besl and R.C. Jain, "Three-Dimensional Object Recognition", *Computing Surveys* 17:1 (March 1985) 75-145

[40] M. Betke and N.C. Makris, "Information-conserving object recognition", *Proc. Int. Conf. on Computer Vision (ICCV'98)*, Bombay, India, Jan. 4-7, 1998, Narosa Publishing House, New Delhi Madras 1998, 145-152

[41] J. Bigün and G.H. Granlund, "Optimal orientation detection of linear symmetry", *Proc. Int. Conf. on Computer Vision (ICCV'87)*, London, England, June 8-11, 1987, IEEE Computer Society Press, Washington, D.C., 1987, 433-438

[42] L. Binder, K. Rohr, R. Sprengel, and H.S. Stiehl, "Bildregistrierung mit interpolierenden 'Thin-Plate Splines' und Bezüge zur linearen Elastizitätstheorie", *18. DAGM-Symposium Mustererkennung*, Sept. 1996, Heidelberg/Germany, *Informatik aktuell*, B. Jähne, P. Geißler, H. Haußecker, and F. Hering (Eds.), Springer-Verlag Berlin Heidelberg 1996, 281-288

[43] T.O. Binford, "Visual perception by computer", *IEEE Conf. on Systems and Control*, Dec. 1971

[44] T.O. Binford, "Survey of model-based image understanding systems", *Int. J. of Robotics Research* 1:1 (1982) 18-62

[45] M.J. Black, D.J. Fleet, and Y. Yacoob, "A Framework for Modeling Appearance Change in Image Sequences", *Proc. Int. Conf. on Computer Vision (ICCV'98)*, Bombay, India, Jan. 4-7, 1998, Narosa Publishing House, New Delhi Madras 1998, 660-667

[46] A. Blake and A. Zisserman, *Visual Reconstruction,* MIT Press, Cambridge, MA, 1987

[47] J. Blom, B.M. ter Haar Romeny, and J.J. Koenderink, "Affine invariant corner detection", submitted for publication, see "Topological and Geometrical Aspects of Image Structure", J. Blom, doctoral dissertation, University of Utrecht, May 1992

[48] R.M. Bolle and B.C. Vemuri, "On Three-Dimensional Surface Reconstruction Methods, *IEEE Trans. on Pattern Anal. and Machine Intell.* 13:1 (1991) 1-13

[49] F.L. Bookstein, "Principal Warps: Thin-Plate Splines and the Decomposition of Deformations", *IEEE Trans. on Pattern Anal. and Machine Intell.* 11:6 (1989) 567-585

[50] F.L. Bookstein, "Thin-Plate Splines and the Atlas Problem for Biomedical Images", *Proc. 12th Internat. Conf. Information Processing in Medical Imaging (IPMI'91),* July 1991, Wye/UK, *Lecture Notes in Computer Science* 511, A.C.F. Colchester, D.J. Hawkes (Eds.), Springer-Verlag Berlin Heidelberg 1991, 326-342

[51] F.L. Bookstein, "Four metrics for image variation", *Proc. 11th Internat. Conf. Information Processing in Medical Imaging (IPMI'89),* In *Progress in Clinical and Biological Research,* Vol. 363, D. Ortendahl and J. Llacer (Eds.), Wiley-Liss New York, 1991, 227-240

[52] F.L. Bookstein, *Morphometric tools for landmark data: Geometry and biology,* Cambridge University Press, Cambridge New York 1991

[53] F.L. Bookstein, "Visualizing Group Differences in Outline Shape: Methods from Biometrics of Landmark Points", *Proc. 4th Internat. Conf. Visualization in Biomedical Computing (VBC'96),* Hamburg, Germany, Sept. 22-25, 1996, *Lecture Notes in Computer Science* 1131, K.H. Höhne and R. Kikinis (Eds.), Springer Berlin Heidelberg 1996, 405–410

[54] F.L. Bookstein, "Landmark methods for forms without landmarks: morphometrics of group differences in outline shape", *Medical Image Analysis* 1:3 (1996/7) 225-243

[55] F.L. Bookstein and D.K. Green, "A Feature Space for Edgels in Images with Landmarks", *J. of Mathematical Imaging and Vision* 3 (1993) 231-261

[56] T.E. Boult and J.R. Kender, "Visual surface reconstruction using sparse depth data", *Proc. Conf. on Computer Vision and Pattern Recognition (CVPR'86),* June 22-26, Miami Beach, FL, IEEE Computer Society Press 1986, 68-76

[57] T.E. Boult, S.D. Fenster, and T. O'Donnell, "Physics in a Fantasy World vs Robust Statistical Estimation", *Proc. NSF Workshop 3D Object Recognition,* New York, Nov. 1994

[58] K.W. Bowyer and P.J. Phillips (Eds.), *Empirical Evaluation Techniques in Computer Vision,* IEEE Computer Society Press, Los Alamitos/CA 1998

[59] J.R. Bradshaw, *Neuroradiologie – das Gehirn,* VCH Weinheim 1991

[60] M. Brady and B.K.P. Horn, "Rotationally Symmetric Operators for Surface Interpolation", *Computer Vision, Graphics, and Image Processing* 22 (1983) 70-94

[61] D. Braess, *Finite Elemente,* Springer Berlin Heidelberg 1997

[62] P. Brand and R. Mohr, "Accuracy in Image Measure", *Videometrics III,* Boston/MA, USA, 31 Oct. - 4 Nov. 1994, Proc. SPIE 2350, 218-228

[63] W. Brauer and S. Münch, *Studien- und Forschungsführer Informatik,* Springer Berlin Heidelberg 1996

[64] C. Bregler, "Learning and Recognizing Human Dynamics in Video Sequences", *Proc. Conf. on Computer Vision and Pattern Recognition (CVPR'97),* Puerto Rico, June 17-19, IEEE Computer Society Press 1997, 794-800

[65] C. Bregler and J. Malik, "Tracking People with Twists and Exponential Maps", *Proc. Conf. on Computer Vision and Pattern Recognition (CVPR'98),* Santa Barbara, CA, June 23-25, 1998, IEEE Computer Society Press 1998, 8-15

[66] L. Le Briquer, F. Lachmann, and C. Barillot, "Using Local Extremum Curvatures to Extract Anatomical Landmarks from Medical Images", *Medical Imaging 1993: Image Processing,* 16-19 Febr. 1993, Newport Beach, California/USA, Proc. SPIE 1898, M.H. Loew (Ed.), 549-558

[67] T.J. Broida and R. Chellappa, "Estimation of Object Motion Parameters from Noisy Images", *IEEE Trans. on Pattern Anal. and Machine Intell.* 8 (1986) 90-99

[68] M. Bro-Nielsen, "Finite Element Modeling in Surgery Simulation", *Proc. of the IEEE* 86:3 (1998) 490-503

[69] M. Bro-Nielsen and C. Gramkow, "Fast Fluid Registration of Medical Images", *Proc. 4th Internat. Conf. Visualization in Biomedical Computing (VBC'96),* Hamburg, Germany, Sept. 22-25, 1996, *Lecture Notes in Computer Science* 1131, K.H. Höhne and R. Kikinis (Eds.), Springer Berlin Heidelberg 1996, 267-276

[70] M. Bro-Nielsen, C. Gramkow, and S. Kreiborg, "Non-rigid Image Registration Using Bone Growth Model" *Proc. First Joint Conf. CVRMed-MRCAS'97,* Grenoble/France, March 1997, *Lecture Notes in Computer Science* 1205, J. Troccaz, E. Grimson, and R. Mösges (Eds.), Springer Verlag Berlin Heidelberg 1997, 3-12

[71] I.N. Bronstein and K.A. Semendjajew, *Taschenbuch der Mathematik,* 19. Auflage, Verlag Harri Deutsch, Thun und Frankfurt/Main 1981

[72] D.S. Broomhead and D. Lowe, "Multivariable Functional Interpolation and Adaptive Networks", *Complex Systems* 2 (1988) 321-355

[73] L.G. Brown, "A Survey of Image Registration Techniques", *ACM Computing Surveys* 24:4 (1992) 325-376

[74] K. Brunnström, T. Lindeberg, and J.-O. Eklundh, "Active Detection and Classification of Junctions by Foveation with a Head-Eye System Guided by the Scale-Space Primal Sketch", *Proc. European Conf. on Computer Vision (ECCV'92),* S. Margherita/Italy,

May 18-23, 1992, *Lecture Notes in Computer Science* 588, G. Sandini (Ed.), Springer-Verlag Berlin Heidelberg 1992, 701-709

[75] R.D. Buchholz, D.D. Yeh, J. Trobaugh, L.L. McDurmont, C.D. Sturm, C. Baumann, J.M. Henderson, A. Levy, and P. Kessman, "The Correction of Stereotactic Inaccuracy Caused by Brain Shift Using an Intraoperative Ultrasound Device", *Proc. First Joint Conf. CVRMed-MRCAS'97*, Grenoble/France, March 1997, *Lecture Notes in Computer Science* 1205, J. Troccaz, E. Grimson, and R. Mösges (Eds.), Springer Verlag Berlin Heidelberg 1997, 459-466

[76] M.D. Buhmann, "New Developments in the Theory of Radial Basis Function Interpolation", *Multivariate Approximations: From CAGD to Wavelets*, K. Jetter and F. Utreras (Eds.), World Scientific Singapore 1993, 35-75

[77] P.A. Burrough and R.A. McDonnell, *Principles of Geographical Information Systems*, Oxford University Press 1998

[78] T.W. Calvert and A.E. Chapman, "Analysis and synthesis of human movement", in T.Y. Young (Ed.), *Handbook of Pattern Recognition and Image Processing (Vol. 2): Computer Vision*, Academic Press, San Diego, CA, 1994, 431-474

[79] F. Canny, "A computational approach to edge detection", *IEEE Trans. on Pattern Anal. and Machine Intell.* 8 (1986) 679-698

[80] V. Caselles, F. Catté, T. Coll, and F. Dibos, "A geometric model for active contours in image processing", *Numerische Mathematik* 66 (1993) 1-31

[81] V. Caselles, R. Kimmel, and G. Sapiro, "Geodesic active contours", *Int. J. of Computer Vision* 22 (1997) 61-79

[82] C. Cédras and M. Shah, "Motion-based recognition: a survey", *Image and Vision Computing* 13:2 (1995) 129-155

[83] N. Cerneaz and M. Brady, "Finding Curvilinear Structures in Mammograms", *Proc. First Internat. Conf. Computer Vision, Virtual Reality and Robotics in Medicine (CVRMed'95)*, Nice/France, April 1995, *Lecture Notes in Computer Science* 905, N. Ayache (Ed.), Springer Verlag Berlin Heidelberg 1995, 372-382

[84] Y.T. Chang and S.M. Thomas, "Cramer-Rao Lower Bounds for Estimation of a Circular Arc Center and Its Radius", *Graphical Models and Image Processing* 57:6 (1995) 527-532

[85] H. Chang and J. Fitzpatrick, "A technique for accurate magnetic resonance imaging in the presence of field inhomogeneities", *IEEE Trans. on Medical Imaging* 11 (1992) 319-329

[86] C.-H. Chen, J.-S. Lee, and Y.-N. Sun, "Wavelet Transformation for Gray-Level Corner Detection", *Pattern Recognition* 28:6 (1995) 853-861

[87] G.T.Y. Chen, M. Kessler, and S. Pitluck, "Structure Transfer Between Sets of Three Dimensional Medical Imaging Data", *Proc. 6th Annual Conf. on Computer Graphics*, 1985, 171-177

[88] M.-C. Chiang and T.E. Boult, "Local Blur Estimation and Super-Resolution", *Proc. Conf. on Computer Vision and Pattern Recognition (CVPR'97)*, Puerto Rico, June 17-19, IEEE Computer Society Press 1997, 821-826

[89] R.T. Chin and C.R. Dyer, "Model-Based Recognition in Robot Vision", *Computing Surveys* 18:1 (1986) 67-108

[90] P.C. Chou and N.J. Pagano, *Elasticity: Tensor, Dyadic, and Engineering Approach*, Dover Publ. 1967

[91] G.E. Christensen, M.I. Miller, M. Vannier, and U. Grenander, "Individualizing neuroanatomical atlases using a massively parallel computer", *IEEE Computer* 29:1 (1996) 32-38

[92] G.E. Christensen, S.C. Joshi, and M.I. Miller, "Individualizing Anatomical Atlases of the Head", *Proc. 4th Internat. Conf. Visualization in Biomedical Computing (VBC'96)*, Hamburg, Germany, Sept. 22-25, 1996, *Lecture Notes in Computer Science* 1131, K.H. Höhne and R. Kikinis (Eds.), Springer Berlin Heidelberg 1996, 343-348

[93] G.E. Christensen, S.C. Joshi, and M.I. Miller, "Volumetric Transformation of Brain Anatomy", *IEEE Trans. on Medical Imaging* 16:6 (Dec. 1997) 864-877

[94] H.I. Christensen, "Lessons learnt from the last thirty years of research", *Proc. Dagstuhl Seminar "Knowledge Based Computer Vision"*, Dagstuhl-Seminar-Report 196, 8.12.-12.12.1997 (9750), Schloß Dagstuhl, Wadern/Germany, H.I. Christensen, D. Hogg, and B. Neumann (Eds.), IBFI 1997, 1-3

[95] H.I. Christensen and W. Förstner, "Performance characteristics of vision algorithms", *Machine Vision and Applications* 9 (1997) 215-218

[96] P.G. Ciarlet, *Mathematical Elasticity, Vol. I: Three-Dimensional Elasticity*, North-Holland Amsterdam New York 1988

[97] U. Claussen, "Beleuchtungsmodelle und Beleuchtungsalgorithmen in der graphischen Datenverarbeitung", Techn. Report WSI-GRIS 88-3, Univ. Tübingen, Inst. für Informatik, 1988

[98] C. Coelho, A. Heller, J.L. Mundy, D.A. Forsyth, and A. Zisserman, "An Experimental Evaluation of Projective Invariants", *Geometric Invariance in Computer Vision*, J.L. Mundy and A. Zisserman (Eds.), The MIT Press, Cambridge, MA, 1992, 87-104

[99] L.D. Cohen and I. Cohen, "Finite-Element Methods for Active Contour Models and Balloons for 2-D and 3-D Images", *IEEE Trans. on Pattern Anal. and Machine Intell.* 15:11 (1993) 1131-1147

[100] A. Collignon, D. Vandermeulen, P. Suetens, and G. Marchal, "Registration of 3D multimodality medical images using surfaces and point landmarks", *Pattern Recognition Letters* 15 (1994) 461-467

[101] D.L. Collins, G. Le Goualher, and A.C. Evans, "Non-linear Cerebral Registration with Sulcal Constraints", *Proc. First Internat. Conf. on Medical Image Computing and Computer-Assisted Intervention (MICCAI'98)*, Massachusetts Institute of Technology (MIT), Cambridge/MA, USA, Oct. 11-13, 1998, *Lecture Notes in Computer Science*

1496, W.M. Wells, A. Colchester, and S. Delp (Eds.), Springer Verlag Berlin Heidelberg 1998, 974-984

[102] T.F. Cootes and C.J. Taylor, "Combining point distribution models with shape models based on finite element analysis", *Image and Vision Computing* 13:5 (1995) 403-409

[103] T.F. Cootes, G.J. Edwards, and C.J. Taylor, "Active Appearance Models", *Proc. European Conf. on Computer Vision (ECCV'98)*, June 1998, Freiburg, Germany, Vol. II, *Lecture Notes in Computer Science* 1406, H. Burkhardt and B. Neumann (Eds.), Springer Berlin Heidelberg 1998, 484-498

[104] T.F. Cootes, C. Beeston, G.J. Edwards, and C.J. Taylor, "A Unified Framework for Atlas Matching Using Active Appearance Models", *Proc. 16th Internat. Conf. on Information Processing in Medical Imaging (IPMI'99)*, Visegrád, Hungary, June 28 - July 2, 1999, In *Lecture Notes in Computer Science* 1613, A. Kuba, M. Šámal, and A. Todd-Pokropek (Eds.), Springer-Verlag Berlin Heidelberg 1999, 322-333

[105] S. Cotin, H. Delingette, and N. Ayache, "Real time volumetric deformable models for surgery simulation", *Proc. 4th Internat. Conf. Visualization in Biomedical Computing (VBC'96)*, Hamburg, Germany, Sept. 22-25, 1996, *Lecture Notes in Computer Science* 1131, K.H. Höhne and R. Kikinis (Eds.), Springer Berlin Heidelberg 1996, 535-540

[106] R. Courant and D. Hilbert, *Methoden der Mathematischen Physik I*, Springer-Verlag Berlin Heidelberg 1968

[107] N.A.C. Cressie, *Statistics for spatial data*, John Wiley & Sons New York 1991

[108] D. Crevier and R. Lepage, "Knowledge-Based Image Understanding Systems: A Survey", *Computer Vision and Image Understanding* 67:2 (1997) 161-185

[109] C. Cutting, F.L. Bookstein, B. Haddad, D. Dean, and D. Kim, "A spline-based approach for averaging three-dimensional curves and surfaces", *Mathematical Methods in Medical Imaging II*, July 1993, San Diego, California/USA, Proc. SPIE 2035, D.C. Wilson, J.N. Wilson (Eds.), 29-44

[110] C. Cutting, F.L. Bookstein, B. Haddad, D. Dean, and D. Kim, "A Three-Dimensional Smooth Surface Analysis of Untreated Crouzon's Syndrome in the Adult", *J. of Craniofacial Surgery* 6 (1995) 444-453

[111] C. Davatzikos, J.L. Prince, and R.N. Bryan, "Image registration based on boundary mapping", *IEEE Trans. on Medical Imaging* 15:1 (1996) 112-115

[112] C. Davatzikos, J.L. Prince, and R.N. Bryan, "Spatial Transformation and Registration of Brain Images Using Elastically Deformable Models", *Computer Vision and Image Understanding* 66:2 (1997) 207-222

[113] M.H. Davis, A. Khotanzad, D.P. Flamig, and S.E. Harms, "A Physics-Based Coordinate Transformation for 3-D Image Matching", *IEEE Trans. on Medical Imaging* 16:3 (1997) 317-328

[114] D. Dean, P. Buckley, F. Bookstein, J. Kamath, D. Kwon, L. Friedman, C. Lys, "Three Dimensional MR-Based Morphometric Comparison of Schizophrenic and Normal Cerebral Ventricles", *Proc. 4th Internat. Conf. Visualization in Biomedical Computing*

(VBC'96), Hamburg, Germany, Sept. 22-25, 1996, *Lecture Notes in Computer Science* 1131, K.H. Höhne and R. Kikinis (Eds.), Springer Berlin Heidelberg 1996, 363-372

[115] J. Declerck, G. Subsol, J.-P. Thirion, and N. Ayache, "Automatic Retrieval of Anatomical Structures in 3D Medical Images", *Proc. First Internat. Conf. Computer Vision, Virtual Reality and Robotics in Medicine (CVRMed'95)*, Nice/France, April 1995, *Lecture Notes in Computer Science* 905, N. Ayache (Ed.), Springer Verlag Berlin Heidelberg 1995, 153-162

[116] H. Delingette, "Toward Realistic Soft-Tissue Modeling in Medical Simulation", *Proc. of the IEEE* 86:3 (1998) 512-523

[117] E. De Micheli, B. Caprile, P. Ottonello, and V. Torre, "Localization and Noise in Edge Detection", *IEEE Trans. on Pattern Anal. and Machine Intell.* 11 (1989) 1106-1117

[118] R. Deriche and G. Giraudon, "A Computational Approach for Corner and Vertex Detection", *Int. J. of Computer Vision* 10:2 (1993) 101-124

[119] R. Deriche and T. Blaszka, "Recovering and Characterizing Image Features Using An Efficient Model Based Approach", *Proc. IEEE Conf. on Computer Vision & Pattern Recognition*, New York/NY, USA, June 15-17, 1993, 530-535

[120] H. Dickhaus, K. Ganser, A. Staubert, M.M. Bonsanto, C.R. Wirtz, V.M. Tronnier, and S. Kunze, "Quantification of brain shift effects by MR-imaging", *Proc. Int. Conf. IEEE Engineering Medicine Biology Soc.*, 1997, 491-494

[121] M.P. do Carmo, *Differentialgeometrie von Kurven und Flächen*, Friedr. Vieweg & Sohn, Braunschweig 1983

[122] L. Dreschler, "Ermittlung markanter Punkte auf den Bildern bewegter Objekte und Berechnung einer 3D-Beschreibung auf dieser Grundlage", Dissertation, Fachbereich Informatik, Universität Hamburg, Juni 1981

[123] L. Dreschler and H.-H. Nagel, "Volumetric Model and 3D-Trajectory of a Moving Car Derived from Monocular TV-Frame Sequences of a Street Scene", *Proc. IJCAI'81*, Vancouver, BC, 1981, 692-697, see also: *Computer Graphics and Image Processing* 20 (1982) 199-228

[124] C. Drewniok, "Objektlokalisation durch Adaption parametrischer Grauwertmodelle und ihre Anwendung in der Luftbildauswertung", Dissertation, Universität Hamburg, Fachbereich Informatik, published by infix Sankt Augustin 1999

[125] C. Drewniok and K. Rohr, "High-Precision Localization of Circular Landmarks in Aerial Images", *17. DAGM-Symposium Mustererkennung*, Sept. 1995, Bielefeld/Germany, *Informatik aktuell*, G. Sagerer, S. Posch, and F. Kummert (Eds.), Springer-Verlag Berlin Heidelberg 1995, 594-601

[126] C. Drewniok and K. Rohr, "Automatic Exterior Orientation of Aerial Images in Urban Environments", *Proc. ISPRS Congress*, Vienna, July 1996, *Internat. Archives of Photogrammetry and Remote Sensing*, Vol. XXXI, Part B3, 146-152

[127] C. Drewniok and K. Rohr, "Exterior Orientation – An Automatic Approach Based on Fitting Analytic Landmark Models", Special Theme Issue "Automatic Image Orientation", *ISPRS J. of Photogrammetry & Remote Sensing* 52 (1997) 132-145

[128] C. Drewniok and K. Rohr, "Model-Based Detection and Localization of Circular Landmarks in Aerial Images", *Int. J. of Computer Vision* 24:3 (1997) 187-217

[129] C. Drewniok and K. Rohr, "Lokalisation planarer Objekte durch Adaption parametrischer Grauwertmodelle", *16. Wissenschaftlich-Technische Jahrestagung der DGPF: Digitale Bildverarbeitung zur Erfassung geometrischer und thematischer Informationen,* 18.-20. Sept. 1996, Oldenburg, F.K. List (Ed.), Publikationen der Deutschen Gesellschaft für Photogrammetrie und Fernerkundung, Band 5, Berlin 1997, 63-72

[130] J. Duchon, "Interpolation des fonctions de deux variables suivant le principe de la flexion des plaques minces", *R.A.I.R.O. Analyse Numérique* 10:12 (1976) 5-12

[131] J. Duchon, "Splines minimizing rotation-invariant semi-norms in Sobolev spaces", in W. Schempp and K. Zeller (Eds.), *Proc. Constructive Theory of Functions of Several Variables,* Oberwolfach, April 25 - May 1, 1976, *Lecture Notes in Mathematics* 571, Springer-Verlag Berlin Heidelberg 1977, 85-100

[132] R.O. Duda and P.E. Hart, *Pattern classification and scene analysis,* Wiley New York 1973

[133] H.S. Dulimarta and A.K. Jain, "Mobile robot localization in indoor environment", *Pattern Recognition* 30:1 (1997) 99-111

[134] J.S. Duncan and N. Ayache, "Medical Image Analysis: Progress over Two Decades and the Challenges Ahead", *IEEE Trans. on Pattern Anal. and Machine Intell.* 22:1 (2000) 85-106

[135] N. Dyn and G. Wahba, "On the estimation of functions of several variables from aggregated data", *SIAM J. Math. Anal.* 13:1 (1982) 134-152

[136] D. Eberly, *Ridges in Image and Data Analysis,* Computational Imaging and Vision Series, Vol. 7, Kluwer Academic Publishers, Dordrecht Boston London 1996

[137] D. Eberly, R. Gardner, B. Morse, S. Pizer, and C. Scharlach, "Ridges for image analysis", *J. of Mathematical Imaging and Vision* 4:4 (1994) 353-373

[138] P.J. Edwards, D.L.G. Hill, J.A. Little, and D.J. Hawkes, "Deformation for Image Guided Interventions Using a Three Component Tissue Model", *Proc. 15th Internat. Conf. Information Processing in Medical Imaging (IPMI'97),* In *Lecture Notes in Computer Science* 1230, J. Duncan and G. Gindi (Eds.), Poultney, Vermont, USA, June 1997, Springer-Verlag Berlin Heidelberg 1997, 218-231

[139] P.J. Edwards, D.L.G. Hill, J.A. Little, and D.J. Hawkes, "A three-component deformation model for image-guided surgery", *Medical Image Analysis* 2:4 (1998) 355-367

[140] J.O. Eklundh and L. Kjelldahl, "Computer Graphics and Computer Vision – Some Unifying and Discriminating Features", *Computer & Graphics* 9:4 (1986) 339-349

[141] S.R. Ellis and D.R. Begault, "Virtual Environment as Human-Computer Interfaces", in *Handbook of Human-Computer Interaction,* M.G. Helander, T.K. Landauer, and P.V. Prabhu (Eds.), Elsevier Science Amsterdam 1997, 163-201

[142] P.A. van den Elsen, *Multimodality Matching of Brain Images,* Utrecht University Thesis, 1993

[143] P.A. van den Elsen, E-J.D. Pol, and M.A. Viergever, "Medical image matching – A review with classification", *IEEE Engineering in Medicine and Biol.* 12:1 (1993) 26-39

[144] G. Ende, H. Treuer, and R. Boesecke, "Optimization and evaluation of landmark-based image correlation", *Phys. Med. Biol.* 37:1 (1992) 261-271

[145] H. Eschenauer and W. Schnell, *Elastizitätstheorie*, BI Wissenschaftsverlag Mannheim 1993

[146] R.L. Eubank, *Spline Smoothing and Nonparametric Regression*, Marcel Dekker New York Basel 1988

[147] A.C. Evans, W. Dai, L. Collins, P. Neelin, and S. Marrett, "Warping of a computerized 3-D atlas to match brain image volumes for quantitative neuroanatomical and functional analysis", *Medical Imaging V: Image Processing*, 1991, San Jose/CA, USA, Proc. SPIE 1445, M.H. Loew (Ed.), 236-246

[148] A.C. Evans, D.L. Collins, P. Neelin, and T.S. Marrett, "Correlative Analysis of Three-Dimensional Brain Images", in *Computer-Integrated Surgery*, R.H. Taylor, S. Lavallée, G.C. Burdea, and R. Mösges (Eds.), The MIT Press, Cambridge/Massachusetts, 1996, 99-114

[149] O. Faugeras, *Three-Dimensional Computer Vision: A Geometric Viewpoint*, MIT Press Cambridge/MA 1993

[150] J. Feldmar, J. Declerck, G. Malandain, and N. Ayache, "Extension of the ICP Algorithm to Nonrigid Intensity-Based Registration of 3D Volumes", *Computer Vision and Image Understanding* 66:2 (1997) 193-206

[151] M. Ferrant, S.K. Warfield, C.R.G. Guttmann, R.V. Mulkern, F.A. Jolesz, and R. Kikinis, "3D Image Matching Using a Finite Element Based Elastic Deformation Model", *Proc. Second Internat. Conf. on Medical Image Computing and Computer-Assisted Intervention (MICCAI'99)*, Cambridge, England, Sept. 19-22, 1999, *Lecture Notes in Computer Science* 1679, C.J. Taylor and A. Colchester (Eds.), Springer-Verlag Berlin Heidelberg 1999, 202-209

[152] M. Fidrich and J.-P. Thirion, "Stability of Corner Points in Scale Space: The Effects of Small Nonrigid Deformations ", *Computer Vision and Image Understanding* 72:1 (1998) 72-83

[153] M.A. Fischler and R.A. Elschlager, "The Representation and Matching of Pictorial Structures", *IEEE Trans. on Computers* C-22:1 (1973) 67-92

[154] L.M.J. Florack, B.M. ter Haar Romeny, J.J. Koenderink, and M.A. Viergever, "General Intensity Transformations and Differential Invariants", *J. of Mathematical Imaging and Vision* 4 (1994) 171-187

[155] L.M.J. Florack, *Image structure*, Computational Imaging and Vision Series, Vol. 10, Kluwer Academic Publishers, Dordrecht Boston London 1997

[156] J. Flusser, "An adaptive method for image registration", *Pattern Recognition* 25:1 (1992) 45-54

[157] T.A. Foley, "Interpolation and Approximation of 3-D and 4-D Scattered Data", *Comput. Math. Applic.* 13:8 (1987) 711-740

[158] M. Fornefett, K. Rohr, R. Sprengel, and H.S. Stiehl, "Elastic Medical Image Registration using Orientation Attributes at Landmarks", *Proc. Medical Image Understanding and Analysis (MIUA'98)*, Univ. of Leeds/UK, 6-7 July 1998, E. Berry, D.C. Hogg, K.V. Mardia, and M.A. Smith (Eds.), University Print Services Leeds 1998, 49-52

[159] M. Fornefett, K. Rohr, R. Sprengel, and H.S. Stiehl, "Incorporating Orientation Attributes in Landmark-based Elastic Medical Image Registration", *Proc. Image and Multidimensional Digital Signal Processing (IMDSP'98)*, July 12-16, 1998, Alpbach/Austria, H. Niemann, H.-P. Seidel, and B. Girod (Eds.), infix Verlag Sankt Augustin 1998, 37-40

[160] M. Fornefett, K. Rohr, R. Sprengel, and H.S. Stiehl, "Orientation Constraints in Point-Based Elastic Image Registration", *20. DAGM-Symposium Mustererkennung*, 29. Sept.-1. Okt. 1998, Stuttgart/Germany, *Informatik aktuell*, P. Levi, R.-J. Ahlers, F. May, and M. Schanz (Eds.), Springer-Verlag Berlin Heidelberg 1998, 533-539

[161] M. Fornefett, K. Rohr, and H.S. Stiehl, "Elastic Registration of Medical Images Using Radial Basis Functions with Compact Support", *Proc. IEEE Conf. on Computer Vision and Pattern Recognition (CVPR'99)*, Fort Collins, Colorado, USA, June 23-25, 1999, IEEE Computer Society Press 1999, 402-407

[162] M. Fornefett, K. Rohr, and H.S. Stiehl, "Radial Basis Functions with Compact Support for Elastic Registration of Medical Images", *Proc. Internat. Workshop Biomedical Image Registration (WBIR'99)*, Bled, Slovenia, Aug. 30-31, 1999, F. Pernuš, S. Kovačič, H.S. Stiehl, and M. Viergever (Eds.), Slovenian Pattern Recognition Society, Ljubljana 1999, 173-185

[163] M. Fornefett, K. Rohr, and H.S. Stiehl, "Elastic Medical Image Registration Using Surface Landmarks With Automatic Finding of Correspondences", *Proc. Workshop Bildverarbeitung für die Medizin 2000 – Algorithmen, Systeme, Anwendungen –*, München, Germany, 12.-14. März 2000, *Informatik aktuell*, A. Horsch and T. Lehmann (Eds.), Springer-Verlag Berlin Heidelberg 2000, 48-52

[164] M. Fornefett, K. Rohr, and H.S. Stiehl, "Radial Basis Functions with Compact Support for Elastic Registration of Medical Images", *Image and Vision Computing*, 2000, in press

[165] O. Forster, *Analysis 3*, Vieweg Braunschweig 1984

[166] W. Förstner, "On the Geometric Precision of Digital Correlation", *Int. Arch. of Photogrammetry and Remote Sensing* 24-3, Helsinki, 1982, 176-189

[167] W. Förstner, "Quality Assessment of Object Location and Point Transfer Using Digital Image Correlation Techniques", *Int. Arch. of Photogrammetry and Remote Sensing* 25-3a, Rio de Janero, 1984, 197-219

[168] W. Förstner, "A Feature Based Correspondence Algorithm for Image Matching", *Int. Arch. of Photogrammetry and Remote Sensing* 26-3/3 (1986) 150-166

[169] W. Förstner, "Reliability analysis of parameter estimation in linear models with applications to mensuration problems in computer vision", *Computer Vision, Graphics, and Image Processing* 40 (1987) 273-310

[170] W. Förstner, "Image Matching", Chapter 16 in *Computer and Robot Vision*, Vol. II, R.M. Haralick and L.G. Shapiro, Addison-Wesley Publ. Company, Reading Menlo Park New York 1993

[171] W. Förstner, "A framework for low level feature extraction", *Proc. European Conf. on Computer Vision (ECCV'94)*, Stockholm, Sweden, May 2-6, 1994, Vol. B, *Lecture Notes in Computer Science* 802, J.O. Eklundh (Ed.), Springer Berlin Heidelberg 1994, 383-394

[172] W. Förstner, "10 Pros and Cons Against Performance Characterization of Vision Algorithms", *Workshop on Performance Characteristics of Vision Algorithms*, Cambridge/UK, April 1996, in conjunction with ECCV'96

[173] W. Förstner and E. Gülch, "A Fast Operator for Detection and Precise Location of Distinct Points, Corners and Centres of Circular Features", *Proc. ISPRS Intercomission Conf. on Fast Processing of Photogrammetric Data*, Interlaken/Switzerland, June 2-4, 1987, 281-305

[174] A.F. Frangi, W.J. Niessen, K.L. Vincken, and M.A. Viergever, "Multiscale Vessel Enhancement Filtering", *Proc. First Internat. Conf. on Medical Image Computing and Computer-Assisted Intervention (MICCAI'98)*, Massachusetts Institute of Technology (MIT), Cambridge/MA, USA, Oct. 11-13, 1998, *Lecture Notes in Computer Science* 1496, W.M. Wells, A. Colchester, and S. Delp (Eds.), Springer Verlag Berlin Heidelberg 1998, 130-137

[175] R. Franke, "Scattered Data Interpolation: Test of Some Methods", *Mathematics of Computation* 38:157 (1982) 181-200

[176] S. Frantz, K. Rohr, and H.S. Stiehl, "On the Localization of 3D Anatomical Point Landmarks in Medical Imagery Using Multi-Step Differential Approaches", *19. DAGM-Symposium Mustererkennung*, 15.-17. Sept. 1997, Braunschweig/Germany, *Informatik aktuell*, E. Paulus and F.M. Wahl (Eds.), Springer-Verlag Berlin Heidelberg 1997, 340-347

[177] S. Frantz, K. Rohr, and H.S. Stiehl, "Refined Localization of Three-Dimensional Anatomical Point Landmarks Using Multi-Step Differential Approaches", *Medical Imaging 1998 – Image Processing (MI'98)*, Proc. SPIE Internat. Symposium, Vol. 3338, Part One, Febr. 23-26, 1998, San Diego/CA, USA, K.M. Hanson (Ed.), 28-38

[178] S. Frantz, K. Rohr, and H.S. Stiehl, "Multi-Step Procedures for the Localization of 2D and 3D Point Landmarks and Automatic ROI Size Selection", *Proc. European Conf. on Computer Vision (ECCV'98)*, June 1998, Freiburg, Germany, Vol. I, *Lecture Notes in Computer Science* 1406, H. Burkhardt and B. Neumann (Eds.), Springer Berlin Heidelberg 1998, 687-703

[179] S. Frantz, K. Rohr, and H.S. Stiehl, "Multi-Step Differential Approaches for the Localization of 3D Point Landmarks in Medical Images", *J. of Computing and Information Technology (CIT)* 6:4 (1998) 435-447

[180] S. Frantz, K. Rohr, and H.S. Stiehl, "Reducing False Detections in Extracting 3D Anatomical Point Landmarks", *Proc. Workshop Bildverarbeitung für die Medizin 1999 – Algorithmen, Systeme, Anwendungen –*, DKFZ Heidelberg, Germany, 4./5. März 1999,

Informatik aktuell, H. Evers, G. Glombitza, T. Lehmann, and H.-P. Meinzer (Eds.), Springer-Verlag Berlin Heidelberg 1999, 54-59

[181] S. Frantz, K. Rohr, H.S. Stiehl, S.-I. Kim, and J. Weese, "Validating Point-based MR/CT Registration Based on Semi-automatic Landmark Extraction", *Proc. 13th Internat. Congress and Exhibition Computer Assisted Radiology and Surgery (CARS'99),* Paris, France, June 23-26, 1999, H.U. Lemke, M.W. Vannier, K. Inamura, and A.G. Farman (Eds.), Elsevier Science Amsterdam Lausanne 1999, 233-237

[182] S. Frantz, K. Rohr, and H.S. Stiehl, "Improving the Detection Performance in Semi-automatic Landmark Extraction", *Proc. Second Internat. Conf. on Medical Image Computing and Computer-Assisted Intervention (MICCAI'99),* Cambridge, England, Sept. 19-22, 1999, *Lecture Notes in Computer Science* 1679, C.J. Taylor and A. Colchester (Eds.), Springer-Verlag Berlin Heidelberg 1999, 253-262

[183] M. Gabrani and O.J. Tretiak, "Surface-based matching using elastic transformations", *Pattern Recognition* 32 (1999) 87-97

[184] T. Gaens, F. Maes, D. Vandermeulen, and P. Suetens, "Non-rigid Multimodal Image Registration Using Mutual Information", *Proc. First Internat. Conf. on Medical Image Computing and Computer-Assisted Intervention (MICCAI'98),* Massachusetts Institute of Technology (MIT), Cambridge/MA, USA, Oct. 11-13, 1998, *Lecture Notes in Computer Science* 1496, W.M. Wells, A. Colchester, and S. Delp (Eds.), Springer Verlag Berlin Heidelberg 1998, 1099-1106

[185] J.M. Gauch and S.M. Pizer, "Multiresolution Analysis of Vertex Curves and Watershed Boundaries", *Medical Imaging VI: Image Processing,* Febr. 1992, Newport Beach, California/USA, Proc. SPIE 1652, M.H. Loew (Ed.), 226-240

[186] D.M. Gavrila, "The Visual Analysis of Human Movement: A Survey", *Computer Vision and Image Understanding* 73:1 (1999) 82-98

[187] Y. Ge, J.M. Fitzpatrick, R.M. Kessler, M. Jeske-Janicka, and R.A. Margolin, "Intersubject brain image registration using both cortical and subcortical landmarks", *Medical Imaging 1995: Image Processing,* Febr./March 1995, San Diego/CA, USA, Proc. SPIE 2434, M.H. Loew (Ed.), 81-95

[188] J.C. Gee, D.R. Haynor, M. Reivich, and R. Bajcsy, "Finite element approach to warping of brain images", *Medical Imaging 1994: Image Processing,* 15-18 Febr. 1994, Newport Beach, California/USA, Proc. SPIE 2167, M.H. Loew (Ed.), 327-337

[189] J.C. Gee, "On matching brain volumes", *Pattern Recognition* 32 (1999) 99-111

[190] A. Gelb, *Applied Optimal Estimation,* MIT Press, Cambridge/MA, 1974

[191] P. Gerlot and Y. Bizais, "Image Registration: A Review and Strategy for Medical Applications", *Proc. 10th Internat. Conf. Information Processing in Medical Imaging (IPMI'88),* C.N. de Graaf and M.A. Viergever (Eds.), Plenum Press New York/NY 1988, 81-89

[192] F.A. Gerritsen, C.W.M. van Veelen, W.P.Th. Mali, A.J.M. Bart, A.H.W. v. Eeuwijk, M.J. Hartkamp, S. Lobgret, L. Moreira Pereira Ramos, L.J. Polman, P.C. v. Rijen, and C.P. Visser, "Some Requirements for and Experience with COVIRA Algorithms

for Registration and Segmentation", in *Medical Imaging – Analysis of Multimodality 2D/3D Images*, L. Beolchi and M.H. Kuhn (Eds.), IOS Press 1994, 4-28

[193] S. Gibson, C. Fyock, E. Grimson, T. Kanade, R. Kikinis, H. Lauer, N. McKenzie, A. Mor, S. Nakajima, H. Ohkami, R. Osborne, J. Samosky, and A. Sawada, "Volumetric object modeling for surgical simulation", *Medical Image Analysis* 2:2 (1998) 121-132

[194] G. Giraudon and R. Deriche, "On Corner and Vertex Detection", *Proc. IEEE Conf. on Computer Vision and Pattern Recognition (CVPR'91)*, Lahaina, Maui, Hawaii, June 3-6, 1991, 650-655

[195] E. Gladilin, W. Peckar, K. Rohr, and H.S. Stiehl, "Vergleich der Randelemente- mit der Finite-Elemente-Methode zur elastischen Registrierung medizinischer Bilder", Techn. Report FBI-HH-M-287/99, FB Informatik, Universität Hamburg, June 1999

[196] C.A. Glasbey and K.V. Mardia, "A review of image-warping methods", *J. of Applied Statistics* 25:2 (1998) 155-171

[197] A. Goshtasby, "Piecewise Cubic Mapping Functions for Image Registration", *Pattern Recognition* 20:5 (1987) 525-533

[198] A. Goshtasby, "Registration of Images with Geometric Distortions", *IEEE Trans. on Geoscience and Remote Sensing* 26:1 (1988) 60-64

[199] A. Goshtasby, "Image registration by local approximation methods", *Image and Vision Computing* 6:4 (1988) 255-261

[200] A. Goshtasby and W.D. O'Neill, "Surface fitting to scattered data by a sum of Gaussians", *Computer Aided Geometric Design* 10 (1993) 143-156

[201] D. Graham and A. Barrett, *Knowledge-Based Image Processing Systems*, Springer-Verlag London Berlin 1997

[202] P.J. Green and B.W. Silverman, *Nonparametric Regression and Generalized Linear Models*, Chapman & Hall London Glasgow 1994

[203] R.D. Green, L. Guan, and J.A. Burne, "Real-time gait analysis for diagnosing movement disorders", *Medical Imaging 1998 – Image Processing (MI'98)*, Proc. SPIE Internat. Symposium, Vol. 3338, Part One, Febr. 23-26, 1998, San Diego/CA, USA, K.M. Hanson (Ed.), 818-825

[204] W.D.K. Green, "Spline-based deformable models", *Vision Geometry IV*, Proc. SPIE 2573, 1995, 290-301

[205] W.D.K. Green, "The thin-plate spline and images with curving features", *Proc. Image Fusion and Shape Variability Techniques*, Leeds/UK, 3-5 July 1996, K.V. Mardia, C.A. Gill, and I.L. Dryden (Eds.), Leeds University Press 1996, 79-87

[206] U. Grenander and M.I. Miller, "Computational Anatomy: An Emerging Discipline", *Quarterly of Applied Mathematics* LVI:4 (Dec. 1998) 617-694

[207] W.E.L. Grimson, "A Computational Theory of Visual Surface Interpolation", *Phil. Trans. R. London* B 298 (1982) 395-427

[208] W.E.L. Grimson, "An Implementation of a Computational Theory of Visual Surface Interpolation", *Computer Vision, Graphics, and Image Processing* 22 (1983) 39-69

[209] W.E.L. Grimson, "Medical Applications of Image Understanding", *IEEE Expert* 10:5 (1995) 18-28

[210] W.E.L. Grimson, R. Kikinis, F.A. Jolesz, and P. McL. Black, "Image-Guided Surgery", *Scientific American* (June 1999) 54-61

[211] A. Guéziec, P. Kazanzides, B. Williamson, and R.H. Taylor, "Anatomy-Based Registration of CT-Scan and Intraoperative X-Ray Images for Guiding a Surgical Robot", *IEEE Trans. on Medical Imaging* 17:5 (1998) 715-728

[212] A. Guiducci, "Corner characterization by differential geometry techniques", *Pattern Recognition Letters* 8 (1988) 311-318

[213] G. Guiot and P. Derome, "The principles of stereotaxic thalamotomy", in *Correlative Neurosurgery*, Vol. II, R.C. Schneider, E.A. Kahn, E.L. Crosby, and J.A. Taren (Eds.), Charles Thanas, Springfield 1982, 481

[214] B. ter Haar Romeny, L. Florack, J. Koenderink, and M. Viergever (Eds.), *Scale-Space Theory in Computer Vision, Proc. Int. Conf. Scale-Space'97*, Utrecht, The Netherlands, July 1997, *Lecture Notes in Computer Science* 1252, Springer Berlin Heidelberg 1997

[215] A. Hagemann, K. Rohr, and H.S. Stiehl, "Theoretische und experimentelle Untersuchung eines Verfahrens zur Attributschätzung von Grauwertkanten in 2D CT/MR Bildern", *Proc. Workshop Bildverarbeitung für die Medizin 1998 – Algorithmen, Systeme, Anwendungen –*, Aachen, Germany, 26./27. März 1998, *Informatik aktuell*, T. Lehmann, V. Metzler, K. Spitzer, and T. Tolxdorff (Eds.), Springer-Verlag Berlin Heidelberg 1998, 29-33

[216] A. Hagemann, K. Rohr, H.S. Stiehl, U. Spetzger, and J.M. Gilsbach, "Elastic Registration of MR-Images Based on a Biomechanical Model of the Human Head", *Navigated Brain Surgery – Interdisciplinary Views of Neuronavigation from Neurosurgeons and Computer Scientists*, U. Spetzger, H.S. Stiehl, and J.M. Gilsbach (Eds.), Verlag Mainz, Aachen 1999, 203-209

[217] A. Hagemann, K. Rohr, H.S. Stiehl, U. Spetzger, and J.M. Gilsbach, "Nonrigid matching of tomographic images based on a biomechanical model of the human head", *Medical Imaging 1999 – Image Processing (MI'99)*, Proc. SPIE Internat. Symposium, Vol. 3661, Part One, Febr. 22-25, 1999, San Diego/CA, USA, K.M. Hanson (Ed.), 583-592

[218] A. Hagemann, K. Rohr, H.S. Stiehl, U. Spetzger, and J.M. Gilsbach, "A Biomechanical Model of the Human Head for Elastic Registration of MR-Images", *Proc. Workshop Bildverarbeitung für die Medizin 1999 – Algorithmen, Systeme, Anwendungen –*, DKFZ Heidelberg, Germany, 4./5. März 1999, *Informatik aktuell*, H. Evers, G. Glombitza, T. Lehmann, and H.-P. Meinzer (Eds.), Springer-Verlag Berlin Heidelberg 1999, 44-48

[219] A. Hagemann, K. Rohr, H.S. Stiehl, U. Spetzger, and J.M. Gilsbach, "Intraoperative Image Correction Using a Biomechanical Model of the Human Head with Different Material Properties", *21. DAGM-Symposium Mustererkennung 1999*, 15.-17. Sept. 1999, Bonn/Germany, *Informatik aktuell*, W. Förstner, J.M. Buhmann, A. Faber, and P. Faber (Eds.), Springer-Verlag Berlin Heidelberg 1999, 223-231

[220] A. Hagemann, K. Rohr, H.S. Stiehl, U. Spetzger, and J.M. Gilsbach, "Biomechanical Modelling of the Human Head for Physically-Based, Nonrigid Image Registration", *IEEE Trans. on Medical Imaging* 18:10 (1999) 875-884

[221] A. Hagemann, K. Rohr, H.S. Stiehl, "Biomechanically based simulation of brain deformations for intraoperative image correction: coupling of elastic and fluid models", *Medical Imaging 2000 – Image Processing (MI'2000)*, Proc. SPIE Internat. Symposium, Vol. 3979, Part One, Febr. 14-17, 2000, San Diego/CA, K.M. Hanson (Ed.), 658-667

[222] G.D. Hager and P.N. Belhumeur, "Efficient region tracking with parametric models of geometry and illumination", *IEEE Trans. on Pattern Anal. and Machine Intell.* 20:10 (1998) 1025-1039

[223] H. Handels, *Medizinische Bildverarbeitung,* Teubner Stuttgart 2000

[224] R.M. Haralick, "Performance Characterization in Computer Vision", *CVGIP: Image Understanding* 60:2 (1994) 245-249

[225] R.M. Haralick, "Propagating covariance in computer vision," *Proc. 12th Int. Conf. on Pattern Recognition (ICPR'94)*, Jerusalem/Israel, Oct. 9-13, 1994, IEEE Computer Society Press, Los Alamitos/CA, 1994, 493-498

[226] R.M. Haralick and L.G. Shapiro, *Computer and Robot Vision,* Vols. I and II, Addison-Wesley Publ. Company, Reading Menlo Park New York 1992 and 1993

[227] R.M. Haralick, L.T. Watson, and T.J. Laffey, "The Topographic Primal Sketch", *The Int. J. of Robotics Research* 2:1 (1983) 50-72

[228] R.L. Harder and R.N. Desmarais, "Interpolation Using Surface Splines", *J. of Aircraft* 9 (1972) 189-191

[229] R.L. Hardy, "Theory and Application of the Multiquadric-Biharmonic Method", *Computers Math. Applic.* 19:8/9 (1990) 163-208

[230] C. Harris and M. Stephens, "A Combined Corner and Edge Detector", *Proc. Fourth Alvey Vision Conf.,* Manchester/UK, Aug. 1988, 147-151

[231] T. Hartkens, "Untersuchung von 3D-Operatoren zur Detektion von Punktlandmarken in tomographischen Bildern", Diplomarbeit, Universität Hamburg, Fachbereich Informatik, Arbeitsbereich Kognitive Systeme, Juli 1997

[232] T. Hartkens, K. Rohr, and H.S. Stiehl, "Evaluierung von Differentialoperatoren zur Detektion charakteristischer Punkte in tomographischen Bildern", *18. DAGM-Symposium Mustererkennung,* 11.-13. Sept. 1996, Heidelberg/Germany, *Informatik aktuell,* B. Jähne, P. Geißler, H. Haußecker, and F. Hering (Eds.), Springer-Verlag Berlin Heidelberg 1996, 637-644

[233] T. Hartkens, K. Rohr, and H.S. Stiehl, "Evaluierung der Detektionsleistung von 3D-Operatoren zur Ermittlung anatomischer Landmarken in tomographischen Bildern", *Proc. Workshop Bildverarbeitung für die Medizin 1998, – Algorithmen, Systeme, Anwendungen –,* Aachen, Germany, 26./27. März 1998, *Informatik aktuell,* T. Lehmann, V. Metzler, K. Spitzer, and T. Tolxdorff (Eds.), Springer-Verlag Berlin Heidelberg 1998, 93-97

[234]   T. Hartkens, K. Rohr, and H.S. Stiehl, "Untersuchung der Detektionsleistung von 3D-Operatoren zur Ermittlung von Punktlandmarken in MR- und CT-Bildern", *20. DAGM-Symposium Mustererkennung,* 29. Sept.- 1. Okt. 1998, Stuttgart/Germany, *Informatik aktuell,* P. Levi, R.-J. Ahlers, F. May, and M. Schanz (Eds.), Springer-Verlag Berlin Heidelberg 1998, 211-218

[235]   T. Hartkens, K. Rohr, and H.S. Stiehl, "Performance of 3D differential operators for the detection of anatomical point landmarks in MR and CT images", *Medical Imaging 1999 – Image Processing (MI'99),* Proc. SPIE Internat. Symposium, Vol. 3661, Part One, Febr. 22-25, 1999, San Diego/CA, USA, K.M. Hanson (Ed.), 32-43

[236]   U. Hartmann and F. Kruggel, "Erste klinische Untersuchungen mit einem mechanischen Finite-Elemente-Modell des menschlichen Kopfes", *Proc. Workshop Bildverarbeitung für die Medizin 1998 – Algorithmen, Systeme, Anwendungen –,* Aachen, Germany, 26./27. März 1998, *Informatik aktuell,* T. Lehmann, V. Metzler, K. Spitzer, and T. Tolxdorff (Eds.), Springer-Verlag Berlin Heidelberg 1998, 59-63

[237]   N. Hata, T. Dohi, S. Warfield, W. Wells III, R. Kikinis, and F.A. Jolesz, "Multimodality Deformable Registration of Pre- and Intraoperative Images for MRI-Guided Brain Surgery", *Proc. First Internat. Conf. on Medical Image Computing and Computer-Assisted Intervention (MICCAI'98),* Massachusetts Institute of Technology (MIT), Cambridge/MA, USA, Oct. 11-13, 1998, *Lecture Notes in Computer Science* 1496, W.M. Wells, A. Colchester, and S. Delp (Eds.), Springer Verlag Berlin Heidelberg 1998, 1067-1074

[238]   H. Haußecker and B. Jähne, "A Tensor Approach for Local Structure Analysis in Multi-Dimensional Images", *Proc. Workshop 3D Image Analysis and Synthesis,* Erlangen, Nov. 1996, 171-178

[239]   G. Herzog and K. Rohr, "Integrating Vision and Language: Towards Automatic Description of Human Movements", *Proc. 19th Conf. on Artificial Intelligence, KI-95: Advances in Artificial Intelligence,* Sept. 1995, Bielefeld/Germany, *Lecture Notes in Artificial Intelligence* 981, I. Wachsmuth, C.-R. Rollinger, and W. Brauer (Eds.), Springer-Verlag Berlin Heidelberg 1995, 259-268

[240]   H. Heuser, *Funktionalanalysis,* B.G. Teubner Stuttgart 1986

[241]   A. Heyden, "On the Consistency of Line-Drawings, Obtained by Projections of Piecewise Planar Objects", *J. of Mathematical Imaging and Vision* 6:4 (1995) 393-412

[242]   A. Heyden and K. Rohr, "Evaluation of Corner Extraction Schemes Using Invariance Methods", *Proc. 13th Internat. Conf. on Pattern Recognition (ICPR'96),* Vienna, Austria, Aug. 25-29, Vol. I, IEEE Computer Society Press 1996, 895-899

[243]   A. Hill, T.F. Cootes, and C.J. Taylor, "Least-Squares Solution as Absolute Orientation with Non-Scalar Weights", *Proc. 13th Internat. Conf. on Pattern Recognition (ICPR'96),* Vienna, Austria, Aug. 25-29, IEEE Computer Society Press 1996, 461-465

[244]   D.L.G. Hill, D.J. Hawkes, J.E. Crossman, M.J. Gleeson, T.C.S. Cox, E.E.C.M. Bracey, A.J. Strong, and P. Graves, "Registration of MR and CT images for skull base surgery using point-like anatomical features", *The British J. of Radiology* 64:767 (1991) 1030-1035

[245] D.L.G. Hill, D.J. Hawkes, M.J. Gleeson, T.C.S. Cox, A.J. Strong, W-L. Wong, C.F. Ruff, N. Kitchen, D.G.T. Thomas, J.E. Crossman, C. Studholme, A.J. Gandhe, S.E.M. Green, and G.P. Robinson, "Accurate Frameless Registration of MR and CT images of the Head: Applications in Surgery and Radiotherapy Planning", *Radiology* 191 (May 1994) 447-454

[246] D.L.G. Hill, C.R. Maurer, M.Y. Wang, R.J. Maciunas, J.A. Barwise, and J.M. Fitzpatrick, "Estimation of Intraoperative Brain Surface Movement", *Proc. First Joint Conf. CVRMed-MRCAS'97*, Grenoble/France, March 1997, *Lecture Notes in Computer Science* 1205, J. Troccaz, E. Grimson, and R. Mösges (Eds.), Springer Verlag Berlin Heidelberg 1997, 449-458

[247] D.L.G. Hill, C.R. Maurer, R.J. Maciunas, J.A. Barwise, J.M. Fitzpatrick, and M.Y. Wang, "Measurement of Intraoperative Brain Surface Deformation under a Craniotomy", *Neurosurgery* 43:3 (1998) 514-528

[248] F.S. Hill, *Computer Graphics*, Macmillan Publishing Company, New York 1990

[249] C.M. Hoffmann, *Geometric and Solid Modeling – An Introduction*, Morgan Kaufmann Publishers, San Mateo, California, 1989

[250] K.H. Höhne, "3D-Bildverarbeitung und Computer-Graphik in der Medizin", *Informatik-Spektrum* 10 (1987) 192-204

[251] K.H. Höhne, M. Bomans, M. Riemer, R. Schubert, U. Tiede, and W. Lierse, "A Volume-based Anatomical Atlas", *IEEE Computer Graphics & Applications* (July 1992) 72-77

[252] K.H. Höhne (Ed.), "VOXEL-MAN, Part 1: Brain and Skull", Version 1.0, Springer-Verlag Electronic Media, Heidelberg, 1995

[253] K.H. Höhne, "Phantastische Reisen durch den menschlichen Körper", *Spektrum der Wissenschaft*, April 1999, 54-62

[254] B.K.P. Horn, *Robot vision*, MIT Press Cambridge/MA 1986

[255] B.K.P. Horn, "Closed-from solution of absolute orientation using unit quaternions", *J. Opt. Soc. Am. A* 4:4 (1987) 629-642

[256] J. Hoschek and D. Lasser, *Grundlagen der geometrischen Datenverarbeitung*, B.G. Teubner Stuttgart 1989

[257] U. Hübner, F.J. Schuier, and J.A. Newell, "Software applied to multimodal images and education", *Computer Methods and Programs in Biomedicine* 45 (1994) 149-152

[258] M.H. Hueckel, "An Operator Which Locates Edges in Digitized Pictures", *J. of the Association for Computing Machinery* 18:1 (Jan. 1971) 113-125

[259] I.R.H. Jackson, "Radial Basis Functions: a Survey and New Results", *The Mathematics of Surfaces III*, 1989, 115-133

[260] B. Jähne, *Spatio-Temporal Image Processing – Theory and Scientific Applications*, Springer-Verlag Berlin 1993

[261] A.K. Jain, Y. Zhong, and S. Lakshmanan, "Object Matching Using Deformable Templates", *IEEE Trans. on Pattern Anal. and Machine Intell.* 18:3 (1996) 267-278

[262] R.C. Jain and T.O. Binford, "Ignorance, Myopia, and Naiveté in Computer Vision Systems", *CVGIP: Image Understanding* 53:1 (1991) 112-117

[263] Q. Ji and R.M. Haralick, "Breakpoint detection using covariance propagation", *IEEE Trans. on Pattern Anal. and Machine Intell.* 20:8 (1998) 845-851

[264] M.J. Jones and T. Poggio, "Multidimensional Morphable Models", *Proc. Int. Conf. on Computer Vision (ICCV'98)*, Bombay, India, Jan. 4-7, 1998, Narosa Publishing House, New Delhi Madras 1998, 683-688

[265] S.C. Joshi, M.I. Miller, G.E. Christensen, A. Banerjee, T.A. Coogan, and U. Grenander, "Hierarchical brain mapping via a generalized Dirichlet solution for mapping brain manifolds", *Vision Geometry IV,* Proc. SPIE 2573, 1995, 278-289

[266] R. Kakarala and A.O. Hero, "On Achievable Accuracy in Edge Localization", *IEEE Trans. on Pattern Anal. and Machine Intell.* 14:7 (1992) 777-781

[267] R.E. Kalman, "A New Approach to Linear Filtering and Prediction Problems", *Trans. ASME J. Basic Eng.,* Series 82D (March 1960) 35-45

[268] C. Kambhamettu, D.B. Goldgof, D. Terzopoulos, and T.S. Huang, "Nonrigid motion analysis", *Handbook of Pattern Recognition and Image Processing: Computer Vision,* Vol. II, T. Young (Ed.), Academic Press, San Diego/CA, USA, 1994, 405-430

[269] T. Kanade, "Region Segmentation: Signal vs. Semantics," *Proc. Int. Joint Conf. on Pattern Recognition,* Nov. 7-10, 1978, Kyoto/Japan, 95-105, see also: *Computer Graphics and Image Processing* 13 (1980) 279-297

[270] T. Kanade and K. Ikeuchi, "Introduction to the Special Issue on Physical Modeling in Computer Vision," *IEEE Trans. on Pattern Anal. and Machine Intell.* 13:7 (1991) 609-610

[271] K. Kanatani, *Statistical Optimization for Geometric Computation: Theory and Practice,* Elsevier Amsterdam Lausanne 1996

[272] K. Kanatani, "Cramer-Rao Lower Bounds for Curve Fitting", *Graphical Models and Image Processing* 60:2 (1998) 93-99

[273] S.B. Kang, R. Szeliski, and H.-Y. Shum, "A parallel Feature Tracker for Extended Image Sequences", *Computer Vision and Image Understanding* 67:3 (1997) 296-310

[274] M. Kass, A. Witkin, and D. Terzopoulos, "Snakes: active contour models", *Int. J. of Computer Vision* 1 (1988) 321-331

[275] A. Kelemen, G. Székely, and G. Gerig, "Elastic Model-Based Segmentation of 3-D Neuroradiological Sets", *IEEE Trans. on Medical Imaging* 18:10 (1999) 828-839

[276] J.T. Kent and K.V. Mardia, "The Link Between Kriging and Thin-Plate Splines", in *Probability, Statistics and Optimisation,* F.P. Kelly (Ed.), John Wiley & Sons Chichester New York 1994

[277] W.S. Kerwin and J.L. Prince, "Cardiac material markers from tagged MR images", *Medical Image Analysis* 2:4 (1998) 339-353

[278] R. Kikinis, M.E. Shenton, D.V. Iosifescu, R.W. McCarley, P. Saiviroonporn, H.H. Hokama, A. Robatino, D. Metcalf, C.G. Wible, C.M. Portas, R. Donnino, and F.A. Jolesz, "A Digital Brain Atlas for Surgical Planning, Model Driven Segmentation and Teaching", *IEEE Trans. on Visualization and Computer Graphics* 2:3 (1996)

[279] G.S. Kimeldorf and G. Wahba, "Spline Functions and Stochastic Processes", *SANKHYA A* 32:1 (1970) 173-180

[280] L. Kitchen and A. Rosenfeld, "Gray-level corner detection", *Pattern Recognition Letters* 1 (1982) 95-102

[281] R. Klette, H.S. Stiehl, M.A. Viergever, and K.L. Vincken (Eds.), *Performance Characterization and Evaluation of Computer Vision Algorithms*, Proc. Dagstuhl Seminar, March 15-20, 1998, Schloß Dagstuhl, Wadern/Germany, Computational Imaging and Vision Series, Kluwer Academic Publishers, Dordrecht Boston London 2000, in press

[282] H. Knutsson, "Representing local structure using tensors", *Proc. Scandinavian Conf. on Image Analysis*, Oulu, Finnland, June 1989, 244-151

[283] J.J. Koenderink, "The Structure of Images", *Biol. Cybernetics* 50 (1984) 363-370

[284] J.J. Koenderink, *Solid Shape*, The MIT Press Cambridge/MA 1990

[285] J.J. Koenderink and A.J. van Doorn, "The Internal Representation of Solid Shape with Respect to Vision", *Biol. Cybernetics* 32 (1979) 211-216

[286] Th.M. Koller, G. Gerig, G. Székely, and D. Dettwiler, "Multiscale Detection of Curvilinear Structures in 2-D and 3-D Image Data", *Proc. Int. Conf. on Computer Vision (ICCV'95)*, Boston/MA, June 1995, IEEE Computer Society Press, Washington, D.C., 1995, 864-869

[287] A.F. Korn, "Toward a Symbolic Representation of Intensity Changes in Images", *IEEE Trans. on Pattern Anal. and Machine Intell.* 10 (1988) 610-625

[288] S.H. Koslow and M.F. Huerta (Eds.), *Neuroinformatics – An Overview of the Human Brain Project*, Lawrence Erlbaum Associates, Mahwah New Jersey 1997

[289] K. Krissian, G. Malandain, N. Ayache, R. Vaillant, and Y. Trousset, "Model Based Multiscale Detection of 3D Vessels", *Proc. IEEE Workshop on Biomedical Image Analysis*, June 26-27, 1998, Santa Barbara/California, B. Vemuri (Ed.), IEEE Computer Society Press Washington 1998, 202-210

[290] C. Kuhn, U. Kühnapfel, and O. Deussen, "Echtzeitsimulation deformierbarer Objekte zur Ausbildungsunterstützung in der Minimal-Invasiven Chirurgie", *Proc. of Int. Workshop Modeling Virtual Worlds-Distributed Graphics (MVD'95)*, Bad Honnef, Germany

[291] M.H. Kuhn, "Multimodality Image Analysis for COmputer VIsion in RAdiology – Status of the COVIRA Project –", *Proc. Third Internat. Conf. on Image Management and Communication*, June 23-24, 1993, Berlin/Germany, S.K. Mun and H.U. Lemke (Eds.), IEEE Computer Society Press Washington, 99-109

[292] S.K. Kyriacou and C. Davatzikos, "A Biomechanical Model of Soft Tissue Deformation, with Applications to Non-rigid Registration of Brain Images with Tumor Pathology",

Proc. First Internat. Conf. on Medical Image Computing and Computer-Assisted Intervention (MICCAI'98), Massachusetts Institute of Technology (MIT), Cambridge/MA, USA, Oct. 11-13, 1998, *Lecture Notes in Computer Science* 1496, W.M. Wells, A. Colchester, and S. Delp (Eds.), Springer Verlag Berlin Heidelberg 1998, 531-538

[293] S.K. Kyriacou, C. Davatzikos, S.J. Zinreich, and R.N. Bryan, "Nonlinear Elastic Registration of Brain Images with Tumor Pathology Using a Biomechanical Model", *IEEE Trans. on Medical Imaging* 18:7 (1999) 580-592

[294] R.K.-S. Kwan, A.C. Evans, and G.B. Pike, "MRI Simulation-Based Evaluation of Image-Processing and Classification Methods", *IEEE Trans. on Medical Imaging* 18:11 (1999) 1085-1097

[295] M. Lades, J.C. Vorbrüggen, J. Buhmann, J. Lange, C. v.d. Malsburg, R.P. Würtz, and W. Konen, "Distortion Invariant Object Recognition in the Dynamic Link Architecture", *IEEE Trans. on Computers* 42:3 (1993) 300-311

[296] R. Laganière, "Morphological Corner Detection", *Proc. Int. Conf. on Computer Vision (ICCV'98)*, Bombay, India, Jan. 4-7, 1998, Narosa Publishing House, New Delhi Madras 1998, 280-285

[297] S.-H. Lai, C.-W. Fu, and S. Chang, "A Generalized Depth Estimation Algorithm with a Single Image", *IEEE Trans. on Pattern Anal. and Machine Intell.* 14:4 (1992) 405-411

[298] P. Lancaster and K. Šalkauskas, *Curve and Surface Fitting*, Academic Press London San Diego 1986

[299] L.D. Landau and E.M. Lifschitz, *Lehrbuch der Theoretischen Physik*, Band VII, *Elastizitätstheorie*, Akademie-Verlag Berlin 1989

[300] L.J. Latecki, *Discrete Representation of Spatial Objects in Computer Vision*, Computational Imaging and Vision Series, Vol. 11, Kluwer Academic Publishers, Dordrecht Boston London 1998

[301] S. Lavallée, "Registration for Computer-Integrated Surgery: Methodology, State of the Art", in *Computer-Integrated Surgery*, R.H. Taylor, S. Lavallée, G.C. Burdea, and R. Mösges (Eds.), The MIT Press, Cambridge/Massachusetts, 1996, 77-97

[302] E.E. Leamer, *Specification Searches – Ad Hoc Inferences with Nonexperimental Data*, John Wiley & Sons New York Chichester 1978

[303] G. Le Goualher, C. Barillot, L. Le Briquer, J.C. Gee, and Y. Bizais, "3D Detection and Representation of Cortical Sulci", *Proc. Internat. Symposium Computer Assisted Radiology (CAR'95)*, June 1995, Berlin/Germany, H.U. Lemke, K. Inamura, C.C. Jaffe, and M.W. Vannier (Eds.), Springer-Verlag Berlin Heidelberg 1995, 234-240

[304] T. Lehmann, W. Oberschelp, E. Pelikan, and R. Repges, *Bildverarbeitung für die Medizin – Grundlagen, Modelle, Methoden, Anwendungen*, Springer-Verlag Berlin Heidelberg 1997

[305] W. Leister and K. Rohr, "Voruntersuchungen von Bildsynthesemethoden zur Analyse von Bildfolgen", Techn. Report Nr. 25/90, Universität Karlsruhe (TH), Fakultät für Informatik, Sept. 1990

[306] J. Lengyel, "The convergence of Graphics and Vision", *IEEE Computer* 31:7 (1998) 46-53

[307] H. Lester, S.R. Arridge, and K.M. Jansons, "Local deformation metrics and nonlinear registration using a fluid model with variable viscosity", *Proc. Medical Image Understanding and Analysis (MIUA'98)*, Univ. of Leeds/UK, 6-7 July 1998, E. Berry, D.C. Hogg, K.V. Mardia, and M.A. Smith (Eds.), University Print Services Leeds 1998, 45-48

[308] H. Lester and S.R. Arridge, "A survey of hierarchical non-linear medical image registration", *Pattern Recognition* 32 (1999) 129-149

[309] T. Lindeberg, "Feature Detection with Automatic Scale Selection", *Int. J. of Computer Vision* 30:2 (1998) 79-116

[310] T. Lindeberg and J. Gårding, "Shape-Adapted Smoothing in Estimation of 3-D Depth Cues from Affine Distortions of Local 2-D Brightness Structure", *Image and Vision Computing* 15 (1997) 415-434

[311] M.M. Lipschutz, *Differentialgeometrie: Theorie und Anwendung,* Schaum's Outline, McGraw-Hill Düsseldorf New York 1980

[312] J.A. Little, D.L.G. Hill, and D.J. Hawkes, "Deformations Incorporating Rigid Structures", *Computer Vision and Image Understanding* 66:2 (1997) 223-232

[313] S. Lobregt and M.A. Viergever, "A Discrete Dynamic Contour Model", *IEEE Trans. on Medical Imaging* 14:1 (1995) 12-24

[314] G. Lohmann, *Volumetric Image Analysis,* John Wiley & Sons and B.G. Teubner, Chichester New York Weinheim 1998

[315] C. Lorenz, I.-C. Carlsen, T.M. Buzug, C. Fassnacht, and J. Weese, "Multi-scale Line Segmentation with Automatic Estimation of Width, Contrast and Tangential Direction in 2D and 3D Medical Images", *Proc. First Joint Conf. CVRMed-MRCAS'97,* Grenoble/France, March 1997, *Lecture Notes in Computer Science* 1205, J. Troccaz, E. Grimson, and R. Mösges (Eds.), Springer Verlag Berlin Heidelberg 1997, 233-242

[316] L.M. Lorigo, O. Faugeras, W.E.L. Grimson, R. Keriven, R. Kikinis, and C.-F. Westin, "Co-dimension 2 Geodesic Active Contours for MRA Segmentation", *Proc. 16th Internat. Conf. on Information Processing in Medical Imaging (IPMI'99),* Visegrád, Hungary, June 28 - July 2, 1999, In *Lecture Notes in Computer Science* 1613, A. Kuba, M. Šámal, and A. Todd-Pokropek (Eds.), Springer-Verlag Berlin Heidelberg 1999, 126-139

[317] B.D. Lucas and T. Kanade, "An Iterative Image Registration Technique with an Application to Stereo Vision", *Proc. Int. Joint Conf. on Artificial Intell. (IJCAI'81),* Vancouver, BC, 1981, 674-679

[318] K. Lüdeke, P. Röschmann, and R. Tischler, "Susceptibility artifacts in nmr imaging", *MRI* 3 (1985) 329-343

[319] F. Maes, A. Collignon, D. Vandermeulen, G. Marchal, and P. Suetens, "Multimodality Image Registration by Maximization of Mutual Information", *IEEE Trans. on Medical Imaging* 16:2 (1997) 187-198

[320] J.B.A. Maintz, P.A. van den Elsen, and M.A. Viergever, "Comparison of edge-based and ridge-based registration of CT and MR brain images", *Medical Image Analysis* 1:2 (1996) 151-161

[321] J.B.A. Maintz and M.A. Viergever, "A survey of medical image registration", *Medical Image Analysis* 2:1 (1998) 1-36

[322] R. Malladi, J.A. Sethian, and B.C. Vemuri, "Shape Modeling with Front Propagation: A Level Set Approach", *IEEE Trans. on Pattern Anal. and Machine Intell.* 17:2 (1995) 158-175

[323] K.V. Mardia, "Shape Advances and Future Perspectives", *Proc. Current Issues in Statistical Shape Analysis,* Leeds/UK, 5-7 April 1995, K.V. Mardia and C.A. Gill (Eds.), Leeds University Press 1995, 57-75

[324] K. Mardia and J. Little, "Image warping using derivative information", In *Mathematical Methods in Medical Imaging III,* 25-26 July 1994, San Diego/CA, USA, Proc. SPIE 2299, F. Bookstein, J. Duncan, N. Lange, and D. Wilson (Eds.), 16-31

[325] K. Mardia, J.T. Kent, C.R. Goodall, and J. Little, "Kriging and splines with derivative information", *Biometrika* 83:1 (1996) 207-221

[326] D. Marquardt, "An algorithm for least-squares estimation of nonlinear parameters", *J. Soc. Indust. Appl. Math.* 11 (1963) 431-441

[327] D. Marr, "Representing Visual Information – A Computational Approach", in *Computer Vision Systems,* A.R. Hanson and E.M. Riseman (Eds.), Academic Press, New York San Francisco London 1978, 61-80

[328] D. Marr, *Vision: A computational investigation into the human representation and processing of visual information,* Freeman San Francisco/CA 1982

[329] D. Marr and H.K. Nishihara, "Representation and recognition of the spatial organization of three-dimensional shapes", *Proc. R. Soc. Lond.* B 200 (1978) 269-294

[330] D. Marr and E. Hildreth, "Theory of Edge Detection", *Proc. Royal Society of London* B 207 (1980) 187-217

[331] D. Marr and L. Vaina, "Representation and recognition of the movements of shapes", *Proc. R. Soc. Lond.* B 214 (1982) 501-524

[332] J. Martin, A. Pentland, S. Sclaroff, and R. Kikinis, "Characterization of Neuropathological Shape Deformations", *IEEE Trans. on Pattern Anal. and Machine Intell.* 20:2 (1998) 97-112

[333] W. Maurel, Y. Wu, N. Magnenat Thalmann, and D. Thalmann, *Biomechanical Models for Soft Tissue Simulation,* Springer Berlin 1998

[334] C.R. Maurer and J.M. Fitzpatrick, "A Review of Medical Image Registration", *Interactive Image-Guided Neurosurgery,* R.J. Maciunas (Ed.), Park Ridge IL: American Association of Neurological Surgeons, 1993, 17-44

[335] C.R. Maurer, R.J. Maciunas, and J.M. Fitzpatrick, "Registration of Head CT Images to Physical Space Using a Weighted Combination of Points and Surfaces", *IEEE Trans. on Medical Imaging* 17:5 (1998) 753-761

[336] J.C. Mazziotta, A.W. Toga, A. Evans, P. Fox, and J. Lancaster, "Atlases of the Human Brain", in *Neuroinformatics – An Overview of the Human Brain Project*, S.H. Koslow and M.F. Huerta (Eds.), Lawrence Erlbaum Associates, Mahwah New Jersey 1997, 255-308

[337] T. McInerney and D. Terzopoulos, "Deformable Models in Medical Image Analysis: A Survey", *Medical Image Analysis* 1:2 (1996/7) 91-108

[338] E.H.W. Meijering, W.J. Niessen, and M.A. Viergever (Eds.), "Retrospective Motion Correction in Digital Subtraction Angiography: A Review", *IEEE Trans. on Medical Imaging* 18:1 (1999) 2-21

[339] J. Meinguet, "Multivariate Interpolation at Arbitrary Points Made Simple", *J. of Applied Mathematics and Physics (ZAMP)* 30 (1979) 292-304

[340] J. Meinguet, "Surface Spline Interpolation: Basic Theory and Computational Aspects", in *Approximation Theory and Spline Functions*, S.P. Singh, J.W.H. Burry, and B. Watson (Eds.), D. Reidel Publishing Company Dordrecht 1984, 127-142

[341] D. Metaxas and D. Terzopoulos (Eds.), Special Issue on "Physics-Based Modeling and Reasoning in Computer Vision", *Computer Vision and Image Understanding* 65:2 (1997) 111-359

[342] C.R. Meyer, G.S. Leichtman, J.A. Brunberg, R.L. Wahl, and L.E. Quint, "Simultaneous usage of homologous points, lines, and planes for optimal, 3-D, linear registration of multimodality imaging data", *IEEE Trans. on Medical Imaging* 14:1 (1995) 1-11

[343] C.R. Meyer, J.L. Boes, B. Kim, P.H. Bland, K.R. Zasadny, P.V. Kison, K. Koral, K.A. Frey, and R.L. Wahl, "Demonstration of accuracy and clinical versatility of mutual information for automatic multimodality image fusion using affine and thin-plate spline warped geometric deformations", *Medical Image Analysis* 1:3 (1996/7) 195-206

[344] C.A. Micchelli, "Interpolation of scattered data: Distance matrices and conditionally positive definite functions", *Constructive Approximation* 2 (1986) 11-22

[345] J. Michiels, H. Bosmans, P. Pelgrims, D. Vandermeulen, J. Gybels, G. Marchal, and P. Suetens, "On the problem of geometric distortion in magnetic resonance images for stereotactic neurosurgery", *Mag. Res. Imag.* 12 (1994) 749

[346] M.I. Miga, K.D. Paulsen, J.M. Lemery, S.D. Eisner, A. Hartov, F.E. Kennedy, and D.W. Roberts, "Model-Updated Image Guidance: Initial Clinical Experiences with Gravity-Induced Brain Deformation", *IEEE Trans. on Medical Imaging* 18:10 (1999) 866-874

[347] M.I. Miller, G.E. Christensen, Y. Amit, and U. Grenander, "Mathematical textbook of deformable neuroanatomies", *Proc. Natl. Acad. Sci. USA* 90 (Dec. 1993) 11944-11948

[348] J.V. Miller, D.E. Breen, W.E. Lorensen, R.M. O'Bara, and M.J. Wozny, "Geometrically deformed models: A method to extract closed geometric models from volume data", *Computer Graphics* 25:4 (1991) 217-226

[349] R. Möller, B. Neumann, and M. Wessel, "Towards Computer Vision with Description Logics: Some Recent Progress", *Proc. Integration of Speech and Image Understanding*, Sept. 21, 1999, Corfu, Greece, IEEE Computer Society, Los Alamitos 1999, 101-115

[350] F. Mokhtarian and R. Suomela, "Robust Image Corner Detection Through Curvature Scale Space", *IEEE Trans. on Pattern Anal. and Machine Intell.* 20:12 (1998) 1376-1381

[351] O. Monga and S. Benayoun, "Using partial derivatives of 3D images to extract surface features", *Computer Vision and Image Understanding* 61:2 (1995) 171-189

[352] O. Monga, S. Benayoun, and O.D. Faugeras, "From Partial Derivatives of 3D Density Images to Ridge Lines", *Proc. Conf. on Computer Vision and Pattern Recognition (CVPR'92)*, Urbana, Champaign, USA, June 1992, IEEE Computer Society Press 1992, 354-359

[353] O. Monga, R. Lengagne, and R. Deriche, "Extraction of the zero-crossings of the curvature derivatives in volumic 3D medical images: a multi-scale approach", *Proc. Conf. on Computer Vision and Pattern Recognition (CVPR'94)*, Seattle/Washington, USA, June 21-23, IEEE Computer Society Press 1994, 852-855

[354] H.P. Moravec, "Rover Visual Obstacle Avoidance", *Proc. Int. Joint Conf. on Artificial Intell. (IJCAI'81)*, Vancouver, BC, 1981, 785-790

[355] D.D. Morris and T. Kanade, "A Unified Factorization Algorithm for Points, Line Segments and Planes with Uncertainty Models", *Proc. Int. Conf. on Computer Vision (ICCV'98)*, Bombay, India, Jan. 4-7, 1998, Narosa Publishing House, New Delhi Madras 1998, 696-702

[356] M. Moshfeghi, "Elastic Matching of Multimodality Medical Images", *CVGIP: Graphical Models and Image Processing* 53:3 (1991) 271-282

[357] M. Moshfeghi, S. Ranganath, and K. Nawyn, "Three-Dimensional Elastic Matching of Volumes", *IEEE Trans. on Image Processing* 3:2 (1994) 128-138

[358] H. Müller and D. Ruprecht, "Spatial Interpolants for Warping", in *Brain Warping,*, A.W. Toga (Ed.), Academic Press San Diego 1999, 199-220

[359] J.C. de Munck, R. Bhagwandien, S.H. Muller, F.C. Verster, and M.B. van Herk, "The Computation of MR Image Distortions Caused by Tissue Susceptibility Using the Boundary Element Method", *IEEE Trans. on Medical Imaging* 15:5 (1996) 620-627

[360] H. Murase and S.K. Nayar, "Visual Learning and Recognition of 3-D Objects from Appearance" *Int. J. of Computer Vision* 14 (1995) 5-24

[361] D.E. Myers, "Kriging, cokriging, radial basis functions and the role of positive definiteness", *Computers Math. Applic.* 24:12 (1992) 139-148

[362] H.-H. Nagel, "Displacement Vectors Derived from Second-Order Intensity Variations in Image Sequences", *Computer Vision, Graphics, and Image Processing* 21 (1983) 85-117

[363] H.-H. Nagel, "Constraints for the Estimation of Displacement Vector Fields from Image Sequences", *Proc. Int. Joint Conf. on Artificial Intell. (IJCAI'83)*, Karlsruhe/Germany, 8-12 Aug. 1983, 945-951

[364] V.S. Nalwa and T.O. Binford, "On Detecting Edges", *IEEE Trans. on Pattern Anal. and Machine Intell.* 8:6 (1986) 699-714

[365] C. Nastar, B. Moghaddam, and A. Pentland, "Generalized Image Matching: Statistically Learning of Physically-Based Deformations", *Proc. European Conf. on Computer Vision (ECCV'96)*, Vol. I, Cambridge/UK, April 1996, *Lecture Notes in Computer Science* 1064, B. Buxton and R. Cipolla (Eds.), Springer Berlin Heidelberg 1996, 589-598

[366] S. Negahdaripour, "Revised definition of optical flow: integration of radiometric and geometric cues for dynamic scene analysis", *IEEE Trans. on Pattern Anal. and Machine Intell.* 20:9 (1998) 961-979

[367] B. Neumann, "Natural Language Description of Time-Varying Scenes", in *Semantic Structures, Advances in Natural Language Processing*, D.L. Waltz (Ed.), Lawrence Erlbaum, Hillsdale/NJ, 1989, 167-206

[368] B. Neumann, "Künstliche Intelligenz – Anwendungen und Grenzen", Techn. Report LKI-M-2/90, Labor für Künstliche Intelligenz, FB Informatik, Universität Hamburg, 1990

[369] B. Neumann, "Bildverstehen – ein Überblick", in *Einführung in die künstliche Intelligenz*, G. Görz (Ed.), Kapitel 6.1, Addison-Wesley Bonn Paris 1995, 559-582

[370] B. Neumann, "Knowledge-Based Computer Vision: The Issues", *Proc. Dagstuhl Seminar "Knowledge Based Computer Vision"*, Dagstuhl-Seminar-Report 196, 8.12.-12.12.1997 (9750), Schloß Dagstuhl, Wadern/Germany, H.I. Christensen, D. Hogg, and B. Neumann (Eds.), IBFI 1997, 4

[371] H. Neumann and H.S. Stiehl, "Towards a Testbed for Evaluation of Early Vision Processes", *Proc. Internat. Conf. on Computer Analysis of Images and Patterns (CAIP'87)*, Wismar, GDR, Sept. 2-4, 1987, L.P. Yaroslavskii, A. Rosenfeld, and W. Wilhelmi (Eds.), Akademie-Verlag Berlin 1987, 202-208

[372] H. Neumann and H.S. Stiehl, "Modelle der frühen visuellen Informationsverarbeitung", in *Einführung in die Künstliche Intelligenz*, G. Görz (Ed.), Kapitel 6.2, Addison-Wesley Bonn Paris 1995, 583-657

[373] H. Neumann, K. Ottenberg, and H.S. Stiehl, "Accuracy of Regularized Differential Operators for Discontinuity Localization in 1-D and 2-D Intensity Functions", *Proc. First IEEE Int. Workshop on Robust Computer Vision*, Seattle, WA/USA, Oct. 1-3, 1990, R.M. Haralick, W. Förstner (Eds.), 214-252

[374] W.M. Newman and R.F. Sproull, *Grundzüge der interaktiven Computergrafik*, McGraw-Hill Book Company Hamburg 1986

[375] G.M. Nielson "Scattered Data Modeling", *IEEE Computer Graphics & Appl.* (Jan. 1993) 61-70

[376] H. Niemann, "Wissensbasierte Bildanalyse", *Informatik-Spektrum* 8 (1985) 201-214

[377] H. Niemann, *Pattern Analysis and Understanding*, Springer-Verlag Berlin Heidelberg 1990

[378] K. Niemann, R. van den Boom, A. Theilig, G. Berks, G. Matthies, D. Noelchen, D. Graf von Keyserlingk, "Digitale stereotaktische Atlanten des menschlichen Gehirns: Erstellung, Verifikation und Anwendung", *Proc. Aachener Workshop 1996: Bildverarbeitung für die Medizin – Algorithmen, Systeme, Anwendungen –*, Aachen, Germany,

Nov. 8-9, 1996, T. Lehmann, I. Scholl, and K. Spitzer (Eds.), Verlag der Augustinus Buchhandlung, Aachen 1996, 215-221

[379] K. Niemann, R. van den Boom, K. Haeselbarth, and F. Afshar, "A brainstem stereotactic atlas in a three-dimensional magnetic resonance imaging navigation system: first experiences with atlas-to-patient registration", *J. Neurosurgery* 90 (May 1999) 891-901

[380] W.J. Niessen, B.M. ter Haar Romeny, and M.A. Viergever (Eds.), "Geodesic Deformable Models for Medical Image Analysis", *IEEE Trans. on Medical Imaging* 17:4 (1998) 634-641

[381] W.J. Niessen and M.A. Viergever (Eds.), "Guest Editorial", Special Issue on "Model-Based Analysis of Medical Images", *IEEE Trans. on Medical Imaging* 18:10 (1999) 825-827

[382] M. Nitzberg and T. Shiota, "Nonlinear image filtering with edge and corner enhancement", *IEEE Trans. on Pattern Anal. and Machine Intell.* 14:8 (1992) 826-833

[383] J.A. Noble, "Finding Corners", *Proc. Third Alvey Vision Conf.*, University of Cambridge, Cambridge/UK, 15.-17. Sept., 1987, 267-274; see also: *Image and Vision Computing* 6:2 (1988) 121-128

[384] C. Nölker and H. Ritter, "Detection of Fingertips in Human Hand Movement Sequences", in *Gesture and Sign Language in Human-Computer Interaction, Proc. of the International Gesture Workshop 1997*, Bielefeld, Germany, Sept. 17-19, 1997, I. Wachsmuth and M. Fröhlich (Eds.), Springer Verlag Berlin 1998, 209-218

[385] H.J. Noordmans, A.W.M. Smeulders, and M.A. Viergever, "Accurate Tracking of blood vessels and EEG electrodes by Consecutive Cross-Section Matching", *Medical Imaging 1999 – Image Processing (MI'99)*, Proc. SPIE Internat. Symposium, Vol. 3661, Part Two, Febr. 22-25, 1999, San Diego/CA, USA, K.M. Hanson (Ed.), 1637-1645

[386] W.L. Nowinski, A. Fang, B.T. Nguyen, J.K. Raphel, L. Jagannathan, R. Raghavan, R.N. Bryan, and G.A. Miller, "Multiple Brain Atlas Database and Atlas-Based Neuroimaging System", *Computer Aided Surgery* 2:1 (1997) 42-66

[387] M. Okutomi and T. Kanade, "A Locally Adaptive Window for Signal Matching", *Int. J. of Computer Vision* 7:2 (1992) 143-162

[388] C.M. Orange and F.C.A. Groen, "Model Based Corner Detection", *Proc. Conf. on Computer Vision and Pattern Recognition (CVPR'93)*, New York/NY, USA, June 15-17, IEEE Computer Society Press 1993, 690-691

[389] M. Oren, C. Papageorgiou, P. Sinha, E. Osuna, and T. Poggio, "Pedestrian Detection Using Wavelet Templates", *Proc. Conf. on Computer Vision and Pattern Recognition (CVPR'97)*, Puerto Rico, June 17-19, IEEE Computer Society Press 1997, 193-199

[390] F. O'Sullivan, "A Statistical Perspective on Ill-posed Inverse Problems", *Statistical Science* 1:4 (1996) 502-527

[391] D.W. Paglieroni, "A unified transform algorithm and architecture", *Machine Vision and Applications* 5:1 (1992) 47-55

[392] L. Parida, D. Geiger, and R. Hummel, "Junctions: Detection, Classification, and Reconstruction", *IEEE Trans. on Pattern Anal. and Machine Intell.* 20:7 (1998) 687-698

[393] W. Peckar, *Application of Variational Methods to Elastic Registration of Medical Images*, Doctoral dissertation, Fachbereich Informatik, Univ. Hamburg, published by Logos Verlag Berlin 1998

[394] W. Peckar, C. Schnörr, K. Rohr, and H.S. Stiehl, "Two-Step Parameter-Free Elastic Image Registration with Prescribed Point Displacements", *Proc. 9th Internat. Conf. on Image Analysis and Processing (ICIAP'97)*, 17-19 Sept. 1997, Florence/Italy, *Lecture Notes in Computer Science* 1310, A. Del Bimbo (Ed.), Vol. I, Springer-Verlag Berlin Heidelberg 1997, 527-534

[395] W. Peckar, C. Schnörr, K. Rohr, and H.S. Stiehl, "Non-Rigid Image Registration Using a Parameter-Free Elastic Model", *Proc. British Machine Vision Conference (BMVC'98)*, Southampton/UK, Sept. 14-17, 1998, J.N. Carter and M.S. Nixon (Eds.), British Machine Vision Association 1998, 134-143

[396] W. Peckar, C. Schnörr, K. Rohr, H.S. Stiehl, and U. Spetzger, "Linear and Incremental Estimation of Elastic Deformations in Medical Registration Using Prescribed Displacements", *Machine GRAPHICS & VISION* 7:4 (1998) 807-829

[397] W. Peckar, C. Schnörr, K. Rohr, and H.S. Stiehl, "Parameter-Free Elastic Deformation Approach for 2-D and 3-D Registration Using Prescribed Displacements", *J. of Mathematical Imaging and Vision* 10 (1999) 143-162

[398] X. Pennec and J.-P. Thirion, "A Framework for Uncertainty and Validation of 3-D Registration Methods Based on Points and Frames", *Int. J. of Computer Vision* 25:3 (1997) 203-229

[399] A.P. Pentland, "Perceptual Organization and the Representation of Natural Form", *Artificial Intelligence* 28 (1986) 293-331

[400] A.P. Pentland, "A New Sense for Depth of Field", *IEEE Trans. on Pattern Anal. and Machine Intell.* 9:4 (1987) 523-531

[401] A. Pentland and S. Sclaroff, "Closed-Form Solutions for Physically Based Shape Modeling and Recognition", *IEEE Trans. on Pattern Anal. and Machine Intell.* 13:7 (1991) 715-729

[402] B.T. Phong, "Illumination for Computer-Generated Pictures", *Commun. of the ACM* 18:6 (1975) 311-317

[403] T. Poggio and F. Girosi, "Networks for Approximation and Learning", *Proc. of the IEEE* 78:9 (1990) 1481-1497

[404] T. Poggio, V. Torre, and C. Koch, "Computational vision and regularization theory", *Nature* 317 (Sept. 1985) 314-319

[405] A.R. Pope and D.G. Lowe, "Modeling Positional Uncertainty in Object Recognition", Techn. Report 94-32, Dept. of Computer Science, Univ. of British Columbia, Vancouver/Canada, Nov. 1994

[406] M.J.D. Powell, "An efficient method for finding the minimum of a function of several variables without calculating derivatives", *Computer J.* 7 (1964) 155-162

[407] W.H. Press, B.P. Flannery, S.A. Teukolsky, and W.T. Vetterling, *Numerical Recipes*, Cambridge University Press, Cambridge/UK and New York/NY 1988

[408] T. Pun and E. Blake, "Relationships between Image Synthesis and Analysis: Towards Unification", *Computer Graphics Forum* 9:2 (1990) 149-163

[409] R.D. Rabbitt, J.A. Weiss, G.E. Christensen, and M.I. Miller, "Mapping of hyperelastic deformable templates using the finite element method", *Vision Geometry IV,* Proc. SPIE 2573, 1995, 252-265

[410] A. Rangarajan, H. Chui, and J.S. Duncan, "Rigid point feature registration using mutual information", *Medical Image Analysis* 3:4 (1999) 425-440

[411] K. Rangarajan, M. Shah, and D. Van Brackle, "Optimal Corner Detector", *Computer Vision, Graphics, and Image Processing* 48 (1989) 230-245

[412] A.R. Rao and R. Jain, "Knowledge Representation and Control in Computer Vision Systems", *IEEE Expert* 3 (Spring 1988) 64-79

[413] M.H.T. Reinges, H.-H. Nguyen, U. Spetzger, W. Küker, and J.M. Gilsbach, "Beurteilung des präoperativen Brain shift mit Hilfe des Neuronavigationssystems EasyGuide Neuro", *Proc. Workshop Bildverarbeitung für die Medizin 1998 – Algorithmen, Systeme, Anwendungen –*, Aachen, Germany, 26./27. März 1998, *Informatik aktuell*, T. Lehmann, V. Metzler, K. Spitzer, and T. Tolxdorff (Eds.), Springer-Verlag Berlin Heidelberg 1998, 124-128

[414] G. Reinsch, "Smoothing by spline functions", *Numerische Mathematik* 10 (1967) 177-183

[415] C. Rezk-Salama, P. Hastreiter, G. Greiner, and T. Ertl, "Non-linear Registration of Pre- and Intraoperative Volume Data Based On Piecewise Linear Transformations", *Proc. Erlangen Workshop'99 – Vision, Modeling, and Visualization*, Erlangen, Germany, Nov. 17-19, 1999

[416] J.H. Rieger, "Generic properties of edges and "corners" on smooth greyvalue surfaces", *Biol. Cybern.* 66 (1992) 497-502

[417] J.H. Rieger, "On the complexity and computation of view graphs of piecewise smooth algebraic surfaces", *Phil. Trans. R. Soc. Lond.* A 354 (1996) 1899-1940

[418] J.H. Rieger, "Hypersurfaces of extremal slope", Preprint, 1997

[419] J.H. Rieger and K. Rohr, "Report on visibility and detectability of "characteristic view" invariants", Techn. Report FBI-HH-M-232/93, FB Informatik, Universität Hamburg, Nov. 1993

[420] J.H. Rieger and K. Rohr, "Semi-algebraic solids in 3-space: a survey of modelling schemes and implications for view graphs", *Image and Vision Computing* 12:7 (1994) 395-410

[421] R.A. Robb, *Three-Dimensional Biomedical Imaging – Principles and Practice*, VCH Publishers, New York Weinheim 1995

[422] B. Robbins and R. Owens, "2D feature detection via local energy", *Image and Vision Computing* 15 (1997) 353-368

[423] R. Rohling, A. Gee, and L. Berman, "A comparison of freehand three-dimensional ultrasound reconstruction techniques", *Medical Image Analysis* 3:4 (1999) 339-359

[424] K. Rohr, *Untersuchung von grauwertabhängigen Transformationen zur Ermittlung des optischen Flusses in Bildfolgen,* Diplomarbeit, Institut für Nachrichtensysteme, Universität Karlsruhe, 1987

[425] K. Rohr, "Über die Modellierung und Identifikation charakteristischer Grauwertverläufe in Realweltbildern", *12. DAGM - Symposium Mustererkennung,* 24.-26. Sept. 1990, Oberkochen-Aalen, Germany, *Informatik-Fachberichte* 254, R.E. Großkopf (Hrsg.), Springer-Verlag Berlin Heidelberg, 217-224

[426] K. Rohr, "Modelling and Identification of Characteristic Intensity Variations", *Image and Vision Computing* 10:2 (March 1992) 66-76

[427] K. Rohr, "Recognizing Corners by Fitting Parametric Models", *Int. J. of Computer Vision* 9:3 (1992) 213-230

[428] K. Rohr, "Lokalisierungseigenschaften direkter Ansätze zur Ermittlung von Grauwertecken", *15. DAGM-Symposium Mustererkennung,* 27.-29. Sept. 1993, Lübeck, *Informatik aktuell,* S.J. Pöppl and H. Handels (Ed.), Springer-Verlag Berlin Heidelberg 1993, 647-654

[429] K. Rohr, "Towards Model-based Recognition of Human Movements in Image Sequences", *Computer Vision, Graphics, and Image Processing: Image Understanding* 59:1 (1994) 94-115

[430] K. Rohr, "Localization Properties of Direct Corner Detectors", *J. of Mathematical Imaging and Vision* 4:2 (1994) 139-150

[431] K. Rohr, *Modellgestütztes Erkennen charakteristischer Strukturen in Bildern,* Dissertation, Universität Hamburg, Fachbereich Informatik, Juli 1994

[432] K. Rohr, "A Survey on Elastic Registration in Medical Computer Vision", Techn. Report FBI-HH-M-245/95, FB Informatik, Universität Hamburg, Dec. 1994

[433] K. Rohr, "On the Precision in Estimating the Location of Edges and Corners", *J. of Mathematical Imaging and Vision* 7:1 (1997) 7-22

[434] K. Rohr, "On 3D Differential Operators for Detecting Point Landmarks", *Image and Vision Computing* 15:3 (1997) 219-233

[435] K. Rohr, "Human Movement Analysis Based on Explicit Motion Models", Chapter 8 in *Motion-Based Recognition,* M. Shah and R. Jain (Eds.), Computational Imaging and Vision Series, Vol. 9, Kluwer Academic Publishers, Dordrecht Boston London 1997, 171-198

[436] K. Rohr, "Image Registration Based on Thin-Plate Splines and Local Estimates of Anisotropic Landmark Localization Uncertainties", *Proc. First Internat. Conf. on Medical Image Computing and Computer-Assisted Intervention (MICCAI'98),* Massachusetts Institute of Technology (MIT), Cambridge/MA, USA, Oct. 11-13, 1998, *Lecture Notes*

in Computer Science 1496, W.M. Wells, A. Colchester, and S. Delp (Eds.), Springer Verlag Berlin Heidelberg 1998, 1174-1183

[437]   K. Rohr, "Extraction of 3D Anatomical Point Landmarks Based on Invariance Principles", *Pattern Recognition* 32 (1999) 3-15

[438]   K. Rohr, *Geometric and Intensity Models for 2D and 3D Image Analysis,* Habilitation Thesis, Universität Hamburg, Fachbereich Informatik, April 1999

[439]   K. Rohr, "Elastic Registration of Multimodal Medical Images: A Survey", *KI – Künstliche Intelligenz,* 2000, in press

[440]   K. Rohr and C. Schnörr, "An Efficient Approach to the Identification of Characteristic Intensity Variations", *Image and Vision Computing* 11:5 (June 1993) 273-277

[441]   K. Rohr and H.S. Stiehl, "On the Definition and Characterization of 3D Brain Landmarks", Techn. Report FBI-HH-M-268/96, FB Informatik, Universität Hamburg, Dec. 1996

[442]   K. Rohr and H.S. Stiehl, "Characterization and Localization of Anatomical Landmarks in Medical Images", *Proc. 1st Aachen Conf. on Neuropsychology in Neurosurgery, Psychiatry, and Neurology,* Dec. 12-14, 1997, Aachen/Germany, B.O. Hütter and J.M. Gilsbach (Eds.), Verlag der Augustinus Buchhandlung, Aachen 1997, 9-12

[443]   K. Rohr, H.S. Stiehl, R. Sprengel, W. Beil, T.M. Buzug, J. Weese, and M.H. Kuhn, "Point-Based Elastic Registration of Medical Image Data Using Approximating Thin-Plate Splines", *Proc. 4th Internat. Conf. Visualization in Biomedical Computing (VBC'96),* Hamburg, Germany, Sept. 22-25, 1996, *Lecture Notes in Computer Science* 1131, K.H. Höhne and R. Kikinis (Eds.), Springer Berlin Heidelberg 1996, 297-306

[444]   K. Rohr, H.S. Stiehl, R. Sprengel, W. Beil, T.M. Buzug, J. Weese, and M.H. Kuhn, "Nonrigid Registration of Medical Images Based on Anatomical Point Landmarks and Approximating Thin-Plate Splines", *Proc. Aachener Workshop 1996: Bildverarbeitung für die Medizin – Algorithmen, Systeme, Anwendungen –,* Aachen, Germany, Nov. 8-9, 1996, T. Lehmann, I. Scholl, and K. Spitzer (Eds.), Verlag der Augustinus Buchhandlung, Aachen 1996, 41-46

[445]   K. Rohr, H.S. Stiehl, R. Sprengel, W. Beil, T.M. Buzug, J. Weese, and M.H. Kuhn, "Landmark-Based Elastic Matching of Tomographic Images", *Proc. Freiburger Workshop 1997: Digitale Bildverarbeitung in der Medizin,* Freiburg, Germany, March 10-11, 1997, B. Arnolds, H. Müller, D. Saupe, and T. Tolxdorff (Eds.), Albert-Ludwigs-Universität Freiburg, 163-168

[446]   K. Rohr, R. Sprengel, and H.S. Stiehl, "Incorporation of Landmark Error Ellipsoids for Image Registration based on Approximating Thin-Plate Splines", *Proc. Computer Assisted Radiology and Surgery (CAR'97),* Berlin, Germany, June 25-28, 1997, H.U. Lemke, M.W. Vannier, and K. Inamura (Eds.), Elsevier Amsterdam Lausanne 1997, 234-239

[447]   K. Rohr, H.S. Stiehl, M. Fornefett, S. Frantz, and A. Hagemann, "Landmark-Based Elastic Registration of Human Brain Images", *Navigated Brain Surgery – Interdisciplinary Views of Neuronavigation from Neurosurgeons and Computer Scientists,* U. Spetzger, H.S. Stiehl, and J.M. Gilsbach (Eds.), Verlag Mainz, Aachen 1999, 137-148

[448] K. Rohr, M. Fornefett, and H.S. Stiehl, "Approximating Thin-Plate Splines for Elastic Registration: Integration of Landmark Errors and Orientation Attributes", *Proc. 16th Internat. Conf. on Information Processing in Medical Imaging (IPMI'99)*, Visegrád, Hungary, June 28 - July 2, 1999, In *Lecture Notes in Computer Science* 1613, A. Kuba, M. Šámal, and A. Todd-Pokropek (Eds.), Springer-Verlag Berlin Heidelberg 1999, 252-265

[449] K. Rohr, H.S. Stiehl, S. Frantz, and T. Hartkens, "Performance Characterization of Landmark Operators", in *Performance Characterization and Evaluation of Computer Vision Algorithms*, Proc. Dagstuhl Seminar, March 15-20, 1998, Schloß Dagstuhl, Wadern/Germany, R. Klette, H.S. Stiehl, M.A. Viergever, and K.L. Vincken (Eds.), Computational Imaging and Vision Series, Kluwer Academic Publishers, Dordrecht Boston London 2000, in press

[450] K. Rohr, H.S. Stiehl, M. Fornefett, S. Frantz, and A. Hagemann, "Project IMAGINE: Landmark-Based Elastic Registration and Biomechanical Brain Modelling", *KI – Künstliche Intelligenz*, 2000, in press

[451] P.E. Roland and K. Zilles, "Brain atlases: a new research tool", *Trends in Neuroscience* 17:11 (1994) 458-467

[452] J.M. Rosen, A. Lasko-Harvill, and R. Satava, "Virtual Reality and Surgery", in *Computer-Integrated Surgery*, R.H. Taylor, S. Lavallée, G.C. Burdea, and R. Mösges (Eds.), The MIT Press, Cambridge/Massachusetts, 1996, 231-243

[453] A. Rosenfeld, "Computer Vision: Basic Principles", *Proc. of the IEEE* 76:8 (1988) 863-868

[454] P.L. Rosin, "Measuring Corner Properties", *Computer Vision and Image Understanding* 73:2 (1999) 291-307

[455] D. Rueckert, G.I. Sanchez-Ortiz, and P. Burger, "Motion and Deformation Analysis of the Myocardium Using Density and Velocity Encoded MR Images", *Proc. Computer Assisted Radiology and Surgery (CAR'96)*, Paris, June 1996, H.U. Lemke, M.W. Vannier, K. Inamura, and A.G. Farman (Eds.), Elsevier Amsterdam Lausanne 1996, 125-130

[456] D. Rueckert, L.I. Sonoda, C. Hayes, D.L.G. Hill, M.O. Leach, and D.J. Hawkes, "Non-rigid Registration Using Free-Form Deformations: Application to Breast MR Images", *IEEE Trans. on Medical Imaging* 18:8 (1999) 712-721

[457] D. Ruprecht, R. Nagel, and H. Müller, "Spatial Free-From Deformation with Scattered Data Interpolation Methods", *Computers and Graphics* 19:1 (1995) 63-71

[458] T.W. Ryan, R.T. Gray, and B.R. Hunt, "Prediction of correlation errors in stereo-pair images", *Optical Engineering* 19:3 (1980) 312-322

[459] K.B. Sarachik and W.E.L. Grimson, "Gaussian Error Models for Object Recognition", *Proc. Conf. on Computer Vision and Pattern Recognition (CVPR'93)*, New York/NY, USA, June 15-17, IEEE Computer Society Press 1993, 400-406

[460] Y. Sato, S. Nakajima, N. Shiraga, H. Atsumi, S. Yoshida, T. Koller, G. Gerig and R. Kikinis, "Three-dimensional multi-scale line filter for segmentation and visualization of curvilinear structures in medical images", *Medical Image Analysis* 2:2 (1998) 143-168

[461] R.M. Satava and S.B. Jones, "Current and Future Applications of Virtual Reality for Medicine", *Proc. of the IEEE* 86:3 (1998) 484-489

[462] R. Schaback, "Creating Surfaces from Scattered Data Using Radial Basis Functions", *Mathematical Methods in CAGD III*, M. Daehlen, T. Lyche, and L.L. Schumaker (Eds.), 1995, 1-21

[463] G. Schaltenbrand and W. Wahren, *Atlas for Stereotaxy of the Human Brain*, Thieme-Verlag Stuttgart New York 1977

[464] L.L. Scharf, *Statistical Signal Processing: Detection, Estimation, and Time Series Analysis*, Addison-Wesley Reading/Massachusetts 1991

[465] T. Schiemann and K.H. Höhne, "Interaktive Deformation volumenbasierter Körpermodelle," *Proc. Workshop Bildverarbeitung für die Medizin 1998 – Algorithmen, Systeme, Anwendungen –*, Aachen, Germany, 26./27. März 1998, *Informatik aktuell*, T. Lehmann, V. Metzler, K. Spitzer, and T. Tolxdorff (Eds.), Springer-Verlag Berlin Heidelberg 1998, 437-441

[466] C. Schiers, U. Tiede, and K.H. Höhne, "Interactive 3D Registration of Image Volumes from Different Sources", in *Proc. Computer Assisted Radiology (CAR'89)*, H.U. Lemke, M.L. Rhodes, C.C. Jaffe, and R. Felix (Eds.), Springer-Verlag Berlin 1989, 666-670

[467] M. Schill, Ch. Reinhart, T. Günther, Ch. Poliwoda, J. Hesser, M. Schinkmann, H.-J. Bender, and R. Männer, "Simulation of Brain Tissue and Realtime Volume Visualisation", *Proc. Computer Assisted Radiology and Surgery (CAR'97)*, Berlin, Germany, June 25-28, 1997, H.U. Lemke, M.W. Vannier, and K. Inamura (Eds.), Elsevier Amsterdam Lausanne 1997, 283-288

[468] C. Schmid, R. Mohr, and C. Bauckhage, "Comparing and Evaluating Interest Points", *Proc. Int. Conf. on Computer Vision (ICCV'98)*, Bombay, India, Jan. 4-7, 1998, Narosa Publishing House, New Delhi Madras 1998, 230-235

[469] C. Schnörr, "Unique Reconstruction of Piecewise-Smooth Images by Minimizing Strictly Convex Nonquadratic Functionals", *J. of Mathematical Imaging and Vision* 4:2 (1994) 189-198

[470] C. Schnörr, *Variationsansätze zur Bildsegmentation und Merkmalsextraktion*, Habilitationsschrift, Fachbereich Informatik, Universität Hamburg, Okt. 1997

[471] C. Schnörr, "A Study of a Convex Variational Diffusion Approach for Image Segmentation and Feature Extraction", *J. of Mathematical Imaging and Vision* 8:3 (1998) 271-292

[472] I.J. Schoenberg, "Spline functions and the problem of graduation", *Proc. Nat. Acad. Sci. U.S.A.* 52 (1964) 947-950

[473] W. Schöne, *Differentialgeometrie*, Verlag Harri Deutsch, Thun und Frankfurt/Main 1975

[474] T. Schormann, S. Henn, and K. Zilles, "A New Approach to Fast Elastic Alignment with Applications to Human Brains", *Proc. 4th Internat. Conf. Visualization in Biomedical Computing (VBC'96)*, Hamburg, Germany, Sept. 22-25, 1996, *Lecture Notes in Computer Science* 1131, K.H. Höhne and R. Kikinis (Eds.), Springer Berlin Heidelberg 1996, 337-342

[475] W.F. Schreiber, *Fundamentals of Electronic Imaging Systems – Some Aspects of Image Processing*, Springer Berlin 1993

[476] C. Schröder, *Bildinterpretation durch Modellkonstruktion – Eine Theorie zur rechnergestützten Analyse von Bildern*, Dissertation, Universität Hamburg, Fachbereich Informatik, published by infix Sankt Augustin 1999

[477] S. Sclaroff and J. Isidoro, "Active Blobs", *Proc. Int. Conf. on Computer Vision (ICCV'98)*, Bombay, India, Jan. 4-7, 1998, Narosa Publishing House, New Delhi Madras 1998, 1146-1153

[478] K. Sethi and R. Jain, "Finding trajectories of feature points in a monocular image sequence", *IEEE Trans. on Pattern Anal. and Machine Intell.* 9:1 (1987) 56-73

[479] S.A. Shafer, L.B. Wolff, and G.E. Healey, *Physics-Based Vision: Principles and Practice*, 3 Vols., Jones and Bartlett, Cambridge/MA, 1992

[480] M. Shah and R. Jain (Eds.), *Motion-Based Recognition*, Computational Imaging and Vision Series, Vol. 9, Kluwer Academic Publishers, Dordrecht Boston London 1997

[481] R. Shahidi, R. Tombropoulos, and R.P. Grzeszczuk, "Clinical Applications of Three-Dimensional Rendering of Medical Data Sets", *Proc. of the IEEE* 86:3 (1998) 555-568

[482] S.C. Shapiro (Ed.), *Encyclopedia of Artificial Intelligence*, Vol. 1 and 2, John Wiley & Sons New York Chichester 1990

[483] J. Shi and C. Tomasi, "Good Features to Track", *Proc. Conf. on Computer Vision and Pattern Recognition (CVPR'94)*, Seattle/Washington, USA, June 21-23, IEEE Computer Society Press 1994, 593-600

[484] Y. Shirai, *Three-Dimensional Computer Vision*, Springer-Verlag Berlin Heidelberg 1987

[485] R. Sim and G. Dudek, "Learning and Evaluating Visual Features for Pose Estimation", *Proc. Int. Conf. on Computer Vision (ICCV'99)*, Kerkyra, Greece, Sept. 20-27, 1999, Vol. II, IEEE Computer Society Press, Los Alamitos/CA 1999, 1217-1222

[486] E.P. Simoncelli and H. Farid, "Steerable wedge filters for local orientation analysis", *IEEE Trans. of Image Processing* 5:9 (1996) 1377-1382

[487] A. Singh, D. Goldgof, and D. Terzopoulos (Eds.), *Deformable Models in Medical Image Analysis*, IEEE Computer Society Press 1998

[488] O. Škrinjar, D. Spencer, and J. Duncan, "Brain Shift Modeling for Use in Neurosurgery", *Proc. First Internat. Conf. on Medical Image Computing and Computer-Assisted Intervention (MICCAI'98)*, Massachusetts Institute of Technology (MIT), Cambridge/MA, USA, Oct. 11-13, 1998, *Lecture Notes in Computer Science* 1496, W.M. Wells, A. Colchester, and S. Delp (Eds.), Springer Verlag Berlin Heidelberg 1998, 641-649

[489] R. Smith, M. Self, and P. Cheeseman, "Estimating Uncertain Spatial Relationships in Robotics", *Uncertainty in Artificial Intelligence 2*, J.F. Lemmer and L.N. Kanal (Eds.), Elsevier Science Publishers B.V. (North Holland), Amsterdam New York 1988, 435-461

[490] S.M. Smith and J.M. Brady, "SUSAN - A New Approach to Low Level Image Processing", *Int. J. of Computer Vision* 23:1 (1997) 45-78

[491] J. Sobotta, *Atlas der Anatomie des Menschen, 1. Band: Kopf, Hals, Obere Extrem-intäten*, H. Ferner and J. Staubesand (Eds.), Urban und Schwarzenberg, München Wien Baltimore 1988

[492] O. Soligon, A. Le Méhauté, and C. Roux, "Facial expressions simulation with Radial Basis Functions", *Proc. Int. Workshop on Synthetic–Natural Hybrid Coding and Three Dimensional Imaging (IWSNHC3DI'97)*, Sept. 1997, Rhodes/Greece, 233-236

[493] F. Solina and R. Bajcsy, "Recovery of Parametric Models from Range Images: The Case for Superquadrics with Global Deformations", *IEEE Trans. on Pattern Anal. and Machine Intell.* 12:2 (1990) 131-147

[494] H.W. Sorenson, *Parameter Estimation*, Marcel Dekker New York Basel 1980

[495] J. Sporring, M. Nielsen, J. Weickert, and O.F. Olsen, "A Note on Differential Corner Measures", *Proc. Int. Conf. on Pattern Recognition (ICPR'98)*, Brisbane, Australia, Aug. 16-20, 1998, A.K. Jain, S. Venkatesh, and B.C. Lovell (Eds.) IEEE Computer Society Press, Los Alamitos, California, 1998, 652-655

[496] R. Sprengel, K. Rohr, and H.S. Stiehl, "Thin-Plate Spline Approximation for Image Registration" *18th Internat. Conf. IEEE Engineering in Medicine and Biology Society (EMBS'96)*, Oct. 31 - Nov. 3, 1996, Amsterdam, The Netherlands, CD-ROM Proceedings, Track Index 4.7.1 Image Registration

[497] R. Sprengel, K. Rohr, and H.S. Stiehl, "Properties and Extensions of the Thin-Plate Spline Approach for Image Registration", Techn. Report FBI-HH-M-267/96, FB Informatik, Universität Hamburg, Dec. 1996

[498] L.H. Staib and J.S. Duncan, "Boundary finding with parametrically deformable models", *IEEE Trans. on Pattern Anal. and Machine Intell.* 14:11 (1992) 1061-1075

[499] T. Stammberger, M. Michaelis, M. Reiser, and K.H. Englmeier, "A hierarchical filter scheme for efficient corner detection", *Pattern Recognition Letters* 19:8 (1998) 687-700

[500] C. Steger, "An Unbiased Detector of Curvilinear Structures", *IEEE Trans. on Pattern Anal. and Machine Intell.* 20:2 (1998) 113-125

[501] H.S. Stiehl, *On Spatial Image Sequence Understanding*, Habilitation Monograph, Fachbereich Informatik, TU Berlin/FRG, 1987

[502] H.S. Stiehl, "Issues of Spatial Representation in Computational Vision", in *Repräsentation und Verarbeitung räumlichen Wissens*, C. Freksa and C. Habel (Eds.), Springer-Verlag Berlin Heidelberg 1990, 83-98

[503] K.C. Strasters, A. Little, J. Buurman, D.L.G. Hill, and D.J. Hawkes, "Anatomical Landmark Image Registration: Validation and Comparison", *Proc. First Joint Conf. CVRMed-MRCAS'97*, Grenoble/France, March 1997, *Lecture Notes in Computer Science* 1205, J. Troccaz, E. Grimson, and R. Mösges (Eds.), Springer Verlag Berlin Heidelberg 1997, 161-170

[504] M.R. Stytz, G. Frieder, and O. Frieder, "Three-Dimensional Medical Imaging: Algorithms and Computer Systems", *ACM Computing Surveys* 23:4 (1991) 421-499

[505] G. Subsol, J.-P. Thirion, and N. Ayache, "A scheme for automatically building three-dimensional morphometric anatomical atlases: application to a skull atlas", *Medical Image Analysis* 2:1 (1998) 37-60

[506] P. Suetens, P. Fua, and A.J. Hanson, "Computational Strategies for Object Recognition", *ACM Computing Surveys* 24:1 (1992) 5-61

[507] T.S. Sumanaweera, G.H. Glover, T.O. Binford, and J.R. Adler, "MR Susceptibility Misregistration Correction", *IEEE Trans. on Medical Imaging* 12:2 (1993) 251-259

[508] G. Székely, A. Kelemen, C. Brechbühler, and G. Gerig, "Segmentation of 2-D and 3-D objects from MRI volume data using constrained elastic deformations of flexible Fourier contour and surface models", *Medical Image Analysis* 1:1 (1996/7) 19-34

[509] G. Székely and J. Duncan (Eds.), *Int. Workshop on Soft Tissue Deformation and Tissue Palpation*, Cambridge/MA, USA, Oct. 10, 1998, in conjunction with MICCAI'98, Workshop notes

[510] R. Szeliski, *Bayesian Modeling of Uncertainty in Low-level Vision*, Kluwer Academic Publishers Boston Dordrecht 1989

[511] R. Szeliski, "Regularization in Neural Nets", in *Mathematical Perspectives on Neural Networks*, P. Smolensky, M.C. Mozer, and D.E. Rumelhart (Eds.), Lawrence Erlbaum Assoc., Mahurah/New Jersey 1996, 497-532

[512] R. Szeliski and J. Coughlan, "Spline-Based Image Registration", *Int. J. of Computer Vision* 22:3 (1997) 199-218

[513] R. Szeliski and S. Lavallée, "Matching 3-D anatomical surfaces with non-rigid deformations using octree-splines", *Proc. SPIE* 2031, 1993, 306-315

[514] J. Talairach and P. Tornoux, *Co-planar Stereotactic Atlas of the Human Brain*, Georg Thieme Verlag Stuttgart New York 1988

[515] C.-K. Tang and G. Medioni, "Inference of integrated surface, curve, and junction descriptions from sparse 3D data", *IEEE Trans. on Pattern Anal. and Machine Intell.* 20:11 (1998) 1206-1223

[516] R.H. Taylor, S. Lavallée, G.C. Burdea, and R. Mösges (Eds.), *Computer-Integrated Surgery – Technology and Clinical Applications*, The MIT Press, Cambridge/Massachusetts 1996

[517] D. Terzopoulos, "Regularization of Inverse Visual Problems Involving Discontinuities", *IEEE Trans. on Pattern Anal. and Machine Intell.* 8:4 (1986) 413-424

[518] D. Terzopoulos, A. Witkin, and M. Kass, "Constraints on deformable models: recovering 3D shape and nonrigid motion", *Artificial Intelligence* 36:1 (1988) 91-123

[519] D. Terzopoulos and D. Metaxas, "Dynamic 3D models with local and global deformations: Deformable Superquadrics", *IEEE Trans. on Pattern Anal. and Machine Intell.* 13:7 (1991) 703-714

[520] J.-P. Thirion, "Extremal Points: definition and application to 3D image registration", *Proc. Conf. on Computer Vision and Pattern Recognition (CVPR'94)*, Seattle/Washington, USA, June 21-23, IEEE Computer Society Press 1994, 587-592

[521] J.-P. Thirion, "New Feature Points based on Geometric Invariants for 3D Image Registration", *Int. J. of Computer Vision* 18:2 (1996) 121-137

[522] J.-P. Thirion, "Image matching as a diffusion process: an analogy with Maxwell's demons", *Medical Image Analysis* 2:3 (1998) 243-260

[523] J.-P. Thirion, and A. Gourdon, "Computing the differential characteristics of isointensity surfaces", *Computer Vision and Image Understanding* 61:2 (1995) 190-202

[524] P. Thompson and A.W. Toga, "A Surface-Based Technique for Warping Three-Dimensional Images of the Brain", *IEEE Trans. on Medical Imaging* 15:4 (1996) 402-417

[525] J.D. Thurgood and E.M. Mikhail, "Photogrammetric analysis of images", *Proc. ISPRS Commision III*, Helsinki, 1982, 576-590

[526] S. Tieck, S. Gerloff, and H.S. Stiehl, "Interactive Graph-Based Editing of Watershed-Segmented 2D-Images", *Proc. 1st Workshop on Interactive Segmentation of Medical Images (ISMI'98)*, Amsterdam/Netherlands, Sept. 1998

[527] A.N. Tikhonov and V.Y. Arsenin, *Solutions of Ill-Posed Problems*, Winston, Washington/D.C., 1977

[528] K.D. Toennies, "Bildverarbeitung und Computer-Graphik in der Radiologie", Teil A und B, Techn. Report 93/26, TU Berlin, 1993

[529] A.W. Toga (Ed.), *Brain Warping*, Academic Press San Diego 1999

[530] K.E. Torrance and E.M. Sparrow, "Theory for Off-Specular Reflection from Roughened Surfaces", *J. of the Optical Society of America* 57 (1967) 1105-1114

[531] V. Torre and T.A. Poggio, "On Edge Detection", *IEEE Trans. on Pattern Anal. and Machine Intell.* 8:2 (1986) 147-163

[532] D. Tost and X. Pueyo, "Human body animation: a survey", *The Visual Computer* 3 (1988) 254-264

[533] H.L. van Trees, *Detection, Estimation, and Modulation Theory,* Part I, John Wiley and Sons, New York London 1968

[534] J.K. Tsotsos, "Image Understanding", in *Encyclopedia of Artificial Intelligence,* Vol. 1, S.C. Shapiro (Ed.), John Wiley & Sons New York Chichester 1990, 389-409

[535] F. Ulupinar and G. Medioni, "Refining Edges Detected by a LoG Operator", *Computer Vision, Graphics, and Image Processing* 51 (1990) 275-298

[536] B.C. Vemuri and A. Radisavljevic, "Multiresolution Stochastic Hybrid Shape Models with Fractal Priors", *ACM Trans. on Graphics* 13:2 (1994) 177-207

[537] B.C. Vemuri, S. Huang, S. Sahni, C.M. Leonard, C. Mohr, R. Gilmore, and J. Fitzsimmons, "An efficient motion estimator with application to medical image registration", *Medical Image Analysis* 2:1 (1998) 79-98

[538] R. Verbeeck, "Literature overview of model based MR segmentation methods", Internal Report, ESAT-Radiologie, Univ. Hospital Gasthuisberg, Kath. Univ. Leuven, Belgium, July 1994

[539] M.A. Viergever, J.B.A. Maintz, R. Stokking, P.A. van den Elsen, and K.J. Zuiderveld, "Matching and integrated display of brain images from multiple modalities", *Medical Imaging 1995: Image Processing*, Febr./March 1995, San Diego/CA, USA, Proc. SPIE 2434, M.H. Loew (Ed.), 2-13

[540] M.A. Viergever (Ed.), Special Issue on "Image Guidance of Therapy", *IEEE Trans. on Medical Imaging* 17:5 (1998) 669-856

[541] P. Viola and W.M. Wells III, "Alignment by Maximization of Mutual Information", *Int. J. of Computer Vision* 24:2 (1997) 137-154

[542] S.A. Völter, "Virtuelle Realität in der Medizin I", GeSI, Mannheim 1995

[543] L. Voo, S. Kumaresan, F.A. Pintar, N. Yoganandan, and A. Sances, "Finite-element models of the human head", *Medical & Biological Engineering & Computing* 34:5 (1996) 375-381

[544] K. Voss, *Theoretische Grundlagen der digitalen Bildverarbeitung*, Akademie Verlag Berlin 1988

[545] G. Wahba, *Spline Models for Observational Data*, Society for Industrial and Applied Mathematics, Philadelphia, Pennsylvania, 1990

[546] G. Wahba, "Multivariate Function and Operator Estimation, Based on Smoothing Splines and Reproducing Kernels", in *Nonlinear Modeling and Forecasting, SFI Studies in the Sciences of Complexity*, Vol. XII, M. Casdagli and S. Eubank (Eds.), Addison-Wesley 1992, 95-112

[547] G. Wahba and J. Wendelberger, "Some New Mathematical Methods for Variational Objective Analysis Using Splines and Cross Validation", *Monthly Weather Review* 108 (1980) 1122-1143

[548] D. Waltz, "Understanding Line Drawings of Scenes with Shadows", in *The Psychology of Computer Vision*, P.H. Winston (Ed.), McGraw-Hill New York 1975, 19-91

[549] G. Wang, M.W. Vannier, M.W. Skinner, M.G.P. Cavalcanti, and G.W. Harding, "Spiral CT Image Deblurring for Cochlear Implantation", *IEEE Trans. on Medical Imaging* 17:2 (1998) 251-262

[550] S.J. Wang and T.O. Binford, "Local step edge estimation: A new algorithm, statistical model and performance evaluation", *Proc. Image Understanding Workshop (IUW'93)*, Washington/DC, April 18-21, 1993, Morgan Kaufmann, San Mateo/CA, 1993, 1063-1070

[551] Y. Wang, "Smoothing Spline Models With Correlated Random Errors", *J. of the American Statistical Association* 93:441 (1998) 341-348

[552] Y. Wang, W. Guo, and M.B. Brown, "Spline Smoothing For Bivariate Data With Applications To Association Between Hormones", 1997, submitted for publication

[553] S. Warfield, M. Kaus, F.A. Jolesz, and R. Kikinis, "Adaptive Template Moderated Spatially Varying Statistical Classification", *Proc. First Internat. Conf. on Medical Image Computing and Computer-Assisted Intervention (MICCAI'98)*, Massachusetts Institute of Technology (MIT), Cambridge/MA, USA, Oct. 11-13, 1998, *Lecture Notes*

in Computer Science 1496, W.M. Wells, A. Colchester, and S. Delp (Eds.), Springer Verlag Berlin Heidelberg 1998, 431-438

[554] S. Warfield, A. Robatino, J. Dengler, F.A. Jolesz, and R. Kikinis, "Nonlinear Registration and Template Driven Segmentation", in *Brain Warping*, A.W. Toga (Ed.), Academic Press San Diego 1999, 67-84

[555] J. Weickert, "Multiscale Texture Enhancement", *Proc. Internat. Conf. on Computer Analysis of Images and Patterns (CAIP'95)*, Prague, Szech Republic, Sept. 6-8, 1995, V. Hlaváč and R. Šára (Eds.), Springer Berlin Heidelberg 1995, 230-237

[556] J. Weickert, *Anisotropic Diffusion in Image Processing*, Teubner Stuttgart 1998

[557] H. Wendland, "Piecewise polynomial, positive definite and compactly supported radial functions of minimal degree", *Advances in Computational Mathematics* 4 (1995) 389-396

[558] J. West, J.M. Fitzpatrick, et al. "Comparison and Evaluation of Retrospective Inter-modality Brain Image Registration Techniques", *J. of Computer Assisted Tomography* 21:4 (1997) 554-566

[559] C.-F. Westin, A. Bhalerao, H. Knutsson, and R. Kikinis, "Using Local 3D Structure for Segmentation of Bone from Computer Tomography Images", *Proc. Conf. on Computer Vision and Pattern Recognition (CVPR'97)*, Puerto Rico, June 17-19, IEEE Computer Society Press 1997, 794-800

[560] B. Widrow, "The "Rubber-Mask" Technique – I. Pattern Measurement and Analysis", *Pattern Recognition* 5 (1973) 175-197

[561] R. Wiemker, K. Rohr, L. Binder, R. Sprengel, and H.S. Stiehl, "Application of Elastic Registration to Imagery from Airborne Scanners" *Proc. ISPRS Congress*, Vienna, July 1996, *Internat. Archives of Photogrammetry and Remote Sensing*, Vol. XXXI, Part B4, 949-954

[562] R. Wilhelm, *Informatik – Grundlagen, Anwendungen, Perspektiven*, Verlag C.H. Beck 1996

[563] J. Wilhelms, "Toward Automatic Motion Control", *IEEE Computer Graphics & Appl.* 7:4 (April 1987) 11-22

[564] P.H. Winston, *Artificial Intelligence*, Third Edition, Addison-Wesley 1992

[565] L. Wiskott, J.-M. Fellous, N. Krüger, and C. v.d. Malsburg, "Face Recognition by Elastic Bunch Graph Matching", *IEEE Trans. on Pattern Anal. and Machine Intell.* 19:7 (1997) 775-779

[566] A. Witkin, "Scale-Space Filtering", *Proc. Int. Joint Conf. on Artificial Intell. (IJCAI'83)*, Karlsruhe/Germany, 8-12 Aug. 1983, Vol. 2, 1019-1022

[567] A. Witkin, M. Kass, D. Terzopoulos, and K. Fleischer, "Physically Based Modeling for Vision and Graphics", *Proc. Image Understanding Workshop*, Cambridge/MA, April 6-8, 1988, Morgan Kaufmann, San Mateo, 1988, 254-278

[568] G. Wolberg, *Digital Image Warping*, IEEE Computer Society Press Washington 1990

[569] G. Wolberg, "Image morphing: a survey", *The Visual Computer* 14 (1998) 360-372

[570] C. Wren, A. Azarbayejani, T. Darrell, and A. Pentland, "Pfinder: Real-time tracking of the human body", *IEEE Trans. on Pattern Anal. and Machine Intell.* 19:7 (1997) 780-785

[571] J.V. Wyngaerd, L. Van Gool, R. Koch, and M. Proesmans, "Invariant-based registration of surface patches", *Proc. Int. Conf. on Computer Vision (ICCV'99)*, Kerkyra, Greece, Sept. 20-27, 1999, Vol. I, IEEE Computer Society Press, Los Alamitos/CA 1999, 301-306

[572] M.M. Yeung, B.-L. Yeo, S.-P. Liou, and A. Banihashemi, "Three-Dimensional Image Registration for Spiral CT Angiography", *Proc. Conf. on Computer Vision and Pattern Recognition (CVPR'94)*, Seattle/Washington, USA, June 21-23, IEEE Computer Society Press 1994, 423-429

[573] A. Yezzi, S. Kichenassamy, A. Kumar, P. Olver, and A. Tannenbaum, "A Geometric Snake Model for Segmentation of Medical Imagery", *IEEE Trans. on Medical Imaging* 16:2 (1997) 199-209

[574] W.C. Yu, K. Daniilidis, and G. Sommer, "Rotated Wedge Averaging Method for Junction Classification", *Proc. Conf. on Computer Vision and Pattern Recognition (CVPR'98)*, Santa Barbara, CA, June 23-25, 1998, IEEE Computer Society Press 1998, 390-395

[575] A.L. Yuille, P.W. Hallinan, and D.S. Cohen, "Feature extraction from faces using deformable templates", *Int. J. of Computer Vision* 8:2 (1992) 99-111

[576] D. Zeltzer, "Motor Control Techniques for Figure Animation", *IEEE Computer Graphics & Appl.* 2:9 (Nov. 1982) 53-59

[577] W. Zhang and F. Bergholm, "An extension of Marr's "signature" based edge classification", *7th Scandinavian Conf. on Image Analysis*, Aug. 13-16, Aalborg/Denmark, 1991

[578] W. Zhang and F. Bergholm, "Multi-Scale Blur Estimation and Edge Type Classification for Scene Analysis", *Int. J. of Computer Vision* 24:3 (1997) 219-250

[579] G. Zhou, E. Uzi, W. Feng, and B. Yuan, "CCD Camera Calibration Based on Natural Landmarks", *Pattern Recognition* 31:11 (1998) 1715-1724

[580] B. Zitova and J. Flusser, "Landmark recognition using invariant features", *Pattern Recognition Letters* 20:5 (1999) 541-547

[581] O.A. Zuniga and R.M. Haralick, "Corner detection using the facet model", *Proc. IEEE Conf. on Computer Vision and Pattern Recognition (CVPR'83)*, Washington/D.C., June 19-23, 1983, 30-37

Index

2D corner operator, 60, 74, 112
2D landmark, 43
3D corner operator, 63, 74
3D landmark, 36, 45, 99

active contours, 20
active vision, 2, 9
aerial image, 97, 104, 138, 143
affine transformation, 171, 184, 193, 208
analytic model, 20, 88, 93, 112
anatomical landmark, 36, 42, 47
anisotropic errors, 216
appearance-based approach, 19
approximating thin-plate splines, 205, 216
artificial intelligence (AI), 4

bending energy, 192, 197, 198, 207
bias, 22, 101, 112, 143
biharmonic equation, 199, 201
biomechanical model, 33, 190, 248, 254
blob, 98, 136, 149
boundary condition, 196, 199, 200
box landmark, 148
brain shift, 189, 248

central limit theorem, 91
circular landmark, 97, 136, 143
computational theory, 10
computer graphics, 13, 34
computer vision, 1, 13
conceptual descriptions, 6, 8
conditionally positive definite, 196
contour model, 12, 19, 48
corner, 93, 95, 113, 129, 146
corner model, 89, 93, 100, 113, 129
corner operator, 89
Cramér-Rao bound (CRB), 80, 81, 119, 128, 227
CT image, 93, 180, 236
curvature, 54

curvature extremum, 49, 50, 113

data term, 24, 207
deformable models, 11, 19, 180
detection, 35
detection performance measure, 152, 157
detection region, 154
differential corner operator, 51, 58
differential geometry, 19, 47
differential model, 19
differential operator, 52, 58, 113, 151
digital atlas, 180, 181, 190, 239
Dirac delta function, 195, 200
discrete template, 20, 88

edge, 89, 95, 120, 144
edge attributes, 102
elastic body splines (EBS), 203, 253
elastic registration, 257
elastic transformation, 16, 168, 180, 185
error ellipse, 135, 227, 229
error ellipsoid, 80, 228, 230, 232
Euclidean distance, 22, 200, 206
Euclidean space, 23
evaluation, 13, 14, 109, 110, 177
explicit knowledge, 5, 7, 9
exterior orientation, 105

feature-based approach, 26
finite differences, 20, 24, 204, 253
finite element method (FEM), 20, 24, 204, 248, 253
Fisher information matrix, 80, 128, 144
fluid model, 180, 185, 249
functional, 23, 181, 192, 206, 217, 242
fundamental solution, 200

Gaussian curvature, 53, 54, 199
Gaussian noise, 91, 93, 118
generic method, 2

301

generic model, 6, 8, 21
geographic information system (GIS), 33
geometric model, 15, 16
geometric transformation, 16, 179
Green's function, 195, 200
ground truth, 13, 14, 111, 158, 173

Hessian matrix, 49, 50
high-level vision, 6
Hilbert space, 23, 191
homologous points, 235, 241
human-computer interaction, 3, 16
hypothesize-and-test, 8, 105

ill-posed, 24, 207
image, 1
image analysis, 2, 4, 13
image blur, 91, 101, 113
image correspondences, 14, 28, 36, 179,
    191
image features, 9, 20, 26
image formation, 11, 14, 18, 90
image fusion, 179, 238
image matching, 179
image noise, 91, 93, 118
image processing, 2, 4
image registration, 12, 16, 36, 171, 179,
    180, 183
image synthesis, 13
image warping, 34
image-atlas registration, 181, 190, 239
implicit function theorem, 53
implicit knowledge, 5
intensity model, 18, 47, 87, 93, 112
intensity-based approach, 26
intensity-based registration, 187, 253
interpolating thin-plate splines, 191
intraoperative image correction, 190, 248,
    254
intraoperative navigation, 189, 248
invariants, 53, 81, 173
isocontour, 50, 52, 53, 63
isointensity surface, 50, 54
isometric transformation, 53
isotropic errors, 205

junction, 95

Kalman filter, 22
knowledge-based approach, 8, 12

knowledge-based process, 4
kriging, 197, 252

L-corner, 84, 93, 113, 116, 129
landmark, 26, 35, 93, 184, 217, 220, 229
landmark-based image analysis, 26
landmark-based registration, 186, 191
Laplacian operator, 49, 64, 195, 199
large deformations, 249, 254
least-squares method, 22, 85, 101, 139
levels of representation, 6, 9
line, 126, 146
local transformation, 185
localization, 35
localization accuracy, 112, 169
localization precision, 80, 117, 139, 226
localization uncertainty, 80, 117, 139, 226
low-level vision, 6

maximum-likelihood estimation, 22, 101,
    118, 140
mean curvature, 53, 54, 199
medical diagnosis, 188, 237
membrane splines, 202
minimal error, 80, 119, 128, 227
minimal uncertainty, 80, 119, 128, 227
minimal-invasive surgery, 189
model deviation, 101
model fitting, 88, 100, 139
model-based approach, 8, 12, 180
model-based registration, 180
modelling of movements, 15
motion analysis, 15, 179, 254
MR image, 93, 180, 236
multi-step approach, 84, 169
multimodality images, 12, 43, 179
multiquadric splines, 197
mutual information, 187, 254

Navier equation, 187, 201, 205, 249
neural network, 34, 188
nonhomogeneous material, 248, 254
nonlinear diffusion, 173
nonlinear optimization, 22, 101
nonparametric model, 23, 181
nonrigid transformation, 184
nullspace, 193, 196, 200

operator response, 55, 151, 156
optic flow estimation, 254

optimal ROI size, 86
orientation tensor, 61, 230
orientations at landmarks, 241
orthoview images, 38

parametric model, 21, 87, 93, 139
performance characterization, 5, 14, 109, 257
photogrammetry, 29, 97, 104, 138, 143
photometric model, 18, 90
physically-based, 181, 205, 248
physically-motivated, 20, 181, 188, 205
physics-based vision, 11
piecewise transformation, 185
pix, 106, 141, 143
pixel, 1
point landmark, 26, 35, 36, 42, 47, 187, 217, 220, 229
point-based registration, 186, 191
positive definite, 79, 247
positive semidefinite, 128, 231
principal curvature directions, 47
principal curvatures, 47, 53, 54, 199
principal invariants, 81
projective invariants, 173
projective transformation, 17, 18, 173, 186
propositional descriptions, 6

quasi-landmark, 217, 220, 229, 233

radial basis functions (RBF), 194, 197, 250
radiometric model, 14, 18, 90
rectangular landmark, 98, 135
region-of-interest (ROI), 41, 86, 154
registration, 179
regularization, 24, 207, 208
regularization parameter, 24, 208, 213
remote sensing, 29, 97, 104, 138, 143
ridge, 51, 52, 145
rigid transformation, 53, 184

saddle point, 45, 48, 52, 54

scale space, 85, 86, 101, 116, 164
scattered data interpolation, 15, 24, 191, 197, 250
segmentation, 11, 16, 19, 181, 187, 241
semi-automatic localization, 40
semi-global approach, 87
signal-to-noise ratio (SNR), 140, 141, 143
similarity measure, 9, 22, 186
similarity transformation, 82, 192
splines with compact support, 247, 253
splines with tension, 253
statistical performance measure, 152
structure tensor, 61, 230
subpixel localization, 88
subvoxel localization, 84, 170
surface interpolation, 24, 191, 197, 206, 250
surface splines, 191
surgery planning, 189
surgery simulation, 248, 255

T-corner, 92, 100, 133
Talairach reference system, 217, 238, 256
template matching, 20, 140
template model, 20, 88
thin-plate smoothing splines, 209
thin-plate splines (TPS), 24, 182, 188, 191, 205, 216
tip, 45, 52, 54
tomographic image, 93, 180

unbiased, 22, 101, 119, 128, 143, 188, 198
uncertainty ellipse, 135, 229
uncertainty ellipsoid, 230

validation, 13, 14, 109, 110, 177
virtual reality (VR), 16, 33
vox, 171
voxel, 1

weight matrices, 216, 224, 226
well-posed, 188

Computational Imaging and Vision

1. B.M. ter Haar Romeny (ed.): *Geometry-Driven Diffusion in Computer Vision.* 1994
   ISBN 0-7923-3087-0
2. J. Serra and P. Soille (eds.): *Mathematical Morphology and Its Applications to Image Processing.* 1994
   ISBN 0-7923-3093-5
3. Y. Bizais, C. Barillot, and R. Di Paola (eds.): *Information Processing in Medical Imaging.* 1995
   ISBN 0-7923-3593-7
4. P. Grangeat and J.-L. Amans (eds.): *Three-Dimensional Image Reconstruction in Radiology and Nuclear Medicine.* 1996
   ISBN 0-7923-4129-5
5. P. Maragos, R.W. Schafer and M.A. Butt (eds.): *Mathematical Morphology and Its Applications to Image and Signal Processing.* 1996
   ISBN 0-7923-9733-9
6. G. Xu and Z. Zhang: *Epipolar Geometry in Stereo, Motion and Object Recognition. A Unified Approach.* 1996
   ISBN 0-7923-4199-6
7. D. Eberly: *Ridges in Image and Data Analysis.* 1996
   ISBN 0-7923-4268-2
8. J. Sporring, M. Nielsen, L. Florack and P. Johansen (eds.): *Gaussian Scale-Space Theory.* 1997
   ISBN 0-7923-4561-4
9. M. Shah and R. Jain (eds.): *Motion-Based Recognition.* 1997 ISBN 0-7923-4618-1
10. L. Florack: *Image Structure.* 1997
    ISBN 0-7923-4808-7
11. L.J. Latecki: *Discrete Representation of Spatial Objects in Computer Vision.* 1998
    ISBN 0-7923-4912-1
12. H.J.A.M. Heijmans and J.B.T.M. Roerdink (eds.): *Mathematical Morphology and its Applications to Image and Signal Processing.* 1998
    ISBN 0-7923-5133-9
13. N. Karssemeijer, M. Thijssen, J. Hendriks and L. van Erning (eds.): *Digital Mammography.* 1998
    ISBN 0-7923-5274-2
14. R. Highnam and M. Brady: *Mammographic Image Analysis.* 1999
    ISBN 0-7923-5620-9
15. I. Amidror: *The Theory of the Moiré Phenomenon.* 2000 ISBN 0-7923-5949-6;
    Pb: ISBN 0-7923-5950-x
16. G.L. Gimel'farb: *Image Textures and Gibbs Random Fields.* 1999 ISBN 0-7923-5961
17. R. Klette, H.S. Stiehl, M.A. Viergever and K.L. Vincken (eds.): *Performance Characterization in Computer Vision.* 2000
    ISBN 0-7923-6374-4
18. J. Goutsias, L. Vincent and D.S. Bloomberg (eds.): *Mathematical Morphology and Its Applications to Image and Signal Processing.* 2000
    ISBN 0-7923-7862-8
19. Z.C. Li: *Numerical Algorithms for Digital Images and Patterns Under Geometric Transformations.* 2000
    ISBN 0-7923-6476-7
20. A. Jaklič, A. Leonardis and F. Solina: *Segmentation and Recovery of Superquadrics.* 2000
    ISBN 0-7923-6601-8
21. K. Rohr: *Landmark-Based Image Analysis.* Using Geometric and Intensity Models. 2001
    ISBN 0-7923-6751-0

Kluwer Academic Publishers – Dordrecht / Boston / London